AN ILLUSTRATED COLOUR TEXT

ALLERGY

AN ILLUSTRATED COLOUR TEXT

ALLERGY

S HASAN ARSHAD DM MRCP

Consultant Physician in Respiratory Medicine and Allergy, and Director
The David Hide Asthma & Allergy Research Centre
St Mary's Hospital
Newport
Isle of Wight

Hon. Consultant Physician and Senior Lecturer
Department of Medical Specialities
Southampton University Hospitals Trust
University of Southampton
Southampton

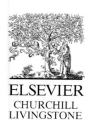

ELSEVIER
CHURCHILL
LIVINGSTONE

EDINBURGH LONDON NEW YORK OXFORD PHILADELPHIA ST LOUIS SYDNEY
TORONTO 2002

CHURCHILL LIVINGSTONE
An imprint of Elsevier Limited

First published 2002
Reprinted 2005

ISBN 0 443 06271 4

British Library Cataloguing in Publication Data
A catalogue record for this book is available from the British Library

Library of Congress Cataloging in Publication Data
A catalog record for this book is available from the Library of Congress

Note
Medical knowledge is constantly changing. As new information becomes available, changes in treatment, procedures, equipment and the use of drugs become necessary. The author and the publishers have, as far as it is possible, taken care to ensure that the information given in this text is accurate and up to date. However, readers are strongly advised to confirm that the information, especially with regard to drug usage, complies with the latest legislation and standards of practice.

Cover photograph
The montage on the cover of this book includes a false coloured photograph of a dustmite, taken using a scanning electron microscope.
© K.H. KJELDSON/SCIENCE PHOTO LIBRARY

 your source for books, journals and multimedia in the health sciences
www.elsevierhealth.com

For Churchill Livingstone

Commissioning Editior: Tim Horne
Project Development Manager: Sarah Keer-Keer
Project Manager: Frances Affleck
Designer: Sarah Russell
Page Layout: Jim Hope

The publisher's policy is to use **paper manufactured from sustainable forests**

Printed in China

PREFACE

Allergy, An Illustrated Colour Text, is written for those involved in the care of patients with allergic disease. It intends to provide a practical, but scientific and evidence based, approach for the management of these patients. It is primarily aimed at medical students and doctors-in-training. However, family practitioners, paediatricians, internists, pulmonologists, otolaryngologists, dermatologists and opthalmologists may find an allergy and immunology perspective helpful in dealing with these disorders. Similarly nurses, dietitians and pharmaceutical industry personnel, working in the field of allergy and immunology, will hopefully benefit from the concise description of allergy related topics.

Each topic is covered on a double-page spread facilitating reference and accessibility to all the relevant facts. The format of the book relies on the clear, concise text, supported by colour illustrations including photographs, line drawings, tables and a bulleted summary of each topic. The book is divided into three sections: the first section provides a background knowledge of the prevalence and pathogenesis of allergic diseases, the second section reviews diagnostic and treatment strategies and major allergic disorders are described in the third section.

S.H.A
Isle of Wight 2002

ACKNOWLEDGEMENTS

I am indebted to Mrs. Sharon Matthews, Allergy Service Co-ordinator at the David Hide Asthma and Allergy Research Centre, for reviewing the manuscript and providing clinical photographs. Also Dr. Susan Wilson and Mr. John Ward for providing photographs of immunohistochemistry preparations of bronchial mucosa and sputum cytology. The contribution of the publishing staff at Harcourt Health Sciences, particularly Sarah Keer-Keer and Mr. Alastair Christie, is gratefully acknowledged. Finally, I must thank my wife Zahida for her remarkable patience and tireless support.

CONTENTS

BASIC CONCEPTS AND HISTORY OF ALLERGY

BASIC CONCEPTS

WHAT IS ALLERGY?

Allergy is a word that is as often misused as it is used correctly. Many people will say they are allergic to something when this is not strictly the case. In scientific terms, allergy is usually caused by proteins called allergens. These allergens enter the body through the airways, the gastrointestinal tract or the skin. Most commonly, allergy is due to proteins that we inhale such as pollens or faeces of the house-dust mite (Fig. 1). These aero-allergens cause diseases such as asthma and allergic rhino-conjunctivitis. Foods are also important allergens, particularly in childhood, causing diseases such as atopic eczema. Other common sources of allergens are domestic animals, insects, moulds, medicines and industrial chemicals.

'Allergy is an inappropriate and harmful immune response to a normally harmless substance'.

Pollens, for example, are quite harmless unless you are allergic to them, in which case they can cause symptoms from mild sneezing and nasal congestion to extreme shortness of breath and wheezing.

SENSITIZATION AND SYMPTOMS

For an allergic reaction to occur, a person needs to become sensitized to an allergen. One, or several, previous encounters with the offending allergen are required before sensitization develops. Subsequent exposure to the allergen then leads to an allergic reaction. The clinical outcome depends on the system or part of the body involved. Allergic reaction may lead to maculopapular, urticarial or eczematous rash on the skin, asthma in the lungs, congestion and watering in the nose and eyes or mucosal swelling and increased motility may lead to diarrhoea and vomiting in the gastrointestinal tract. Sometimes, a systematic allergic reaction occurs leading to widespread vasodilatation, hypotension and shock.

ATOPY AND ALLERGY

Atopy refers to an inherited predisposition to produce IgE antibodies. The exact mode of inheritance is still unknown but is probably multifactorial and at least 25–30% of the population is atopic. Not everybody with this genetic disposition develops allergy and the environment plays a significant role in the development of clinical disease. Allergens stimulate the cells of the immune system to produce IgE antibodies. Recent evidence suggests that exposure to allergens in early infancy is crucial to phenotypic manifestation in those who are genetically predisposed.

THE ALLERGIC REACTION

When an allergen, usually a protein, gains entry to the body, it is recognized as foreign by the immune system. In the IgE-mediated (Type I) immune reaction, the allergen stimulates B cells to proliferate and produce specific IgE antibodies. These antibodies bind to surface receptors of mast cells, which are found in most tissues. On subsequent exposure, the allergens react with the antibodies leading to lysis of the mast cell. This causes the release of histamine and other substances which cause immediate symptoms and also initiate a chain reaction involving various cells and cytokines, which leads to allergic inflammation (Fig. 2).

HISTORY OF ALLERGY

The clinical symptoms and signs of asthma were well described by ancient Greek scholars, although several other types of breathing difficulty were probably attributed to asthma. In 1665 Philipp Jacob Sachs described a case of generalized urticaria following ingestion of strawberries, and of shock after eating fish. During the 17th century, German authors wrote of weakness, fainting and asthma produced in certain subjects by cats, mice, dogs and horses. In the middle of the 17th century, William Cullen witnessed an asthma attack in the wife of a pharmacist while her husband was preparing ipecacuanha. This may be the first reported incidence of drug allergy. Dr Brostock, in 1819, described his own 'periodical affection of eyes and chest'

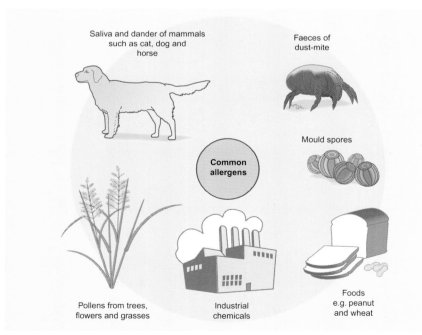

Saliva and dander of mammals such as cat, dog and horse

Faeces of dust-mite

Mould spores

Common allergens

Pollens from trees, flowers and grasses

Industrial chemicals

Foods e.g. peanut and wheat

Fig. 1 **Common allergens include dust mite faeces, pollens, animal dander, food and drugs.**

Initial sensitization

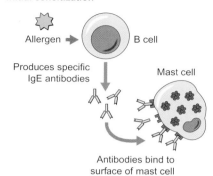

Allergen → B cell

Produces specific
IgE antibodies

Mast cell

Antibodies bind to
surface of mast cell

Subsequent exposure

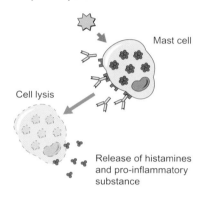

Mast cell

Cell lysis

Release of histamines
and pro-inflammatory
substance

Fig. 2 **Basic allergic reaction.**

which was a good description of hayfever. The classic experiments of Charles Blackley, in his paper of 1873, provided undeniable proof that grass pollen was the cause of hayfever.

ALLERGY AND ANAPHYLAXIS

The word allergy is derived from Greek, meaning 'altered reactivity'. The term was coined by Von Pirquet in 1906 to describe the cause of strange symptoms such as fever and rash observed in some patients after receiving antitoxic serum. In 1901 the French scientist Charles Richet described anaphylaxis as a severe systemic reaction sometimes observed after repeated injection of a substance. In the subsequent years, the mechanism of anaphylactic reaction was further explored by the experiments of Schultz and Dale and the pathogenesis of allergic disease was further elucidated with the demonstration that a shock-like syndrome can be induced by an intravenous administration of histamine. This added to the knowledge of the role of histamine in mediating many of the typical local symptoms of allergic reaction. In 1906, Wolff-Eisner made the connection between hayfever and allergy. In 1910, Meltzer made the connection between asthma and allergy.

ATOPY

The first study of genetic predisposition to allergy was published by Cooke and Vander Veer in 1916. They concluded that inheritance is a definite factor in human sensitization and the antibody responsible for this was named reagin. They also suggested that sensitization is inherited as an unusual capacity to react to foreign proteins. In 1923, Coca and Cooke used the term 'atopy' to designate those human hypersensitivity conditions that are genetically inherited.

REAGIN AND IgE

A significant contribution to the understanding of human allergy came in 1921 from Carl Prausnitz (Fig. 3) and Heinz Küstner. Serum from Küstner, who was allergic to fish, was transferred to the arm of Prausnitz. A typical weal and erythema reaction was observed on the site after local administration of the appropriate allergen. This passive transferability strongly implicated an antibody-mediated reaction. The nature of this antibody or reagin remained unknown until the Ishizakas in the USA and Johansson and Bennich in Sweden independently identified it in 1967. In a WHO conference in 1968, the antibody was named immunoglobulin E or IgE.

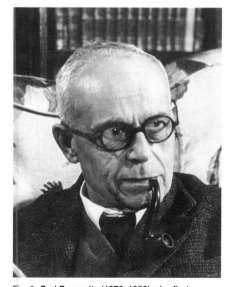

Fig. 3 **Carl Prausnitz (1876–1963) who first demonstrated the existence of a transferable substance in the serum, responsible for allergic reaction, named 'reagin'.** The reaction was called Prausnitz–Küstner reaction and the transferable substance was later proven to be antibody immunoglobulin E, or IgE.

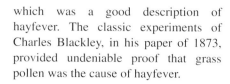

Basic concepts and history of allergy

Basic concepts
• Allergy is an inappropriate and harmful response to a normally harmless substance.
• Allergy is usually caused by proteins called allergens.
• Common allergens are pollens, dust mites, animals, moulds, food, medicines and chemicals.
• Allergy develops after several encounters with the offending allergen.
• Common allergic diseases include asthma, allergic rhinitis, and atopic eczema.

History of allergy
• Asthma and hayfever were well described by the middle of the 19th century.
• In 1873 Charles Blackley proved that grass pollen was the cause of hayfever.
• In 1901 Charles Richet described anaphylaxis.
• In 1906 the term 'allergy' was coined by Von Pirquet.
• In 1921 Prausnitz and Küstner showed passive transfer of allergy.
• In 1923 Coca and Cooke used the term 'atopy' to describe inherited human hypersensitivity conditions.
• The immunoglobulin E or IgE was discovered in 1967.

THE IMMUNE SYSTEM IN HEALTH AND DISEASE

Skin and mucosal surfaces form the body's first line of defence, but they are often broken, which allows microorganisms and other biological substances to enter the body. The immune system is the body's second line of defence. The immune system consists of cells, antibodies and other chemical substances ready to attack and eliminate foreign substances that have entered the body. To do this efficiently the immune system must differentiate between self and non-self substances. It recognizes protein macromolecules of the body as self and does not react against them (immunological tolerance).

The immune defence is organized into two complementary systems, non-specific and specific immunity (Fig. 1).

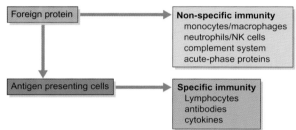

Fig. 1 **The immune system.**

NON-SPECIFIC IMMUNITY

When an organism penetrates the skin or mucosal barrier, it is attacked, engulfed and destroyed by phagocytic cells. These are monocytes, which become macrophages as they move into the tissues, and neutrophils. Neutrophils kill bacteria by releasing toxic substances. These cells are aided in their task by proteins of the complement system. Once activated by the presence of a microorganism, complement system proteins bind to the organism and lyse the cell membrane. They also enhance phagocytosis by making bacteria more palatable for phagocytes (opsonization) and attract other phagocytes to the battlefield (chemotaxis). Some of the acute-phase proteins, such as C-reactive protein, promote complement binding. When a cell becomes infected by a virus it produces interferon, which activates natural killer cells (a type of leukocyte) to engage and kill these cells, thus preventing the spread of virus.

SPECIFIC IMMUNITY

Antigens are large protein molecules that are taken up by monocytes and macrophages, the antigen-presenting cells (APC), and broken down to reveal the part of the molecule called the antigenic determinant, or epitope. Once processed in this way, the antigen is bound to the MHC class II molecules on the surface of these APCs, and the complex is presented to the T lymphocyte cell receptor.

The specificity of the immune system comes from the lymphocytes. Each lymphocyte recognizes only one or a few antigens, i.e. it is specific for these particular antigens. Every moment, trillions of lymphocytes pass through the tissues in search of foreign proteins (immunological surveillance). However, they will only recognize their particular antigen when it has been processed and presented by the APCs.

The antigen, upon entering the body, combines with the T cell receptor, via APC, and thus induces proliferation and production of identical lymphocytes of the same specificity (T cell clones). Some of them develop into cytotoxic cells and destroy the antigen-containing cells (T cell-mediated immunity), while others develop into T helper cells which stimulate B cells (B cell clones) and promote their transformation into plasma cells. Plasma cells then produce antibodies specific to the antigen (B cell-mediated immunity). This is the primary immune response.

Once the antigen is removed, further proliferation ceases and most of these immune cells die. However, a few T and B cells remain and continue to patrol the blood and lymphatic circulation (memory cells). On second encounter to the same antigen, the response is quick and strong due to these memory cells (secondary immune response). This immunological memory is crucial to the fight against the invasion of common bacteria and viruses and provides the basis for immunity provided by vaccination.

Immune reaction is not always beneficial and may cause disease when it is inappropriate, such as when it reacts against the body's own antigens (autoimmunity) or against substances which are not harmful to the body, such as pollens (allergy). Sometimes the system overreacts and the tissue damage caused is more than that caused by the infection itself. These abnormal responses produce disease and are termed hypersensitivity reactions.

HYPERSENSITIVITY

Hypersensitivity is the abnormal or exaggerated response of the immune system, resulting in tissue damage. Four types of hypersensitivity reaction were described by Gell and Coombs, but they are not mutually exclusive as more than one type of immune response is often involved in hypersensitivity.

Type I (immediate hypersensitivity)
This is conducted by immunoglobulin E (IgE) antibodies (Fig. 2). During the allergen exposure of the primary immune response, plasma cell clones produce IgE specific for that allergen. The IgE binds to the high-affinity receptors of the mast cells and basophils and low-affinity receptors of the macrophages, eosinophils and platelets.

On further exposure, the allergen reacts with the IgE bound to the mast cell, causing perforation of the membrane and release of preformed mediators such as histamine, tryptase and heparin. These mediators cause the immediate phase of the Type I reaction, which occurs within a few minutes (hence immediate hypersensitivity). Other mediators and cytokines are released and eosinophils are attracted to the site of activity, precipitating the late phase of the Type I reaction, which starts 3–4 h after exposure. Type I reaction occurs in asthma, rhinitis and anaphylaxis.

Type II (cytotoxic reaction)
This reaction is caused by IgG antibodies reacting to the antigens on the cell membrane (Fig. 3). The antigen may be produced by the patient's own cells (autoimmunity) or a foreign protein may be attached to the cell membrane. Examples of the diseases produced are haemolytic anaemia and thrombocytopenia.

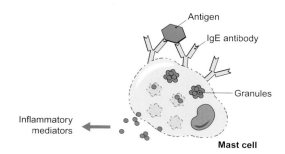

Fig. 2 **Type I or immediate hypersensitivity reaction.** Mast cell degranulation occurs following bridging of two IgE antibodies on the cell surface by antigen.

Type III (immune complex reaction)

IgG or IgM antibodies bind with the antigen in the circulation to form antigen/antibody complexes (Fig. 4). These complexes are then deposited in the tissues where they activate complement cascade, causing tissue necrosis by producing toxic substances.

Type IV (delayed hypersensitivity)

Sensitized T lymphocytes and macrophages play a major role and it is therefore called cell-mediated immune reaction (Fig. 5). T lymphocytes become sensitized on initial exposure. On subsequent contact, the antigen combines with sensitized T lymphocytes, with the release of cytokines resulting in chronic inflammation. Symptoms take 24–48 h to appear following exposure (delayed hypersensitivity). The characteristics of this type of inflammation are the appearance of giant cells and the formation of granulomas. Immune reaction against some of the bacterial or viral proteins and chemicals are due to this type of reaction.

Glossary of terms

- Antigen: a protein molecule capable of stimulating an immune response.
- Antibody: a molecule produced by B cells in response to stimulation by an antigen.
- Antigen-presenting cells: cells, such as macrophages, which process antigen before presenting it to the T lymphocytes.
- Chemotaxis: the process of attraction of immune cells to the site of inflammation.
- Epitope (antigenic determinant): molecular structure of the antigen that combines with the antibody.
- Hypersensitivity: exaggerated immune response producing disease.
- Major histocompatibility complex (MHC): molecules on the cell surface important in recognition and presentation of antigen.
- Memory cells: lymphocytes with long life, sensitized to a specific antigen.
- Phagocytosis: the process by which cells such as macrophages engulf foreign proteins.
- Opsonization: the protein (e.g. complement) coating of a microorganism enhancing phagocytic activity.
- Receptor: a cell-surface molecule that binds to a specific protein.

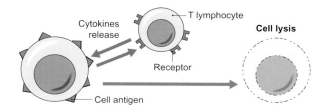

Fig. 5 **Type IV or delayed type reaction.** Receptors on the sensitized T lymphocytes combine with the target cell antigens, releasing cytokines, resulting in cell death.

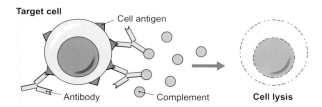

Fig. 3 **Type II or cytotoxic reaction.** Antibodies combine with antigens on the cell surface and bind complement, which leads to cell lysis.

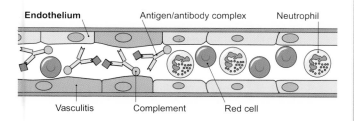

Fig. 4 **Type III or immune complex reaction.** Antigen/antibody complexes are formed in the circulation and, through complement activation, induce inflammation and damage to the endothelium.

The immune system in health and disease

- Phagocytes (macrophages, neutrophils) engulf and destroy microbes (non-specific immunity).
- Lymphocytes proliferate into clones following antigen stimulation (specific immunity).
- An exaggerated or inappropriate immune response may cause disease.
- IgE-mediated immune reaction (Type I) occurs in asthma, rhinitis, atopic eczema and urticaria.
- IgG antibodies react to the antigens on the cell membrane to cause lysis in Type II reaction.
- Antigen/antibody complexes cause tissue damage in Type III reaction.
- An exaggerated T cell response causes damage in Type IV reaction.

CELLS OF THE IMMUNE SYSTEM

Immune system cells originate from the pluripotent stem cells of the bone marrow, which differentiate into lymphocyte stem cells or myeloid stem cells. Lymphoid cells further develop into T lymphocytes or B lymphocytes. The myeloid cell line produces granulocytes (neutrophils, eosinophils, basophils and mast cells) and monocytes/macrophages (Fig. 1).

The immune system attacks foreign particles in two ways. Phagocytes such as neutrophils, monocytes and macrophages engulf and destroy the invaders, while lymphocytes, plasma cells, eosinophils, basophils and mast cells secrete antibodies or mediators which help to eliminate them.

NEUTROPHILS

This is the commonest type of circulating leukocyte and plays a major role in the defence against bacterial infection. Neutrophils have a multilobular nucleus and lysosomal granules. They are quickly attracted to the site of infection by complement fraction or other substances released at the site of inflammation. They engulf bacteria to be destroyed by the lyso-

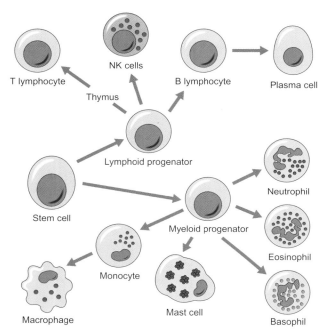

Fig. 1 **Cells of the immune system.**

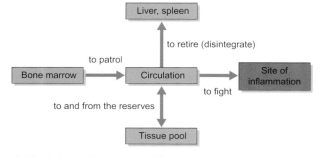

Fig. 2 **Circulation and fate of neutrophils.**

somal enzymes. In the process, however, they do cause some tissue injury, which is usually limited, the process (inflammation) being halted as soon as the infection is controlled. In some situations the process continues in the absence of infection and this chronic inflammation is the basis of many immunological diseases (Fig. 2).

MONOCYTES AND MACROPHAGES

Monocytes and their tissue counterpart, macrophages, have three important functions. By phagocytosis they engulf microorganisms to be destroyed by their lysosomal enzymes. They also secrete cytokines and other proinflammatory mediators and act as antigen-presenting cells.

Macrophages are activated by products of the bacteria, mediators from other cells and complement components. In the activated state receptor expression, phagocytic activity and mediator secretion are all enhanced. Macrophages adapt to local needs and may transform into distinct cells, e.g. Langerhans' cells in the skin, Kupffer cells in the liver and alveolar macrophages in the lung.

EOSINOPHILS

Eosinophils move from the bone marrow into the circulation and then finally migrate into the mucosal surfaces of the gut and to a lesser extent of the lung. However, they are also attracted to sites of inflammation in other tissues. The activated form appears less dense and these hypodense eosinophils are increased in disease states such as parasitic infection and allergic disorders.

Eosinophils have receptors for immunoglobulins and complement on the surface, and the cytoplasm contains granules, with their content of enzymes and mediators. Eosinophils secrete several toxic substances including major basic protein, cationic protein and peroxidase. In addition, they secrete several types of mediators such as platelet activating factor, leukotrienes and cytokines.

Eosinophils are important in defence against parasitic infections, but they also play a central role in allergic inflammation. Release of cationic proteins causes epithelial damage and increases bronchial lability in bronchial asthma. Activation and degranulation of eosinophils is also seen in other allergic diseases such as rhinitis, atopic dermatitis, urticaria and angioedema.

BASOPHILS AND MAST CELLS

Mast cells reside mainly in the tissues exposed to the external environment, such as intestinal and respiratory mucosa and the skin. Two different types of mast cells exist, with somewhat different functions. Those containing the enzyme tryptase are called MCT while others which contain chymase are designated MCTC. Basophils normally circulate in the blood and are only called into the site of inflammation by chemotactic mediators.

Mast cells are the first to respond in allergic reactions. They have high-affinity receptors for IgE on their surface. When anti-

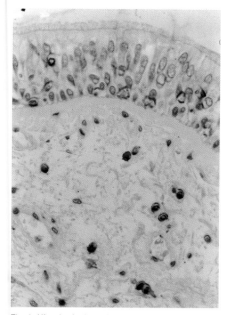

Fig. 3 **Histological section of bronchial mucosa.**
Lymphocytes orchestrate allergic inflammation and can be demonstrated by immunnohisto-chemical stain using antibody labelled against one of its surface markers, CD3.

Table 1 **Mast cell mediators and their effects**

Mediators	Effects
Histamine, PGD2, LTC4	Vasodilatation, bronchoconstriction, increased permeability and mucous secretion
PAF, IL-5	Migration and activation of eosinophils
IL-4	T cell activation and promotion of IgE synthesis from B cells
IL-3, IL-4	Activation of basophils and mast cells
IL-4, LTC4	Promotion of adhesion of leukocytes to endothelium

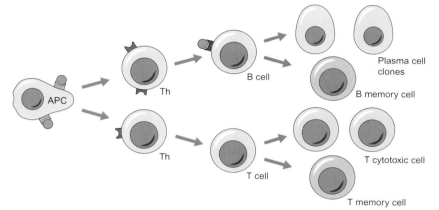

Fig. 4 **Following exposure to antigen, T and B cell clones are produced and sensitization occurs through memory cells, ensuring an augmented response on re-exposure.**

gen combines with the surface-bound IgE, degranulation of the mast cells occurs, with the release of mediators (Table 1). Histamine, prostaglandin D2, leukotrienes (LTC4) and platelet-activating factor, with their effects on blood vessels and bronchial smooth muscles, cause symptoms of immediate hypersensitivity such as bronchoconstriction, oedema and vasodilatation. In addition, the production of various cytokines attracts and activates eosinophils and basophils and upregulates IgE production.

T LYMPHOCYTES

Unlike most other cells, lymphocytes recognize and bind to the antigen directly, through their surface receptors. They develop from their progenitor in the bone marrow and go through the thymus to mature and develop specificity for antigens early on.

All lymphocytes look similar under the light microscope, with a rounded cell and large nucleus. They are differentiated using monoclonal antibodies that recognize markers on their surface. These markers are numbered with a prefix 'cluster of differentiation' (CD). All T lymphocytes have CD2 and CD3 molecules on their surface (Fig. 3).

T lymphocytes primarily orchestrate immunological responses through release of cytokines. T lymphocytes can be divided into those having CD4 molecules on the surface (CD4+) and those with CD8 molecules (CD8+). CD8+ lymphocytes recognize MHC class I molecules on the cell surface and kill those containing appropriate antigens, such as infected and malignant cells (cytotoxic function). CD4+ lymphocytes recognize antigen in conjunction with the MHC class II molecules on antigen-presenting cells and serve a helper function (T helper or Th). There are three types of Th cells. Th0 are uncommitted cells producing a wide range of cytokines. Th1 promote inflammation to fight against microbes and produce cytokines such as IL-2 and interferon γ. Th2 cells promote allergic inflammation by producing cytokines such as IL-4, IL-5, IL-6, and IL-13.

The effects of Th cells on other inflammatory cells are to:

- Promote accumulation at the site of inflammation.
- Induce proliferation.
- Prolong their survival.
- Activate and prime for further action.
- Stimulate the production of immunoglobulins by B cells.

B LYMPHOCYTES

B lymphocytes develop and mature in the bone marrow. This cell initially expresses non-specific IgM or IgD antibodies on its surface. Following exposure to its specific antigen, it assimilates and processes the antigen, then presents the peptide, in combination with MHC class II molecule on its surface, to the Th lymphocyte (CD4+). The Th lymphocyte induces proliferation of B lymphocytes into plasma cells to produce antibodies (IgG, IgA or IgE) of the same specificity as the antigen. Some sensitized B lymphocytes remain as memory cells and mount an augmented response on re-exposure to the same antigen (Fig. 4).

Cells of the immune system

- All immune system cells originate from stem cells in bone marrow.
- Immune cells can kill microbes either by engulfing (phagocytosis) or by secretion of toxic substances.
- Macrophages act as phagocytes and antigen-presenting cells.
- Eosinophils are important in the production of allergic inflammation.
- Mast cells initiate the allergic response when an antigen combines with IgE bound to its receptors.
- Lymphocytes promote and regulate the immune response.

CYTOKINES

Cytokines are proteins secreted by cells to influence or regulate the activity of other cells in the immediate micro-environment. They perform many physiological functions and are crucial in regulation of immune responses. Cytokine is the general term but sometimes lymphokine or monokine is used to denote the origin of these mediators. Some of the cytokines are named interleukins with a number (such as interleukin-1 or IL-1). The numbers relate to the order of their discovery and have no relation to function. Others are named to reflect their function, such as tumour necrosis factor (TNF). More cytokines are still being discovered.

Each type of inflammatory cell may secrete many different cytokines and each cytokine may influence many different cells. A cytokine may promote one type of inflammation and in the process may inhibit another. It has therefore been difficult to classify the cytokine network according to origin or function. They are important in every step of the inflammatory cells; their growth, differentiation, maturation, activation, movement, secretion and death (apoptosis). Lymphocytes control and direct the immune response through these cytokines.

Cytokines are generally proinflammatory and regulate the response of the immune system in a very complex way. A cytokine may stimulate or inhibit the release of its own kind and other cytokines from various different cells. They may also influence receptor expression on the cell surface, thereby potentiating or minimizing their effects on the cell. The effect of one cytokine may be opposed by other cytokines, thus ensuring an effective but controlled response.

The complexity of cytokine function and regulation can be highlighted by interleukin-1. IL-1 is secreted by mononuclear and others cells and influences T cells and fibroblasts, among others. It is generally regarded as a proinflammatory cytokine but there are inherent mechanisms to control its effects. There are three different peptides, IL-1α, IL-1β and IL-1γ and two different receptors for IL-1 (type I and

type II). IL-1α and IL-1β bind to type I receptors to induce the proinflammatory effects of IL-1, while type II receptors capture these cytokines without any effect (minimizing the overall effect). IL-1γ binds to the type I receptor but again without any effect, thus acting as a receptor blocker.

Functions of cytokines include (see Tables 1 and 2):

- Growth, differentiation, survival and activation of cells.
- Haemopoiesis.
- Fibrosis.
- Antibody production and specificity.
- Mediator/cytokine synthesis and release.
- Chemotaxis.

- Receptor expression.
- Killing of tumour cells and bacteria.
- Inhibition of viral replication.
- Production of acute phase proteins.
- Adhesion molecule expression.
- Fever, cachexia, vasodilatation.

T CELL-MEDIATED IMMUNITY

Mononuclear cells present the antigen to Th lymphocytes and release IL-1 (Fig. 1). This combination stimulates Th cells to produce IL-2, which causes proliferation and production of clones of T lymphocytes of the same specificity, against that particular antigen. Th cells also secrete IFN-γ which activates macrophages to augment the reaction in a

Table 1 **The cytokine family: primary cell source and functions of various cytokines.** The list is not exhaustive as many other cytokines are known and still being discovered

Cytokine	Primary source	Main effects
IL-1	Mono/macro	Activation and proliferation of lymphocytes, proliferation of bone marrow stem cells, synthesis of acute phase proteins, systemic effects such as fever, vasodilatation and hypotension, anti-viral and antitumour activity
IL-2	T cells	Clonal T cell proliferation, also activates B cells, cytotoxic T cells, natural killer cells and macrophages
IL-3	T cells	Differentiation and growth of granulocytes, especially basophils and mast cells, activates and prolongs eosinophil survival
IL-4	T and mast cells	Promotes B cells towards IgE production and inhibits cell-mediated immunity
IL-5	T cells	B cell maturation and facilitates IgE production and attracts eosinophils
IL-6	Mono/macro, T cells	Differentiation of B cells into plasma cells and T cells into cytotoxic cells, proliferation of bone marrow stem cells, synthesis of acute phase proteins and anti-viral and anti-tumour activity
IL-7	Stromal cells	Proliferation, prolongs survival and activation of eosinophils
IL-8	Mono/macro	Attracts neutrophils and other cells to the site of inflammation
IL-9	T cells	Growth of T lymphocytes and mast cells
IL-10	Mono/macro	Suppresses T cells and stimulates B cells to produce IgG antibodies
IL-11	Stromal cells	B cell maturation in bone marrow
IL-12	Mono/macro	Proliferation and activation of natural killer (NK) cells, proliferation of bone marrow stem cells
IL-13	T cells	Promotes B cells towards IgE production and inhibits cell-mediated immunity
IL-14	T cells	Facilitates IgE production
IL-15	Mono/macro	Growth and differentiation of T and B lymphocytes
GM-CSF	T cells, epithelium	Promotes growth and differentiation of granulocytes and monocytes
IFN-γ	T cells	Attracts, stimulates and activates monocytes and macrophages, neutrophils and NK cells, inhibits IL-4 mediated effects on B cells and also inhibits viral replication
TGF-β	Mesenchymal cells	Inhibits both T and B lymphocytes, stimulates fibroblasts and promotes B cells towards IgA production
TNF	Mono/macro	Proliferation and activation of T and B cells, attraction and activation of neutrophils, mononuclear and NK cells, synthesis of acute phase proteins and anti-viral and anti-tumour activity

Table 2 **Cytokines involved in different types of immune response**

Immune response	Stimulatory cytokines	Inhibitory
T cell-mediated	IL-1, IL-2, IL-6, IL-8, IL-12, IL-15, IFN-γ, TNF	IL-10, IL-4, TGF-β
B cell-mediated	IL-1, IL-2, IL-5, IL-6, IL-7, IL-10, IL-11, IFN-γ	TGF-β
Allergic	IL-3, IL-4, IL-5, IL-13, IL-14	IFN-γ, IL-12

positive feedback system. IL-2, IFN-γ and TNF-β secreted by activated T lymphocytes also cause stimulation and activation of NK cells, cytotoxic lymphocytes and neutrophils, and attract granulocytes to the site of inflammation. IL-1 and TNF-β directly kill tumour cells and IFN-γ inhibits viral replication. Other proinflammatory cytokines such as TNF-α, IL-6, IL-8 and IL-12, secreted by mononuclear cells, also activate T lymphocytes and other cells, while IL-10 inhibits cytokine production by T cells.

B CELL-MEDIATED IMMUNITY

In the bone marrow, B lymphocytes proliferate from the progenator cells under the influence of IL-7 and IL-11 (Fig. 2). T lymphocytes control their further growth and differentiation by direct contact through CD40 ligand and secretion of cytokines. IL-10 promotes differentiation to IgG-producing cells. IL-4 and IL-13 cause switching to IgE-producing B cells and TGF-β produces IgA-producing B cells. Other cytokines including IL-1, IL-2, IL-5, IL-14 and IFN-γ promote growth and maturation but not differentiation of B cells.

INHIBITORY CYTOKINES

Most cytokines have some modulatory role on the growth and activity of inflammatory cells and the production of mediators. These may be stimulatory, inhibitory or merely a change in the type of activity. Two cytokines are primarily inhibitory in nature. IL-10 is produced by mononuclear cells, T and B lymphocytes, and mast cells and inhibits proliferation and production of cytokines from Th1 lymphocytes and mononuclear cells. It also inhibits eosinophil survival and IgE synthesis. However, it stimulates B lymphocytes and IgG production. Thus it suppresses T cell-mediated and allergic reactions in favour of B cell-mediated reactions. Another cytokine with a primary inhibitory activity is TGF-β. It is produced by mesenchymal cells and inhibits both T and B lymphocytes and allergic inflammation, while stimulating fibroblasts, thus promoting fibrosis. Tumour necrosis factor (TNF), IL-1 (IL-1 receptor antagonist) and IFN-γ also have inhibitory properties.

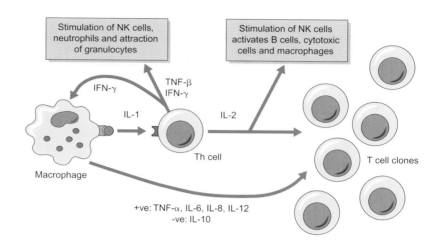

Fig 1 **T cell-mediated immunity.**

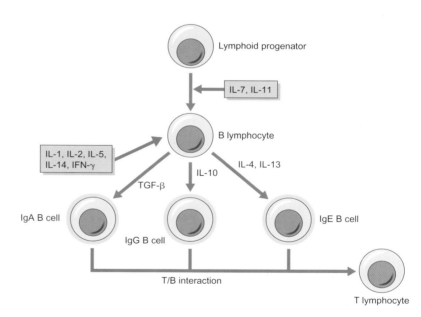

Fig 2 **B cell-mediated immunity.**

Cytokines

- Cytokines are proteins which regulate the immune response.
- They act as local hormones in their microenvironment.
- They are produced by lymphocytes, mononuclear cells and other cells.
- They influence growth, maturation and activity of the inflammatory cells.
- They can be stimulatory or inhibitory.
- Some may have a direct effect to kill bacteria, viruses and tumour cells.
- Some may also cause pyrexia, cachexia and hypotension.

IMMUNOGLOBULINS

Immunoglobulins, or antibodies, are glycoproteins produced by B lymphocytes (or plasma cells) mainly in response to exposure to antigens. They are an essential part of the immune defence system. There are five classes of immunoglobulins; IgG, IgA, IgM, IgD and IgE. These antibodies differ greatly in the size and shape of their molecules between each class, but less so within the group. The antibodies, specific to the antigens that induced their production, are identical.

STRUCTURE

An antibody molecule is Y-shaped and has two heavy chains and two light chains. The heavy chains form the stem of the Y (Fc fragment; c = crystaline) and the two forks (Fab fragments; ab = antigen binding) are made by light chains (Fig. 1). These chains are joined to each other by disulphide bonds. If these disulphide bonds are broken, two heavy chains and two light chains will be produced. The Fc fragment binds to the cell surface receptor and the Fab fragment binds to the antigen. Thus, each antibody can bind to two antigenic sites.

Light chains are of two varieties, named κ and λ. They are found in all classes of antibodies, but in any one antibody both light chains are of the same variety. Heavy chains differ considerably in size between different classes. Both light and heavy chains have a proximal constant (light chain = C_L, heavy chain = C_H) region and a distal variable (V_L and V_H) region. In each antibody, the variable region has a different amino acid constituent, which forms a structure specific for its antigen.

FUNCTIONS

Immunoglobulins are an essential part of the immune defence (Table 1). They play a key role in the B cell-mediated (humoral) immune responses by combining to the antigen, for example, at the cell surface of the bacteria. They activate complement and cell lysis. They also promote cell-mediated immune defence by coating the bacteria, which facilitates phagocytosis by macrophages and neutrophils. They may produce disease by reacting against self antigens (autoimmunity) or by forming antigen/antibody complexes which can deposit in the blood vessels causing vasculitis. IgE antibodies, bound to the mast cells, cause degranulation when combined with the appropriate allergen.

Table 1 **Immunoglobulin classes and their properties**

	Cell binding	Complement fixation
IgG-1	Mononuclear, lymphocyte, neutrophils, platelets	++
IgG-2	Lymphocytes, platelets	+
IgG-3	Mononuclear, lymphocyte, neutrophils, platelets	+++
IgG-4	Lymphocytes, neutrophils, platelets, mast cells	–
IgA	Lymphocytes, neutrophils	–
IgM	Lymphocytes	+++
IgD	–	–
IgE	Mast cells and basophils, lymphocytes	–

CLASSES OF IMMUNOGLOBULINS

IgG is the commonest immunoglobulin, accounting for 75% of the total immunoglobulins in the circulation. It is also widely distributed in the tissues and crosses the placental barrier to confer immunity on the foetus. It has four subclasses (IgG-1–4), which differ in their structure and function. IgG is most important in the defence against bacterial infections.

About 15% of the circulating immunoglobulins are IgA. However IgA is present abundantly in the secretions of the mucosal surfaces such as saliva, bronchial secretion and milk. In this situation it is mainly present as a dimer – two molecules joined together (Fig. 2). This IgA (called secretory IgA or sIgA) is combined with a secretory protein component, which protects it from enzyme digestion. IgA thus forms a forward line of defence combating microorganisms on the mucosal surface.

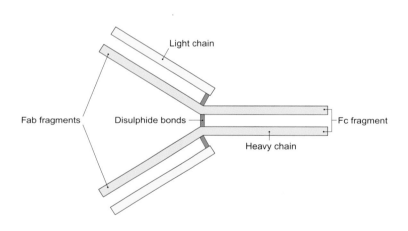

Fig. 1 **Immunoglobulin molecule.**

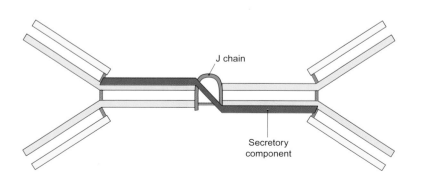

Fig. 2 **Secretory IgA: Fc fragments are joined together by a J chain and the molecule has a secretory component.**

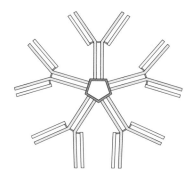

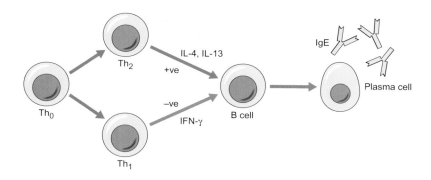

Fig. 3 **IgM: five IgM antibodies are joined together to form a macromolecule (pentamer).**

Fig. 4 **Regulation and synthesis of IgE.** In an atopic subject the positive influence from Th2 cells is strong, leading to switching of B cells towards IgE production.

IgM accounts for about 10% of the immunoglobulin pool. It is present as pentamer, that is, Fc portions of five antibody molecules join together to make a large molecule (Fig. 3). It is mainly present intravascularly and acts against microbes which have invaded the circulation.

IgD is present in small amounts (less than 1%) in the circulation. It is present on the surface of the naïve B cells. The function of IgD is not known.

IMMUNOGLOBULIN E OR IgE

IgE is the principal immunoglobulin involved in allergic reactions. Compared to other immunoglobulins, IgE is present in trace quantities only (< 0.01%). It is slightly larger, having five domains in its heavy chain (other immunoglobulins have four). Its serum half-life is only 2.5 days but is present, bound to mast cells and basophils with their high-affinity receptors (FcεR1), on the cell surface. Some other cells (macrophages, lymphocytes and eosinophils) have low-affinity receptors (FcεR2).

IgE and atopy

IgE has a physiological role in protecting against parasitic infection. In the presence of parasites the levels of IgE are very high. In the absence of these infections the levels remain very low. However, some people have a tendency to produce IgE in response to exposure to foreign proteins called allergens. This tendency, called atopy, is inherited, although the exact mode of inheritance is not yet known. Approximately 25–30% of the population is atopic. In these subjects, IgE levels are high and the high-affinity receptors on mast cells and basophils are increased.

Regulation of IgE synthesis

B cell proliferation and switching, to produce a particular type of immunoglobulin, is under the control of Th lymphocytes. Once the Th lymphocyte is activated by an antigen (through antigen-presenting cells), it makes contact with the B cell to induce proliferation and production of antibodies specific to the antigen. There are two types of Th lymphocytes, Th1 and Th2. Th1 cells produce cytokines such as IFN-γ and TNF-β, whereas Th2 cells produce IL-4, IL-5 and IL-13. Regulation of IgE synthesis is dependent upon the stimulatory influence of IL-4 and IL-13 and the inhibitory influence of IFN-γ. Thus, Th2 cells promote IgE synthesis and allergy and Th1 cells oppose it (Fig. 4).

In atopic subjects Th2/Th1 balance leans towards Th2 cells, i.e. Th0 cells differentiate more towards Th2 type. On allergen stimulation these produce IL-4 and IL-13, promoting IgE synthesis. This Th2 predominance is primarily determined by heredity. However, environmental influences early in life contribute significantly towards the eventual phenotype. The foetus makes IgE from the eleventh week of gestation. Therefore, its synthesis can be affected by maternal influences through the placenta, such as maternal exposure to allergens and maternal smoking. IgE levels are detectable at birth, when measured in the cord blood, in the majority of children. Thereafter, in atopic subjects, its levels are dependent upon the balance of positive influences (exposure to allergens) and negative influences (infection).

Immunoglobulins

- Immunoglobulins are glycoproteins secreted from the B lymphocytes and plasma cells.
- An antibody molecule has two heavy and two light chains.
- There are five types of immunoglobulins; IgG, IgA, IgM, IgD and IgE.
- IgA is present in secretions, thus preventing invasion of the mucosa.
- IgM remains in the circulation and fights intravascular microbes.
- IgG is important in defence against bacterial infections in the tissues.
- IgE plays a key role in allergy.
- IgE synthesis is promoted by Th2 cytokines; IL-4 and IL-13 and inhibited by Th1 cytokine; IFN-γ.

ALLERGIC INFLAMMATION

Although initiated by IgE antibodies, allergic inflammation is more complex than a simple type I allergic reaction (Table 1). T cells play a central role in orchestrating a chain reaction involving antibodies, cells and mediators. This mechanism is activated by allergens in sensitized individuals (Fig. 1).

Allergic inflammation is a combination of an antibody- and cell-mediated reaction. An immediate response, typical of an immediate hypersensitivity reaction, is seen following allergen exposure. This is mediated primarily by the release of histamine from basophils and mast cells. In addition, a delayed response occurs several hours later with an influx of inflammatory cells, characteristic of cell-mediated hypersensitivity. This late-phase response (LPR) is dominated by eosinophils and causes chronic inflammation.

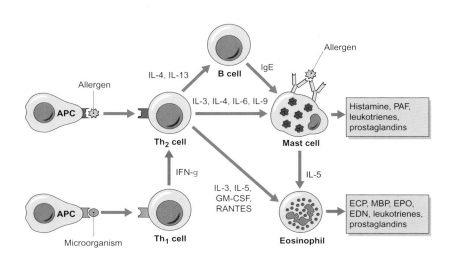

Fig. 1 **Mechanism of allergic inflammation.**

SENSITIZATION

Antigens enter the body through the respiratory and gastrointestinal mucosa and the skin. The antigen-presenting cells engulf the antigens and, after processing, present these to the naïve T cells (Th0). In atopic individuals, this process stimulates the production of Th2 cells, which then secrete cytokines, IL-4 and IL-13. These cytokines cause proliferation and switching of B cells to IgE-producing B and plasma cells, specific to the antigen. Some of these cells have a long life and are called memory cells. The IgE circulates in the blood in small quantities but is mostly present in the tissues bound to high-affinity receptors (FcεR1) on the surface of mast cells and low-affinity receptors (FcεR2) on eosinophils, macrophages and platelets. This IgE can be detected in the serum by immune assays or in the skin by allergy skin tests.

IL-4 promotes synthesis of IgE. It also stimulates T cells and macrophages, and

enhances the expression of FcεR2 on B cells, and adhesion molecules on endothelial cells. IL-13 has similar but weaker biological activity though it lasts longer than IL-4. Interferon-γ (FN-γ) inhibits allergic responses and its effects are opposite to IL-4 and IL-13. Other cytokines which inhibit allergic responses are IL-12 and TGF-β (Table 2). In atopic individuals the balance is tilted towards the production of Th2 type cytokines (IL-4 and IL-13) as opposed to Th1 type, such as IFN-γ.

EARLY RESPONSE

Early response is usually initiated by the interaction between the allergen and the IgE antibodies on the mast cells. Mast cell proliferation is dependent on T cell-derived cytokines, especially IL-9. When the person is sensitized, IgE specific to the allergen is bound to the mast cell receptors. Bridging of the two Fab fragments of adjacent IgE molecules results

in mast cell degranulation and the secretion of mediators such as histamine, prostaglandins, leukotrienes, platelet activating factor and bradykinin. These mediators cause vascular dilatation, increased permeability and attract cells into the tissues, thus leading to inflammation. The immediate effects on the bronchi include bronchoconstriction and increased bronchial responsiveness. In the skin they lead to erythema and induration, and in the nose to sneezing and rhinorrhoea. Mast cells also release cytokines such as IL-3, IL-4, IL-5 and IL-6 which activate T and B lymphocytes, stimulate mast cells and attract eosinophils, further augmenting the allergic reaction (Fig. 2).

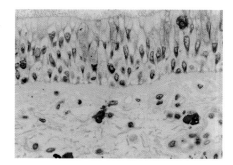

Fig. 2 **Mast cells play a significant role in the pathogenesis of allergic diseases.** Bronchial mucosa showing mast cells. Immunohistochemical staining (× 550).

Table 1 **Components of allergic inflammation**

Cells	Cytokines	Antibodies	Mediators
Mast cells, basophils, eosinophils, Th2 lymphocytes, B lymphocytes and plasma cells, monocytes and macrophages	IL-1, IL-2, IL-3, IL-4, IL-5, IL-6, IL-9, IL-13, GM-CSF, RANTES, TNF	IgE, IgG-4	Histamine, tryptase, chymase, leukotrienes, prostaglandins, PAF, ECP, MBP, EPO

LATE RESPONSE

A few hours after the allergen exposure, events initiated during the early response result in hypersecretion, oedema formation and the accumulation of cells. Eosinophils are the most important cells at this stage but lymphocytes, mononuclear cells and neutrophils are also involved. IL-5, secreted from mast cells, lymphocytes and eosinophils, is the most important cytokine for eosinophils. Besides attracting them to the site of inflammation it also causes their proliferation, activation and increased survival (Fig. 3). Other eosinophilic cytokines are IL-3, GM-CSF and chemokines.

Upon activation, eosinophils release pre-formed and newly synthesized mediators such as eosinophilic cationic protein (ECP), major basic protein (MBP), leukotrienes and prostaglandins. These and other mediators enhance inflammation and cause epithelial damage. Further secretion of a host of cytokines, including IL-3, IL-4 and IL-5, contribute to an ongoing inflammation. Clinically, this results in prolonged mucus secretion, oedema formation and in persistent bronchial hyperresponsiveness.

CHRONIC ALLERGIC INFLAMMATION

With continued or repeated exposure to allergen, a state of chronic inflammation persists, essentially a continued late-phase reaction. This inflammatory reaction, however, is not IgE-dependent and other mechanisms exist which may lead to a similar inflammatory state.

There is evidence of increased numbers of activated Th2 cells, expressing mRNA for the secretion of IL-3, IL-4, IL-5 and GM-CSF. These cytokines are important in the continuation of inflammation and the attraction of mast cells and eosinophils. Increased numbers of mast cells are found with increased histamine and prostaglandin secretion. Similarly, activated eosinophils are found in the mucosa with a parallel increase in their toxic products, causing epithelial damage (Fig. 3). There is up-regulation of intercellular adhesion molecules in the blood vessels promoting stickiness of the endothelium to leukocytes and facilitating their passage across, into the tissues. Increased permeability and cellular infiltration causes mucosal oedema. There is also glandular hyperplasia with increase secretion.

Lungs

Inflammatory changes result in mucosal oedema, bronchoconstriction, mucous plugging and increased bronchial reactivity. These changes are responsible for reversible bronchial constriction. However, in chronic asthma there is evidence of basement membrane thickening and smooth muscle hyperplasia, which may cause irreversible narrowing of the airways.

Nose

Inflammatory changes in nasal mucosa cause symptoms of allergic rhinitis, which include nasal obstruction, rhinorrhoea and sneezing. Histamine plays a significant role in nasal inflammation.

Conjunctiva

Mast cells are increased in allergic conjunctivitis but histological changes are usually mild. More prominent changes are seen in vernal conjunctivitis where mast cells, eosinophils and T lymphocytes are seen supported by Th2 type cytokines.

Skin

In atopic dermatitis, Langerhans cells, lymphocytes and mast cells are seen in increased numbers with a cytokine profile supporting an allergic inflammation.

MINIMAL PERSISTENT INFLAMMATION

Exposure to low allergen concentration, as happens in many patients with house-dust mite or pollen allergy, leads to a state of persistent inflammation without causing symptoms. These patients with mild asthma or allergic rhinitis are usually symptom-free, but respond to a higher allergen dose with severe symptoms. Histologically, increased numbers of inflammatory cells and cytokines can be shown in the mucosa and secretions.

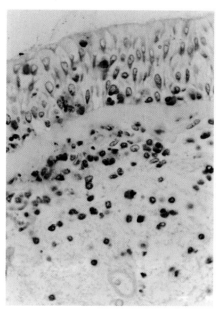

Fig. 3 **Bronchial biopsy showing infiltration of activated eosinophils.** Immunohistochemical staining using monoclonal antibody against EG2 ($\times$ 550).

Table 2 **Some important cytokines with positive and negative influence on allergic inflammation**

Cytokine	Actions
IL-4	IgE synthesis, proliferation of Th2 lymphocytes
IL-13	IgE synthesis
IL-5	Eosinophil stimulation, proliferation, chemoattraction and increased survival, proliferation of Th2 lymphocytes
IL-3	Eosinophil activation and increased survival, mast cell proliferation
GM-CSF	Eosinophil activation and increased survival, inhibits mast cell growth
RANTES	Eosinophil activation and chemoattraction
IL-9	Mast cell growth factor
INF-γ	Inhibits IL-4 and IL-13, neutrophil and macrophage activation
IL-12	Stimulates IFN-γ production by T cells
TGF-β	Inhibits IL-4 and IL-13 and monocytes and T cell function
IL-10	Inhibits cytokine production and monocyte and T cell function

Allergic inflammation

- Allergic inflammation is a combination of antibody and cell-mediated reactions.
- Predominance of Th2 lymphocyte, with its cytokine profile (IL-4, IL-13), is crucial for the development of allergic inflammation.
- Sensitization is the first stage, with the stimulation and proliferation of IgE-producing B cells.
- Early response is IgE-mediated and histamine, secreted from the mast cells, is the principal mediator.
- Delayed response is cell-mediated and eosinophils play an important role.
- Chronic inflammation is demonstrable in all patients with allergic disease, including those with minimal symptoms.

DEVELOPMENT OF ALLERGIC DISEASE

ALLERGY AND ATOPY

Atopy is defined as the genetic propensity to mount an IgE response on exposure to allergens. Atopic status is confirmed by positive skin-test reactions to one or more allergens or the presence of specific IgE antibodies in the blood. Allergy is the clinical manifestation of atopy due to the exaggerated and harmful response of the immune system to normally harmless substances (allergens). Allergic diseases include asthma, atopic eczema, rhinoconjunctivitis and food allergy. Not all atopic individuals manifest clinical disease. A minority (20–30%) of asthma and rhinitis is non-allergic. Eczema is often atopic in early childhood but thereafter it is often not due to any obvious allergies. Acute urticaria is an allergic phenomenon but chronic recurrent urticaria is a non-atopic disease.

NATURAL HISTORY

Eczema and food allergy

Allergic diseases are common in infancy and early childhood (Fig. 1). The prevalence of cow's milk intolerance is reported to be 2–7% in various studies, whereas cow's milk allergy (IgE mediated) occurs in 2–3% of children. Other food allergies are also common, such as egg and wheat. These are usually transient and by the age of 2 years most children tolerate cow's milk and wheat, though egg allergy tends to last a bit longer. Allergy to peanut and other nuts is less common but stays longer and may be lifelong. Atopic eczema is also very common in infancy and early childhood and often occurs together with egg and milk allergy where a cause and effect relationship may exist. In the majority of children atopic eczema is mild and transient, but in some cases it can be generalized, severe and persist into adult life.

Respiratory allergy

Recurrent wheezing is very common in infancy. Most are transient early-life wheezers, in whom the predisposing factors are reduced airway calibre, exposure to tobacco smoke and viral infections. Most of these children are not atopic and do not develop asthma. Recurrent wheez-

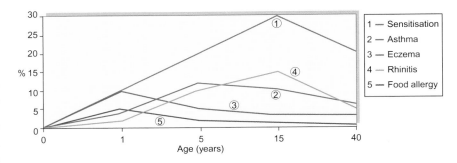

Fig. 1 **Natural history of allergic manifestations in childhood to adult life.**

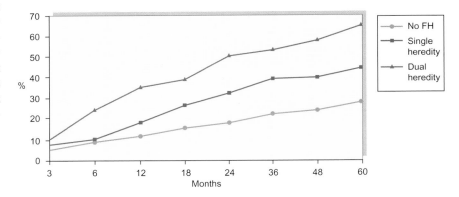

Fig. 2 **Cumulative incidence of atopic eczema in children in relation to eczema in the immediate family** (from: Wahn U, Bergmann RL, Nickel R 1998, Early life markers of atopy and allergy. Clinical and Experimental Allergy 28, supp. 1, pp 20–21).

ing often persists in those with a positive family history of allergy and evidence of other allergic diseases such as eczema and/or sensitization on skin test. Eczema and food allergies often improve between the ages of 2 and 5 years but many of these children develop symptoms of cough and wheeze suggestive of asthma. Allergic rhinitis is uncommon below the age of 5 years. The prevalence gradually increases to a peak at 15–20 years and then declines gradually during adult life.

Sensitization

The natural course of sensitization to common allergens is similar to that of clinical disorders. During the first years of life sensitization to food allergens, such as cow's milk and egg, are common, and inhalant allergens e.g. dust mite, pollens and cat are less common. Between 2 and 5 years, IgE to food allergens disappears in most children as tolerance develops. However this is replaced by sensitization to inhalant allergens.

Adult life

Total IgE level reaches a peak at 10–15 years of age but, on average, declines steadily to low levels in late adult life. The size and number of positive reactions to common allergens on skin-prick test also decrease with age. It was thought that almost 50% of children grow out of their asthma by the age of 20. However, they often continue to have increased bronchial responsiveness and symptoms may return after a period of several years. The prevalence and severity of allergic rhinitis declines considerably in later years.

RISK FACTORS

Genetics of allergy

Although genetic factors have long been associated with the development of allergic disease, the exact mode of inheritance remains controversial. Autosomal dominant trait with variable penetrance and multifactorial inheritance have been suggested as possible mechanisms.

Table 1 **Risk factors for the development of asthma**

Predisposing factor	Atopy
	Gender
Causal factors	Indoor allergens (dust mite, cat, cockroach, fungi, etc.)
	Outdoor allergens (pollen, mould, etc.)
Contributing factors	Exposure to smoking
	Air pollution
	Small size at birth
	Dietary factors
	Air pollution

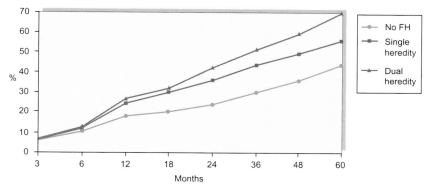

Fig. 3 **Cumulative incidence of recurrent wheezing in children in relation to atopy in the immediate family.**

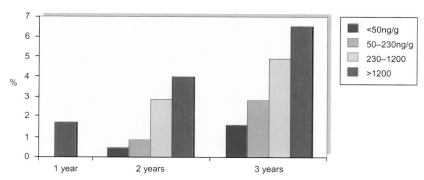

Fig. 4 **Sensitization to house-dust mite at 1, 2 and 3 years of age in relation to levels of dust-mite allergens at home.**

It is likely that IgE responses and related organ-specific disorders (asthma, rhinitis, etc.) are inherited through different, though possibly overlapping mechanisms. Gene loci at chromosome 11 and 5 have been suggested to be associated with atopy and asthma. The genetic risk is indicated by a higher incidence of allergy in those with a positive family history. To some extent this is disease-specific so that the risk for asthma in children is highest if the parents have asthma rather than rhinitis or atopic eczema (Figs 2 and 3).

Environmental factors

Atopic disease manifests itself when the genetically predisposed individual is exposed to various triggering factors (Table 1). Many such triggering factors are allergens to which the individual has become sensitized, usually by ingestion or inhalation. Although such sensitization can occur at any time during life, including the prenatal period, the infant appears particularly vulnerable.

During pregnancy

Maternal smoking during pregnancy is associated with increased IgE levels at birth and increased bronchial responsiveness in infancy. Infants born to smoking mothers tend to have impaired lung growth. The effect of consumption of highly allergenic foods, such as egg and peanut during pregnancy, is not yet clear.

Infancy

There is even stronger evidence linking exposure to allergen and adjuvants in infancy with the development of atopy in later life. A higher level of exposure to house-dust mite (Fig. 4), animal epithelium and pollen have all been proposed as risk factors for the development of allergic disease in genetically susceptible children. Cow's milk protein constitutes a major allergen in bottle-fed babies. However, many studies have not been able to demonstrate a protective effect of breast feeding on the development of allergy. Exposure to passive smoking is a risk factor for infantile wheezing, though the symptoms are usually transient.

A number of studies have concluded that children from large families have a reduced risk of developing atopic disorders, with the risk being lowest for the youngest child. A possible explanation is that infections in early life (a younger child being at a higher risk of respiratory infections from an older sibling) might inhibit the proliferation of Th2 cell clones and thus protect against the development of allergy. Contrary to general belief, some recent reports suggest that a higher exposure to pets and pollen during early childhood may actually induce tolerance and reduce the risk of asthma and rhinitis.

It seems that environmental factors play a significant role in determining phenotypic expression in children who are genetically predisposed. The influence of these factors is greatest during infancy. Any intervention thus has to be from birth, if not earlier. Precise identification of at-risk children is yet another challenge. A better understanding of the genetics of allergic disorders should achieve this goal.

Development of allergic disease

- Atopy is the genetic propensity to mount an exaggerated IgE response.
- Allergy is the clinical manifestation of atopy.
- Food allergy and eczema are common in early childhood.
- Infantile wheezing is often transient.
- Incidence of asthma reaches a peak in late childhood and declines thereafter.
- The genetic predisposition is for atopy as well as for the disease itself.
- Development of allergy depends on the genetic predisposition and environmental exposure to allergens in early life.
- Exposure to highly allergenic foods during early infancy may increase the risk of food allergy and eczema.
- Maternal smoking increases the risk of infantile wheezing.

EPIDEMIOLOGY OF ALLERGIC DISEASE

The percentage of a population affected by a condition at any one time is the 'prevalence'. Estimation of prevalence depends on the criteria used to diagnose the condition. Comparison between allergy prevalence quoted in various studies in different geographical areas has been marred by a lack of consistency and uniformity in diagnosis.

Almost 30% of the population develop one or more allergic disorders, ranging from transient eczema or mild hayfever symptoms to life-threatening asthma or systemic anaphylaxis (Table 1). Several studies have shown an increasing prevalence of asthma and other allergic disorders during the last few decades in the Western world. The International Study of Asthma and Allergy in Childhood (ISAAC) obtained comparable information on the prevalence of asthma and allergy from different parts of the world (Fig. 1).

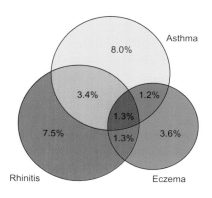

Fig. 1 **Overall prevalence of symptoms of asthma, rhinitis or atopic eczema or a combination of symptoms (ISAAC study).**

PREVALENCE OF ALLERGIC DISEASES

Asthma

Prevalence of wheezing in early childhood is 10–20% (Fig. 2). Most children improve, but others may develop, so that, by the age of 5 years, almost 40% of children have experienced wheezing at some stage. Wheezing in early childhood is often non-atopic and associated with viral upper respiratory infection. After 5 years, a diagnosis of asthma can confidently be made in most children. Previous studies have shown prevalence rates of 10–15% in the Western world. In the ISAAC study the prevalence of self-reported asthma at the age of 13–14 years varied from 1.6–36.8% in different countries. The highest prevalence was in the UK and New Zealand (30–35%) and the lowest in some East European countries (2–3%).

There is a male preponderance with a ratio of 2:1 in children, which disappears in adolescents. In adults, women may have a slightly higher overall prevalence but severe or life-threatening asthma is almost twice as common in women. Repeated studies with similar methods indicate at least a two-fold increase in the prevalence of asthma during the last two decades (Table 2). Hospital admission rates for asthma increased during the 1970s and 1980s but seems now to have stabilized. Despite this increase, the asthma mortality rates have remained at around 10–15 per million population in the Western world.

Allergic rhinitis

Rhinitis is inflammation of the nose, and symptoms are similar whatever the aetiology. Seasonal allergic rhinitis is caused by pollens of grass, trees, weeds or flowers and is easier to diagnose. Perennial allergic rhinitis is often difficult to differentiate from other causes and mild symptoms of rhinitis are often not reported. For these reasons, it is difficult to estimate an accurate prevalence.

The prevalence of seasonal allergic rhinitis (hayfever) is said to be around 10–12% and a similar figure is quoted for perennial allergic rhinitis. In the ISAAC study there was a 30-fold variation (1.4–39.7%) in symptoms of rhinitis between countries. Nigeria and Paraguay had the highest prevalence and some East European countries the lowest. The prevalence of seasonal allergic rhinitis is increasing. The best evidence comes from Switzerland where it was estimated to be 1% in 1926. Later studies indicated a gradually increasing prevalence in the same population to 4.4% in 1958, 9.6% in 1985 and 13.5% in 1993.

Atopic eczema

The prevalence rate of atopic eczema in early childhood is 10–12%. It was thought that infantile eczema clears in the vast majority (80%) but more recent studies indicate a much higher persistence rate (50%) of some eczema lesions into adulthood. In the ISAAC study, there was a 60-fold variation in the prevalence of symptoms of atopic eczema (0.3–20.5%). Highest prevalence was in the UK and Finland and lowest in Albania and China.

Contact dermatitis

Allergic contact dermatitis is due to a delayed-type reaction to contact with chemicals such as dyes, metals and detergents, detected on patch test. It is rare in

Table 1 **Overall prevalence of allergic diseases in the west**

Prevalence of allergic diseases	%
Asthma	10–15
Seasonal allergic rhinitis (hayfever)	10–12
Perennial allergic rhinitis	10
Atopic eczema	10–12
Cow's milk allergy (infancy)	3
Sensitization	35–40

Table 2 **Changes in the prevalence of asthma in same population studied with the same methods on two occasions**

Country	Study year	Age	n	Diagnosed asthma (%)	Author
Australia	1982	8–11	769	12.9	Britton 1986
	1992	8–11	795	19.3	Peat 1993
New Zealand	1975	12–18	715	26.2	Shaw et al 1990
	1989	12–18	435	34.0	
USA	1971–74	6–11	Large	4.8	Gergen 1988
	1976–80	6–11	27,275	7.6	
France	1968	21	814	3.3	Perdrzet et al 1987
	1982	21	10,559	5.4	
Tahiti	1979	16	3,870	11.5	Perdrzet et al 1987
	1984	13	6,731	14.3	

(Adapted from GINA, NHLBI/WHO Workshop report, 1995)

children. In adults the overall prevalence is around 1%, with no significant change noted in recent years. Contact sensitivity without clinical disease is much more common. On patch testing nearly 10% of the population is found to react to one or more common chemicals.

Food allergy

Food allergy is defined as an adverse reaction to food with an immunological basis. Other adverse reactions to foods may be termed food intolerance. Perception of food allergy is much higher than can be proved with tests. In one survey, almost 20% of the population believed they had a food allergy.

The type of food allergen varies according to the region and the eating habits of the population studied. Cow's milk, egg, fruits, nuts, fish, and wheat are the commonest food allergens. Symptoms of food allergy include gastrointestinal disturbance, urticaria/angioedema, worsening of asthma or eczema and rarely anaphylactic shock. Allergy to cow's milk (3–4%) and egg (2–3%) is common in infancy but persists beyond 3 years of age in a minority of these children. Increasing prevalence of peanut, soya and wheat allergy has been reported. No reliable data are available for food allergy in adults.

Anaphylaxis

The number of people who have suffered from one or more anaphylactic shocks in their life is less than 1 per 1000. Common causes of anaphylaxis include drugs, insect venom and foods, especially nuts. Allergy to latex has been reported increasingly in the last decade. Drugs implicated in the causation of anaphylactic shock include antibiotics, non-steroidal antiinflammatory drugs, anaesthetics and radio-contrast media.

PREVALENCE OF SENSITIZATION

Sensitization is assessed with either skin test or the presence of specific IgE in the serum. The type of allergen causing sensitization depends on the age of the subject and the distribution of allergens in the environment. In early childhood, egg and milk are common allergens. In older children and adults, house-dust mite, grass pollen and animals such as cats form the major allergenic sensitizers (Fig. 3). Although mono-sensitization occurs, most subjects are sensitized to several allergens.

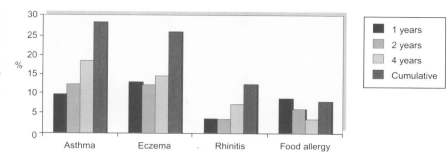

Fig. 2 **Prevalence of allergic disorders in early childhood** (data from Tariq S, Mathews S, Stevens M, Hakim E, Arshad SH 1998 The prevalence of and risk factors for atopy in early childhood: A whole population birth cohort study. J. Allergy Clin. Immunol. 101, p587–93.).

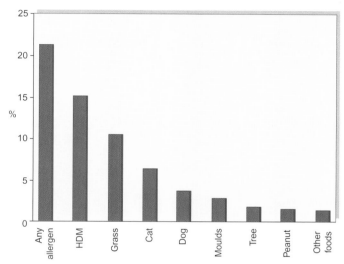

Fig. 3 **Sensitization to common allergens in an unselected population of 10-year-old children** (data from Isle of Wight Birth Cohort Study).

Between 30–40% of the population is sensitized to one or more allergen. This figure was less than 20% two decades ago. A significant proportion of sensitized individuals do not have symptoms of allergy (latent atopy) but they may develop symptoms at a later date.

RISING PREVALENCE OF ALLERGY

There is now compulsive evidence, even accounting for increased awareness, that allergic diseases have increased during the last few decades, primarily observed in the developed world. The reason for this is largely unknown. An upsurge in exposure to allergens and adjuvants has been proposed as a plausible explanation. A Western lifestyle with insulated homes, high indoor humidity and wall-to-wall carpets promotes dust mite proliferation. Dietary habits have also changed, with increased consumption of processed foods. There is little evidence to incriminate air pollution as a possible cause. Reduction in the incidence of infections may be one of the explanations. Infections stimulate Th1 type of immunity with the secretion of IFN-γ and IL-12, which suppress Th2 type reactions responsible for allergic responses.

Epidemiology of allergic disease
- Almost 30% of the population develop one or more allergic disorders.
- Nearly 40% of the population is sensitized to one or more allergens.
- In the Western world the prevalence of allergic disorders is rising.
- The prevalence of asthma varies from 2–36% in different countries.
- In the ISAAC study there was a 30-fold variation in the symptoms of rhinitis and 60-fold in the symptoms of eczema, between countries.
- Allergy to cow's milk and eggs is common in infancy but rare in adults.

PREDICTION AND PREVENTION OF ALLERGIC DISEASE

The recent increase in the prevalence of asthma and other atopic diseases has highlighted the need for primary prevention (preventing the future development of disease in healthy individuals). A history of allergic disease in the immediate family (genetics) is the most important risk factor, and recent studies have focused attention on the role played by environmental factors (environment). The concept that the interaction of genetic and environmental factors is responsible for phenotypic expression of disease in genetically predisposed infants is attractive because children at high risk can be identified and intervention should lead to a reduction in disease prevalence.

Epidemiological and experimental evidence indicates that a critical period exists early in life, when exposure to allergens and adjuvants may be crucial in determining if an atopic phenotype develops. It is therefore important to identify markers which can reliably predict infants at risk of developing atopy. Prophylactic intervention (by allergen avoidance or medication) can then be directed toward the infants at very high risk who will benefit most (Fig. 1).

PREDICTION OF ATOPY

It has long been recognized that a family history of asthma and/or allergy in a young child is strongly associated with an increased risk of developing allergic disease. Approximately 40% of children with single heredity (one parent or sibling) and 60% with dual heredity (two or more first-degree relatives) will develop allergic disease. Family history of atopy is used to predict the risk in clinical settings and as a screening test to identify at-risk children in studies. However, only 70% of subjects with allergic disease have a positive family history. By using family history as the sole criteria for intervention, almost 50% will be subjected to prophylactic measures unnecessarily and 30% will still be missed.

The measurement of cord blood IgE was thought to be a useful screening test and this was advocated before instituting any prevention programme. Unfortunately, more recent studies have shown that its sensitivity is too low for it to be useful (Fig. 2).

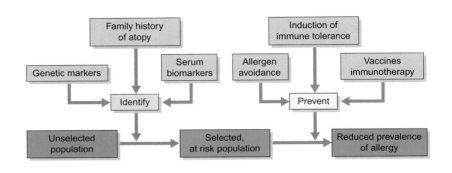

Fig. 1 **A schematic presentation of strategy to predict and prevent allergic disease**.

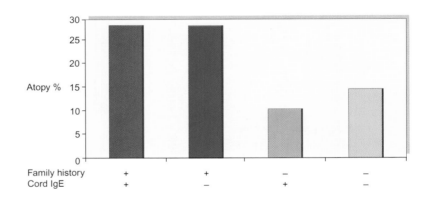

Fig. 2 **Comparison of family history and cord IgE as predictor of atopy in early childhood.** The addition of cord IgE did not add to the predictive capacity of family history. A + indicates a positive history of atopy or of IgE in the umbilical cord. (data from: Hide DW, Arshad H, Twiselton R and Stevens M. 1991 Cord serum IgE: An insensitive method for prediction of atopy. Clin Exp Allergy 21, p739–43).

Sensitization, as assessed by a positive skin-prick test or the presence of specific IgE antibodies, may herald the development of clinical disease. The presence of a positive skin-prick test to egg and milk and to dust mite increases the risk for later development of asthma. However, as the sensitization has already developed, preventive measures may not be very successful.

Current understanding of the immunological mechanisms underlying inflammation has identified a number of bio-markers. Several such markers have been proposed as predictors for the development of allergic disease, but they have not yet been shown to be useful as a screening test (Table 1).

At present only family history appears to have some worthwhile predictive value in the development of asthma and allergic disease. The search goes on for biomarkers that can reliably identify infants at risk of developing atopy in later life. Until markers are shown to have high specificity, sensitivity and predictive value, and are easy to perform, it is unlikely that they will be incorporated into clinical practice as predictors.

Table 1 **Proposed bio-markers in infancy as predictors of allergy**

- High IgE levels at birth
- Presence of serum IgG antibodies to food allergens during infancy
- Presence of specific IgE antibodies or positive skin-prick test to egg and dust mites
- Reduced response of cord blood mononuclear cells to produce IFN-γ
- Low IL-12 production by stimulated peripheral blood mononuclear cells
- Elevated serum levels of IL-4
- Eosinophilic products in serum and urine

Table 2 **Prevention of allergy**

	Target population	Aims	Methods
General measures	Whole population	Reduce prevalence of disease in the community	Reduce pollution and allergens in the environment, encourage breast feeding and healthy eating
Primary prevention	At-risk but healthy or sensitized but without clinical disease	Prevent the development of sensitization and symptomatic disease	Reduce exposure to allergens and pollution, exclusive breast-feeding, preventive medications
Secondary prevention	Diagnosed disease	Prevent symptoms and complications	Optimal treatment, avoidance of triggers, monitoring

Table 3 **Recommended prevention programme for children at high risk of allergic disease**

- Exclusive breast-feeding for 6–12 months
- Maternal avoidance of highly allergenic foods (milk, egg, nuts and fish) during lactation
- Hypoallergenic formula as a substitute for up to 9 months
- Solid foods introduced only after 6 months
- Cow's milk, egg, nuts and fish introduced gradually from 9 months
- Mite avoidance programme with covered mattresses from birth
- No smoking inside the house
- No pets inside the house

GENERAL MEASURES

Measures targeted at the whole population can be effective in reducing the prevalence of a disease in the community. In the early part of this century, improvements in hygiene and sanitation, in addition to vaccination, reduced the incidence and prevalence of infections. For allergy prevention we do not yet know of any measures that can be directed at the whole population, which are safe and effective.

PRIMARY PREVENTION

Any primary preventive programme for infants at high risk requires highly motivated parents and close cooperation with the physician and other health care workers.

Experimental evidence indicates that the child can be sensitized in utero. It is sometimes advised that an atopic mother should avoid highly allergenic foods such as egg, nuts, fish and cow's milk during pregnancy, but this is not recommended because of the concern that this might adversely affect the growth of the foetus.

Avoidance of allergens during early infancy has been shown to reduce the development of allergy in at-risk infants (Fig. 3). Among food allergens, cow's milk is an important allergen at this stage, and exclusive breast-feeding has been advocated (Table 2). Although some studies have reported benefit, others have been inconclusive. As protein ingested by the lactating mother can be detected in the breast milk (a potential source of sensitization) a maternal diet that excludes allergenic foods during lactation has been advised. Delayed (after 6 months) introduction of solid foods and a further (1–2 years) delay of more allergenic foods such as eggs, fish and nuts have also been recommended. The diet of the mother and child should be carefully monitored in any such prevention programme (Table 3).

There is evidence that higher exposure to aeroallergens such as house-dust mites and cats during infancy may result in a higher incidence of sensitization and perhaps asthma. A reduction in exposure to indoor allergens during infancy has been shown to reduce sensitization to these allergens. Maternal smoking during pregnancy and the early years of a child's life may increase the incidence of sensitization and wheezing and this should be avoided.

Children with eczema or those who are sensitized to food allergens have a very high risk of developing asthma and aeroallergen sensitization. Reducing the exposure of these children to aeroallergens may be helpful, and some drugs such as non-sedating antihistamines have been investigated as a preventative strategy in this group.

SECONDARY PREVENTION

Environmental control, focusing on reducing exposure to allergens to which the individual is sensitized, should always be advised. Avoidance of irritants such as cigarette smoke and other triggers help to reduce symptoms and exacerbations. The use of anti-inflammatory drugs such as sodium cromoglicate and topical steroids as preventive medication cannot be overlooked. Specific immunotherapy for allergic rhinitis and asthma may also be considered as prophylactic treatment. Optimal treatment of asthma, eczema and rhinitis should prevent the development of complications.

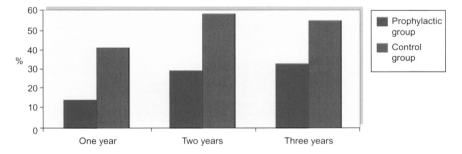

Fig. 3 **Prevention of allergic disease in children at high risk of atopy at ages 1, 2 and 4 years.** Children were protected from allergenic foods and dust mites during infancy.

Prediction and prevention of allergic disease

- In children with atopic heredity, environmental factors in early life determine the development of allergy.
- Family history of atopy is used as a screening test to identify at-risk children.
- Cord blood IgE is not a useful screening test for atopy.
- Several inflammatory bio-markers have been proposed as predictors for atopy, but none has yet proven useful.
- Avoidance of allergens during infancy has been shown to reduce the development of allergy.
- Any prevention programme which includes the diet of the mother and child should be carefully monitored.

AEROALLERGENS 1 – INTRODUCTION

Antigens are protein molecules capable of stimulating an immune response. Allergens are antigens with a specific type of immune response, i.e. the production of IgE antibodies. All of us are exposed to a vast number of allergens in our environment. However, the allergic response occurs only in 20–30% of the population who are genetically predisposed (atopics). Even atopic individuals are not sensitized to every allergen. Why they get sensitized to some allergens and develop tolerance to others is not entirely clear (Fig. 1). Moreover, sensitization does not always cause clinical disease. The factors responsible for this are also not clearly understood.

ALLERGEN SOURCES

Aeroallergens are allergens present in the air and mostly cause symptoms of the respiratory tract. Common indoor allergens include those originating from house-dust mites, animals and moulds. Pollens of grasses, trees, weeds and flowers and some types of mould spores are major outdoor allergens. In the last decades major allergens from most common allergen sources have been purified and characterized (Table 1).

RECOMBINANT ALLERGENS

Molecular biologic techniques have permitted identification of antigenic determinants or epitopes for most allergens. The epitope is the part of the allergen molecule which recognizes and interacts with T or B cell receptors.

Expression cloning of allergen complimentary cDNA enables the production of recombinant proteins which are identical to the native allergen. Recombinant allergens with comparable immunoreactivity to the natural allergen have been

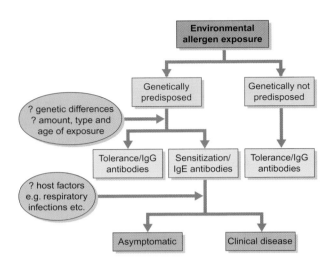

Fig. 1 **Environmental exposure to allergens and development of sensitization.**

produced for most common allergens. The molecular cloning of an allergen allows for the identification of all the epitopes on the allergen. Some epitopes are highly immunoreactive, whereas others are of minor importance. Recombinant allergens are extremely useful in understanding the functional characteristics of these allergens and may become useful in clinical practice (Fig. 2).

ALLERGENS AND ALLERGIC DISEASE

The pattern of sensitization to a specific allergen reflects the mean level of that allergen found in the community (Table 2). Sensitization is a risk factor for the development of allergic diseases. This lends support to the view that increased prevalence of allergic disease is a result of an increase in allergen, especially

Table 1 **Some common allergen sources and their major allergens**

Common name	Species	Allergens
Dust mites	*Dermatophagoides pteronyssinus*	Der-p-1–11
	Dermatophagoides farinae	Der-f-1–4
Cat	*Felix domesticus*	Fel-d-1
Dog	*Canis familiaris*	Can-f-1,2
German cockroach	*Blattella germanica*	Bla-g-1–6
Pollens		
Rye grass	*Lolium perenne*	Lol-p-1–5
Timothy grass	*Phleum pratense*	Phl-p-1,4–6
Bermuda grass	*Cynodon dactylon*	Cyn-d-1
Birch	*Betula verrucosa*	Bet-v-1–4
Ragweed (short)	*Ambrosia artemisiifolia*	Amb-a-1–7,10
Ragweed (giant)	*Ambrosia trifida*	Amb-t-5
Olive	*Olea europaea*	Ole-e-1,2
Moulds	*Alternaria Alternata*	Alta-1,2,3,6,7,10
	Aspergillus fumigatus	Asp-f-1,2,6
Stinging insects		
Honeybee	*Apis melifera*	Api-m-1,2,4
Wasp	*Polistes annularis*	Pol-a-1,2,5
Latex	*Hevea brasiliensis*	Hev-b-1–7
Foods		
Cow's milk	*Caseins*	Group 1–5
Egg white	*Gallus domesticus*	Gal-d-1–3
Peanut	*Arachis hypogea*	Ara-h-1,2
Cod (fish)	*Gadus callarias*	Gad-c-1
Allergen nomenclature as recommended by WHO		

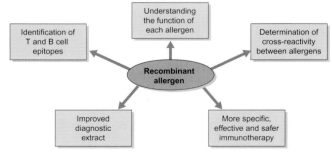

Fig. 2 **Uses of recombinant proteins and peptide allergens.**

Table 2 **Evidence for exposure to indoor allergen in relation to the development of sensitization and development of allergic disease**

- A dose–response relationship exists between exposure to indoor allergens and sensitization
- Sensitization to dust mite, cat and cockroach allergen is a risk factor for asthma and allergic rhinitis
- Allergen bronchial provocation causes bronchial constriction in sensitized subjects with asthma
- Allergen nasal provocation causes nasal inflammation in sensitized subjects with rhinitis
- Provocation with dust mite allergen in patients with atopic dermatitis causes worsening of the condition
- Avoidance of allergen leads to improvement in symptoms of asthma and rhinitis and bronchial reactivity
- The evidence linking allergen exposure and development of allergic disease is best demonstrated for dust mite

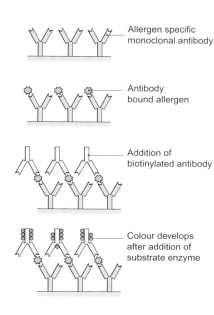

Allergen specific monoclonal antibody

Antibody bound allergen

Addition of biotinylated antibody

Colour develops after addition of substrate enzyme

Fig. 3 **Schematic diagram of enzyme-linked immunoassay using monoclonal antibody for the quantification of allergen in the dust sample.**

ASSESSMENT OF EXPOSURE

Indoor allergens

Indoor allergens such as house-dust mite, cat, dog and cockroach allergens can be measured in the dust with samples collected from a vacuum cleaner, or in the air with the help of an air sampler. Various methods are used, but commonly dust is collected from a 1 m² area of carpet or mattress for 1 min. Enzyme-linked immunoassays (EIA) using monoclonal antibodies have been developed to measure the amount of major allergens, and give a fairly accurate indication of exposure to the respective allergen (Fig. 3). The results are expressed per unit weight of dust (μg/g of dust) or per unit of area (μg/m²). Mites can also be counted and the results expressed as mite density per unit weight of dust, however this is cumbersome and requires experience in identifying and counting the mites. As a rough guide, 10 μg/g of dust is approximately equal to 500 mites per g of dust.

For assessment of exposure the allergen level in the air may be more relevant, but in the absence of major disturbance such as vacuuming or bed-making, the level of dust mite allergen is very low and difficult to detect. The major cat allergen, Fel-d-1, can be measured relatively easily in both dust and air samples, as the particles are generally less than 5 μm in diameter and remain suspended in the air. The major dog allergen Can-f-1 has similar properties. The highest concentration of cockroach allergen is found in dust samples from the kitchen. Like house-dust mite, allergens of German cock-

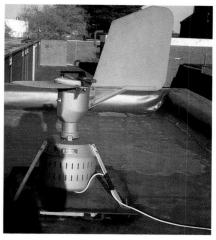

Fig. 4 **Pollen trap located on the roof of a hospital.**

roach, Bla-g-1 and Bla-g-2, are only airborne in significant quantities during disturbance of the dust.

Outdoor allergens

Important outdoor allergens are pollens of grass, trees and weeds. Several methods are available for the assessment of exposure to these allergens. A pollen sampler can be used to trap pollen particles on a slide (Fig. 4). The pollen is then counted under the microscope to give a quantitative assessment of the amount of pollen present in the air.

Mould spores can be grown on culture plates placed indoors or outdoors. Measurement of fungal antigens, for example those from *Alternaria* and *Aspergillus*, is possible, but their usefulness in assessing allergen exposure has not been demonstrated.

indoor allergen, levels. Most important among these is the dust mite, but other allergens assume importance in areas where conditions are less favourable to dust mites. For example, in Northern Scandinavia and mountain areas of the USA, cat and dog allergens are the primary cause of asthma. Similarly, in Arizona and central Australia, *Alternaria* is the dominant allergen associated with asthma. Exposure to pollen does not correlate with prevalence or severity of asthma.

Aeroallergens – Introduction

- Allergens are antigens which evoke an IgE-mediated allergic response in genetically predisposed subjects.
- A number of major and minor allergens have been found for house-dust mites, pollens and moulds.
- Each allergen molecule contains several antigenic determinants or epitopes.
- Recombinant allergens are useful in understanding the functional characteristics of these allergens.
- The pattern of sensitization to a specific allergen reflects the mean level of that allergen found in the community.
- Indoor allergens such as dust mite, cat, dog and cockroach allergens can be measured in the dust.
- Allergens of dust mite and cockroach are airborne in significant quantities only during disturbance of the dust.
- The amount of pollen in the air can be estimated with the help of a pollen trap.

AEROALLERGENS 2 – COMMON ALLERGENS

HOUSE-DUST MITES

The common name 'house-dust mite' includes members of the family *pyroglyphidae*. Two of the commonest species, *pteronyssinus* and *farinae*, belong to the genus *Dermatophagoides*. Approximately 20% of the adult population in Europe are sensitized to *D. pteronyssinus* (Fig. 1). The most important indoor allergen (Der-p-1) is the major allergen from *D. pteronyssinus*. This allergen is essentially a proteolytic enzyme present in the faecal particles of the dust mite. Exposure to allergens from house-dust mite can cause asthma, rhinitis and atopic dermatitis in sensitized subjects.

Habitat

Comfortable home environments and energy-efficient houses with reduced ventilation and high humidity have resulted in an extremely favourable environment for the proliferation of house-dust mites. Mites are found in areas which collect dust, such as mattresses/bedding, carpets, soft furnishings, soft toys and curtains. They thrive in a high-humidity environment (> 60% relative humidity at 20°C). Most of the exposure to dust mite allergen occurs in bed with close proximity to the mite-infested material.

Assessment of exposure

Dust samples are collected with a vacuum cleaner to estimate the burden of mites in the house. Major allergens (group 1 and group 2) of the common species of house-dust mite should be used for the monitoring of dust mite allergen exposure. The faecal pellets (source of the allergen) are relatively heavy and settle quickly from the air. As yet, immunoassays are not sensitive enough to reliably measure the very small amount of allergen present in the air.

Dust mite and disease

The risk of sensitization and development of clinical disease is directly related to the level of exposure. Levels of 2 μg/g dust

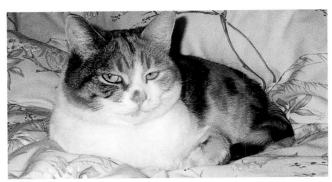

Fig. 2 **Cats (*Felix domesticus*) produce potent allergens in their sebaceous gland secretions.** Once dried, it comes off the skin and hair and is then distributed widely in the house.

and 10 μg/g dust have been suggested as risk factors for sensitization and asthma symptoms respectively. The evidence of exposure to dust mite and allergic disease is strongest for asthma. A dose–response relationship has been suggested in epidemiological and clinical studies between the levels of dust mite and severity of asthma symptoms. Dust mites are also the most important causal factor for perennial allergic rhinitis. Recent studies have demonstrated exacerbation of eczema on bronchial challenge with dust mite allergen.

DOMESTIC ANIMALS

In Europe, nearly 50% of homes have a cat and/or dog (Fig. 2). It is common knowledge that cats and dogs can provoke symptoms of asthma and rhinitis in sensitized individuals. There is no relationship between the species of animal (long or short hair) and allergenicity. In some communities 70% of children with asthma are sensitized to cat and/or dog. Cats are more allergenic than dogs, and the primary source of major cat allergen, Fel-d-1 is the sebaceous glands of the skin. In dogs, major allergen has been identified in saliva, epidermal scales and urine. In houses with cats, a large amount of cat allergen accumulates in the carpet, upholstered furniture and other dust reservoirs. Cat allergen particles are small and remain airborne for a long time. Fel-d-1 can be measured, both in the dust and in the air, using monoclonal antibody-based immunoassays, and can be detected for months after the cat has been removed from the house.

Table 1 **Ecology of common pollens of tree, grasses and weeds**

Common pollens	Distribution
Trees:	
Birch, hazel, alder, oak and elm	North Europe, North America and Asia
Olive	Mediterranean
Japanese cedar	Japan
Grasses:	
Timothy, rye, orchard blue, Bermuda	World-wide
Weeds:	
Ragweed	North America
Parietaria	Mediterranean
Mugwort	North Europe

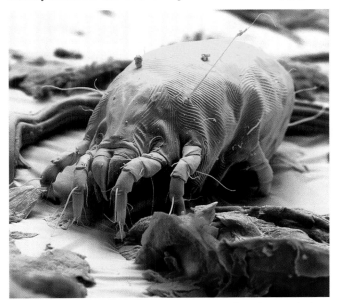

Fig. 1 **House-dust mites: *Dermatophagoids pteronyssinus* photographed with a scanning electron microscope.** © Eye of Science – Science Photo Library

OTHER ANIMALS

Sensitization to cockroach allergens among patients with asthma and rhinitis is common in some inner city areas in the USA. Major cockroach allergens Bla-g-1–4 come from the body parts, saliva and faeces. The highest levels of these allergens are found on kitchen floors.

Mice, rats, guinea pigs and hamsters are used in medical research and they are also increasingly being kept as pets. The urine of these animals is a potent source of allergen. The dust in the cage becomes heavily contaminated with the allergen and when airborne it causes symptoms of asthma and rhinitis. Allergy to horses, cows and birds occasionally becomes a problem in those who are exposed. An IgE-mediated response to bird droppings causes asthma, but an IgG response may result in extrinsic allergic alveolitis.

POLLENS

Pollens of grasses, trees and weeds are the main cause of seasonal allergic rhinitis (Table 1 & Fig. 3). They have a different seasonal distribution (Fig. 4). They are light and spread over a wide area with air currents. Grass pollen counts are high on hot and dry days and low on a rainy day. The exposure is highest in the morning and in the late afternoon. As the grains are 15–50 μm in diameter, they get trapped in the upper respiratory tract and conjunctiva causing nasal and eye symptoms. Flower pollens are usually carried by insects, and are a less common cause of allergy.

There is extensive cross-reactivity between many species of grasses, and among trees. Therefore, a mixture of grass pollens (such as timothy, rye, orchard, etc.) and of trees (birch, hazel and alder) can be used. This limits the number of extracts required for diagnosis and therapy.

MOULDS

Moulds or microfungi grow in damp areas, as they require a high relative humidity. Damp houses may contain large numbers of mould spores. Moulds are perennial allergens although their number may be highest during autumn months.

Table 2 **Common occupational allergens and sensitizing agents**

Allergen	Occupation / Industry
Isocyanates	Plastic and synthetic material industry and painters
Anhydrides	Plastic and paint industry
Rats, mice, guinea-pigs	Laboratory workers
Latex	Health care workers
Fish, crabs, prawns	Fish industry
Enzymes	Pharmaceutical and food industry
Organic dust	Farmer
Wheat flour	Bakers
Chromium	Cement users
Colophony	Electricians
Nickel salts	Metal plating
Platinum salts	Photographers, metal refineries

Alternaria, Cladosporium and Aspergillus are common moulds. The spores are present in the air both indoors and outdoors. As the size of the spores is 2–5 μm, they are inhaled, causing asthma. Sometimes a combined IgE and IgG response occurs (bronchopulmonay aspergillosis), and a predominantly IgG response causes extrinsic allergic alveolitis. In those with immune deficiency, invasive fungal infections may occur.

OCCUPATIONAL SENSITIZERS

The prevalence of occupational asthma has increased in recent years. Both proteins (allergens) and low molecular weight chemicals (haptens) can initiate IgE-mediated allergic reactions (Table 2). Atopy, bronchial hyper-responsiveness and smoking are recognized risk factors.

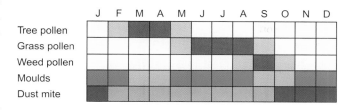

Fig. 4 **Seasonal variation in the level of airborne allergens throughout the year.** Pollens are shown in green; mould in orange and dust mites in red. Darker colours indicate periods of high levels.

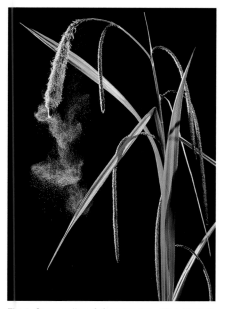

Fig. 3 **Grass pollen.** © Getty Images – Mark Mattlock

Aeroallergens – Common allergens

- House-dust mite is the most important allergen for asthma and perennial allergic rhinitis.
- Dust mites are found in places which collect dust, such as mattresses, carpets and upholstery.
- Dust mite allergen is contained in mite faecal and body particles, which become airborne during disturbance of the dust.
- The major allergen of cat and dog is found in saliva and skin, and becomes airborne as the secretions dry.
- Cat/dog allergen is distributed widely in the indoor environment.
- Wind-pollinating plants such as grasses, trees and weeds cause seasonal allergic rhinitis.
- Insect-pollinating plants (flowers) do not often cause allergic symptoms.
- The grass pollen count is low on cold rainy days and high on hot, dry days.
- Moulds are microscopic fungi that grow in damp conditions.
- Mould spores are small and are found both indoors and outdoors.

SKIN TESTS 1 – METHODS

BACKGROUND

In 1873 Charles Blackley rubbed pollens on abraded skin to give us the first description of an allergy skin test. Skin tests are now used as the first-line diagnostic tool in the management of allergic disorders. Although the technique is simple, the indications and interpretations of allergy skin tests require the expertise of well-trained allergists. Skin tests should be considered as a laboratory aid and interpreted with reference to the information available from history and physical examination.

TYPES OF SKIN TESTS

Several methods are in use, but prick test or its modifications are the most commonly employed. The volar surface of the arm is commonly used for convenience, although the test can be done on the back. The area should be marked with a pen to indicate the site for each test. The only other type of skin test in common use is intradermal (intracutaneous) test, which may be useful in specific situations.

CHOICE OF ALLERGEN EXTRACTS

The choice of allergen to be tested depends on the history. Purified allergen extracts are supplied by the manufacturers (Fig. 1). For respiratory allergy a standard battery of common aeroallergens is used with the addition of other allergens, as indicated by the history (Table 1). The standard battery varies according to the prevalence of allergens in the local environment. For example, in the UK grass pollen should always be included, whereas in Scandinavia birch pollen and in Southern Europe olive, should be part of the standard battery. In

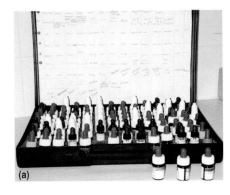
(a)

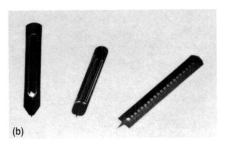
(b)

Fig. 1 (a) Box of allergen extracts used for skin prick tests. (b) Lancets for skin-prick testing.

the UK, more than 90% of atopics would react to one or more of the three most common allergens, dust mite, grass pollen and cat. The choice of allergens in skin tests to food depends largely on the history, but common allergens include cow's milk, eggs, peanuts, fish and shellfish.

ALLERGEN EXTRACTS

It is preferable to use standardized allergen extracts for skin testing. This requires all major allergens from the allergen source (such as dust mites) to be present and the potency tested with both in vitro and in vivo methods. The in vitro method involves techniques such as RAST inhibition, where the allergen is tested against sera from subjects known to be sensitized to that allergen, to confirm the presence of major allergens, and to assess the reactivity of the extract. The potency should also be assessed biologically by skin testing with serial 10-fold dilutions of the extract.

For prick test a concentrated solution (100 000 SQU or AU/ml) is used with the content of the major allergen documented

for each allergen. Unfortunately, standardized extracts are available for only common inhalant allergens, such as pollens and dust mites. Food extracts are not standardized and in many cases, especially for fruits, it is better to use fresh fruits as the allergen source for prick test.

For intradermal test, aqueous extracts are stabilized in human serum albumin and for prick test in 50% glycerine. They are stored refrigerated at −4°C. Positive and negative controls should always be used. Normal saline or diluents used to preserve the extracts may be used as negative control. A reaction to this indicates dermographism (non-specific reaction to trauma). Histamine, 1–10 mg/ml for prick testing, and 0.01–0.1 mg/ml for intradermal testing, is used as positive control. Other mast cell secretory agents, such as codeine phosphate, may also be used as positive control.

METHOD

Skin-prick test

Two methods are in common use. In the modified prick test, a drop of allergen solution is placed on the skin and the

Table 1 **Common allergens used in skin-prick test for the diagnosis of allergy**

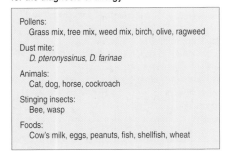

Pollens:
   Grass mix, tree mix, weed mix, birch, olive, ragweed

Dust mite:
   D. pteronyssinus, D. farinae

Animals:
   Cat, dog, horse, cockroach

Stinging insects:
   Bee, wasp

Foods:
   Cow's milk, eggs, peanuts, fish, shellfish, wheat

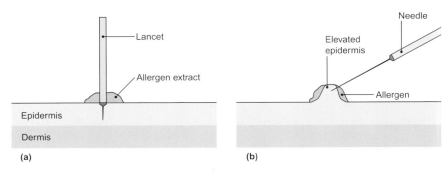

Fig. 2 **Prick test methods** (a) Prick-puncture test: the skin is punctured through a drop of allergen extract at 90° and pressed for 1 s. (b) Modified prick test: the needle is inserted in the epidermis, through the allergen. The superficial layers of the epidermis are elevated slightly, before withdrawing the needle.

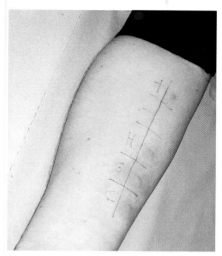

Fig. 3 **An arm with positive skin-prick test reactions:** + = histamine control, − = saline control, H = house-dust mite, G = grass pollen, C = cat.

Histamine	
Saline	
House dust mite	
Grass pollen	
Tree pollen	
Cat	
Dog	
Alternaria	
Cladosporium	

Fig. 4 **A record of skin test reactions, transferred to paper using clear tape.** The test was done to a standard aeroallergen battery.

epidermal surface is pricked through the drop. The needle tip is gently elevated to lift the epidermal layers without causing bleeding. The test solution can then be absorbed with a tissue. Another method (prick-puncture test) is to use a steel lancet with 1 mm tip and shoulders to prevent excessive penetration. The tip is inserted through the drop, into the skin at a right angle, for one second (Fig. 2). This method has a higher reproducibility than modified prick test. Fruits can be tested with the prick-prick method. First the lancet is pierced into the fresh fruit. The skin is then pricked with the same lancet.

After 10–15 min the reactions are seen and recorded (Fig. 3). The largest diameter of the wheal (oedema) and the diameter perpendicular to it are measured and the mean wheal diameter is calculated. A more precise method is to calculate the area of the wheal by planimetry. However, the mean wheal diameter is easy to calculate and correlates well with the area. To obtain a permanent record, the wheal should be encircled with a fine tip pen and the drawing should then be transferred to a sheet by means of translucent tape (Fig. 4).

The coefficient of variation for prick test should not be more than 10–15% if appropriate precautions are taken in performing the test (Table 2). Some authorities recommend that a duplicate skin test should be performed, as the test may be negative in 5% of clearly sensitized patients. For reproducibility of the test, the technician should intermittently perform 20 tests with histamine control solution on the same subject. The reaction size should not vary more than ± 1 mm.

Determination of end-point titration provides a quantitative assessment of reactivity, and is highly reproducible. A series of allergen concentrations are used to determine the lowest concentration that gives a positive reaction.

Intradermal test

A series of allergen dilutions, starting with 1:10 000 of the most concentrated solution, is used. A small amount (0.02–0.03 ml) of each solution is injected in the superficial layers of the dermis, using a 1 ml syringe, to form a small bleb. The reaction is observed after 10–15 min and the size of the wheal and surrounding flare (erythema) noted before injecting the next higher concentration, until a wheal size of 5–10 mm and a flare of 10–30 mm is produced, or the highest concentration reached. Intradermal test is highly reproducible with a coefficient of variation of 5–10%.

Table 2 **Appropriate precautions to take before and during skin test procedure**

Skin test should only be performed where a systemic reaction could be immediately treated

Standardized extracts should be used when possible

Ensure the subject has not taken a drug which may suppress skin reaction

Positive and negative control should always be included in the test panel

Choose an area of healthy skin

The test sites for each allergen should not be too close to each other

Avoid using an area too close to the wrist or antecubital fossa

For prick-puncture test, use the same pressure for test solutions including positive and negative controls

For intradermal test, make sure that the concentrations of extracts and volume injected are appropriate and the injection is not too deep (subcutaneous)

Keep extracts refrigerated between use

Skin tests – Methods

- Skin tests are the most useful diagnostic tool in the management of allergic disorders.
- Allergen extracts for testing are chosen after considering the patient's history and the knowledge of allergens commonly present in the area.
- Standardized extracts should be used whenever possible.
- Positive and negative controls should always be used.
- There are two common methods; prick test and intradermal test.
- In prick test, the allergen is pricked into the epidermis.
- Modified prick and prick-puncture are two methods in common use for prick test.
- In intradermal test, allergen is injected into the dermis.
- Fresh fruits and vegetables can be used as allergen source using prick-prick method.

SKIN TESTS 2 – USES AND INTERPRETATION

Prick-test is generally preferred and is adequate for most diagnostic needs. Intradermal test is more sensitive than prick test and in some situations this may be indicated. If the history is highly suggestive, and the prick-test is negative, an intradermal test may be performed to detect a low degree of sensitization. It may also be used in the evaluation of drug and venom allergy. There is a small risk of systemic reactions including anaphylaxis with intradermal test, whereas prick-test is extremely safe and systemic reactions are rare even in highly sensitized subjects (Fig. 1).

INTERPRETATION

Prick-test is regarded as positive when the wheal size (mean wheal diameter) is at least 3 mm, with a positive control of > 3 mm, in the absence of a reaction to negative control. The reactivity to histamine is less in infants. Therefore, a reaction size of 2 mm or more is regarded as positive. The test is semi-quantitative, in that the size of the reaction correlates with the sensitivity of the patient to that allergen in a logarithmic fashion, i.e. a change of 1 mm in wheal size indicates a 10-fold difference in skin sensitivity. An intradermal test is positive if a wheal size of 5–10 mm is achieved, and the concentration at which this happens is an indicator of the sensitivity.

For inhalant allergens, a good correlation exists between the prick-test, levels of specific IgE and bronchial or nasal allergen challenge. The percentage of agreement between skin test and the presence of specific IgE ranges between 85–95%. Discordance consists primarily of positive skin test in the absence of specific IgE, i.e. skin test is more sensitive but less specific. Although the cut-off for positivity is taken at 3 mm, the correlation with provocation tests is higher with a skin reaction size of 5 mm or more. The correlation is generally low when unstandardized allergen extracts are used and if there is a discrepancy between history and skin test. The correlation of skin test with foods and food challenges is less well documented, except perhaps for peanut and tree nuts. This is due to the unavailability of standardized allergen extracts for foods. Using well-characterized food allergen extracts, a negative test has good predictive value but a positive test does not necessarily indicate clinical reactivity.

False-positive reactions may be due to an irritant reaction. This is less common with a prick-test but may occur more often with an intradermal test. False-negative reactions may occur if the extract has lost potency. Some drugs, particularly antihistamines, and other factors may affect skin-test reaction (Tables 1 and 2). It should be remembered that over-the-counter prepara-

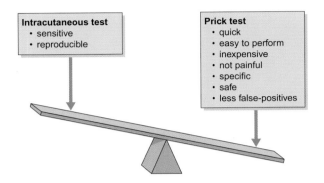

Fig. 1 **Skin prick-tests have more advantages than intracutaneous tests.**

tions and 'cold remedies' may contain antihistamines that may not be obvious from the label. Reaction to positive control gives an indication of the state of skin responsiveness in most conditions. The sensitivity and specificity of prick-test, using standardized allergens, is around 90%.

LATENT ALLERGY

Positive skin-test reactions are commonly noted in patients who do not react clinically to these allergens. In some cases this reaction denotes past allergy, where the patient has become tolerant to the allergen, but skin-sensitivity persists. This often occurs in children with foods such as egg. There are few prospective follow-up studies of patients with sensitization to aeroallergens on skin test without clinical reaction. It seems that nearly 30–50% of these patients will develop clinical allergy over the next 5 years.

MECHANISM

The allergen, when introduced into the skin, reacts with the IgE antibodies bound to the mast cells with the release of mediators. Histamine is the most important mediator in causing the wheal and flare reaction. The wheal is caused by histamine-induced vasodilatation and extravasation of plasma. Flare is a neurovascular response initiated by histamine with the involvement of neuropeptides such as substance P. A skin test is a biological assay of the amount of IgE antibodies present in the blood. The size of the reaction depends on the degree of sensitization, amount of allergen injected, number and releasability of mast cells and the reactivity of dermal tissue to mediators, particularly histamine.

Table 1 **Factors affecting skin-test reactions**

Factors	Comments
Age	Reactivity is reduced in infancy but increases from early childhood to adolescents and declines in older age
Skin surface	Skin of the back is more reactive than the forearm
Allergen exposure	In pollen-sensitive subjects, the reactivity may be higher during, and soon after, the pollen season, but lower outside the season
Dermatological disorders	Eczema and other skin disorders may alter the capacity of the skin to react or the reaction to be read properly
Specific immunotherapy	May inhibit skin reactions to specific allergens

Table 2 **Drugs inhibiting skin-test reaction**

Drugs	Comments
Antihistamines	Inhibitory effect related to the half-life; 24–48 h for classic antihistamines, 3–10 days with most non-sedating antihistamines and 4–8 weeks for astemizole
Corticosteroids	Low-dose systemic or inhaled steroids do not affect skin reactivity but high-dose or topical steroids may inhibit skin responsiveness
Tricyclic antidepressants	May inhibit skin-test reaction for a few weeks
Other drugs	Dopamine and clonidine may inhibit skin reactivity

A late reaction follows the skin test immediate reaction in some individuals, usually in those who are highly sensitized. This consists of a diffuse swelling at the site of the test with surrounding erythema, developing after 2–4 h and resolving within 48 h. The pathogenesis of late-phase skin reaction is the same as late asthmatic reaction seen after bronchial allergen challenge. The reaction is mediated by cytokines and chemotactic factors released from mast cells and lymphocytes. Vascular dilatation with the deposition of fibrin and accumulation of inflammatory cells can be demonstrated.

INDICATIONS AND USES

Clinical

Skin tests are routinely used to standardize allergen extracts for diagnostic and therapeutic uses. They may be used to confirm IgE-mediated disease and identify a causative allergen responsible for the patient's symptoms, so that avoidance measures and, if indicated, specific immunotherapy, can be instituted. Skin test for *Aspergillus* is used to diagnose bronchopulmonary apergillosis. They are of value in monitoring response to venom immunotherapy. They are also of value in drug and occupational allergy.

Research

Skin tests are widely used in clinical research to investigate the pathogenesis of allergic reaction, and the mechanism and effectiveness of new drugs. Prick-tests are used to assess the prevalence of atopy and the pattern of sensitization to common allergens in population studies (Fig. 2). In selected populations (for example, those with respiratory allergic symptoms or those attending an allergy clinic) the prevalence of one or more positive skin tests may be as high as 70% (Fig. 3 & 4). Atopy, as assessed

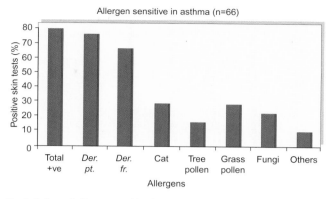

Fig. 4 Pattern of allergen sensitization on skin. Prick tests in patients presenting to an allergy clinic in a city with warm, humid climate (data from Allergy clinic at Aga Khan Hospital, Karachi, Pakistan).

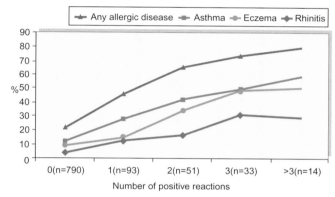

Fig. 5 **The prevalence of allergic disease in children increases linearly with the number of positive skin test reactions** (Data from: Arshad SH, Tariq SM, Mathews SM, Hakim EA 2001 Sensitization to common allergens and its association with allergic disorders at age 4 years: a whole population birth cohort study. Pediatrics 2:e33.).

by positive skin prick test to common allergens, is the most important risk factor for the development of allergic disease (Fig. 5).

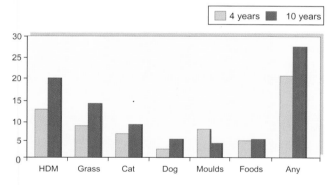

Fig. 2 **Sensitization to common allergens in an unselected population – a birth cohort of children seen at 4 and 10 years.**

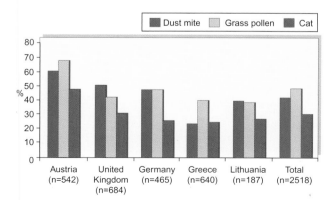

Fig. 3 **Sensitization to common allergens in subjects with symptoms suggestive of allergic disease** – data from five European countries.

Skin tests – Uses and interpretation

- Prick-test is the preferred method as it is quick, reliable, convenient and safe.
- An intradermal test is more sensitive and reproducible, but false-positive reactions are common and anaphylaxis may occur.
- Interpretations of allergy skin tests requires the expertise of a trained allergist.
- Size of prick-test reaction is related to the sensitivity of the subject to that allergen.
- Reaction to aeroallergen correlates with the level of specific IgE and the challenge test.
- Prick-test is more sensitive but less specific than specific IgE measurement.
- Skin tests to food allergens are not as reliable in indicating clinical reactivity as aeroallergens.
- Antihistamines and some other drugs inhibit skin reaction and should be avoided before the test.
- Skin test positivity in asymptomatic subjects is a risk factor for the development of allergic disease.
- Skin test is a biological assay for specific IgE and histamine from mast cells is the most important mediator.
- A late reaction in 2–4 h may follow the immediate reaction in some individuals.

PATCH TESTS

Patch testing was first used in the late 19th century and remains the most useful technique to confirm the diagnosis of allergic contact dermatitis and determine the causative agents. Patch testing should be considered in patients with eczema, where either the distribution (face, hands, feet) or contact with a substance at work or home suggest contact dermatitis. During patch testing patients are exposed to the suspected allergens under controlled conditions. Patch-test reactions are associated with T lymphocyte-mediated allergen-specific immune responses. A high percentage of patients with atopic dermatitis, including children, have relevant contact allergy. Therefore, age or the presence of atopy should not deter the physician from using the patch test.

CHOICE OF ALLERGENS

The choice of allergens depends, to some extent, on the history and examination. However, it is not uncommon for patients to be sensitized to unsuspected allergens. Although the number of possible contact allergens is huge (more than 3000 are known, increasing every year), only a small number of substances are responsible for most reactions. It is therefore recommended that a standard battery containing preparations of common chemical sensitizers (preservatives, cosmetics, drugs, etc.) should be employed (Table 1). The standard batteries used in the USA and Europe identify 70% of cases of allergic contact dermatitis.

Contact allergens relevant in an individual, and not included in the standard battery, may be added. However, a chemical should not be applied to the skin without the knowledge of its properties and safety data. Specialized panels are also available, directed towards specific professions such as gardening, hairdressing and dental work. Personal care products, preservatives and fragrances represent the most common relevant allergens in those diagnosed with facial contact dermatitis. Patients suspected of reacting to a fragrance can be tested to their own products. Rubber products, detergents and occupational allergens are common offenders in hand dermatitis.

Table 1 **European Standard Battery**

No	Allergen	Where found
1	Nickel sulphate	Metal and metal-plated objects such as kitchen utensils, scissors, jewellery, watches, buckles, zippers, coins and some foods
2	Wool alcohols	Ointments, creams, lotions and soaps. Also in technical products such as lubricants, skiwax, cutting fluids and polishes
3	Neomycin sulphate	Topical antibiotic (creams, lotions, drops)
4	Potassium dichromate	Cement, chrome-plating, dyes, chrome glues, paints, safety matches
5	Cain mix	Topical medications, cough syrups and lozenges
6	Fragrance mix	A mixture of eight substances used for scent. These are found in perfumes, cosmetics and other scented household products
7	Colophony	Adhesives, shoe-wax, cosmetics, dental-floss, modelling clay, paints
8	Epoxy resin	Adhesives, surface coatings and paints, cements, electrical parts, dental floss bonding agents
9	Quinoline mix	An antibacterial agent used in medicated creams and paste bandages
10	Balsam of Peru	Cosmetics, perfumes, medical creams and ointments, also used as a flavouring agent for medicines and foods
11	Ethylenediamine dihydrochloride	Antibiotic and antifungal creams and eye and nose drops. Also in industrial products, e.g. textile resins, solvents and antifreezes
12	Cobalt chloride	Metal-plated objects (coins, zippers, etc.), costume jewellery, wet cement and metal alloys
13	p-tert- Butylphenolformaldehyde	A resin used in glues for leather goods and furniture. Also hardboard and fibreglass
14	Paraben mix	Cosmetics, dermatological preparations
15	Carba mix	All rubber products such as shoes, gloves, etc., glues, pesticides
16	Black rubber mix	Tyres, rubber washers, hoses and gloves
17	Kathon CG	Shampoos, creams, lotions and other skin-care products
18	Quaternium-15	Creams, lotions and other cosmetics and skin-care products
19	Mercaptobenzothiazole	Rubber products (e.g. shoes, gloves, elastic and rubber handles), glues for leather and plastic, insulation tape
20	p-Phenylenediamine	Hair dyes, cosmetics, paints and photo ink
21	Formaldehyde	Shampoo, detergents and cleansers, disinfectants
22	Mercapto mix	Rubber products, glues, insulation tape
23	Thiomersal	Cosmetics, topical medicaments
24	Thiuram mix	Rubber products (e.g. gloves, elastics, balloons), glues, pesticides, medications and lubricating oils

METHODS

The test material, in different vehicles (commonly white petroleum), is applied to the skin under a metal disc, called the Finn chamber (Fig. 1). A test battery of 20–24 allergens is used as standard, and additional allergens can be added. The sheet is placed on the upper back and sealed with adhesive tape (Fig. 2). The allergens are numbered on the back with a pen and the patient is asked not to wash the back for 72–96 h. The patch is removed to observe the response after 48 h (Fig. 3). A second observation is performed at 72–96 hours, as some responses are delayed. Laser Doppler perfusion scanning technique has been employed as an objective method of assessing patch-test responses. However, its clinical usefulness is uncertain.

All responses are recorded and graded according to size and intensity (Table 2).

Table 2 **Grading of responses on patch test**

Grades	Reaction	Description
-ve	Negative	No reaction
+/–	Doubtful	Erythema only
+	Weak	Erythema, infiltration, papules
++	Strong	Erythema, infiltration and vesicle formation
+++	Extreme, strong	Coalescing vesicles and ulceration

Doubtful responses (erythema) may be due to an irritant reaction. However, if the index of suspicion is high, the test can be repeated. If there is a history of photosensitivity, standard patch testing may give a negative result unless the test site is exposed to ultraviolet light (photopatch test). Many of these reactions are to fragrance or sunscreen ingredients. Steps should be taken to ensure validity of the results and minimize the risk to patients (Table 3).

Table 3 **Precautions to take during patch test**

- Substances should not be applied to the skin without knowledge of their properties
- Some products such as shampoos and soaps should not be tested under occlusion
- The preferred site is upper back or upper arm
- The skin should be free of dermatitis
- Patch should be removed if there is intense irritation or burning at the site of the test
- After removing the patch, wait for 15–30 min before reading, so that irritant and pressure effects of the patch are cleared

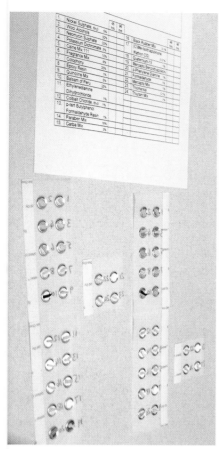

Fig. 1 **Finn chambers used for patch testing, and a chart for recording positive reactions.**

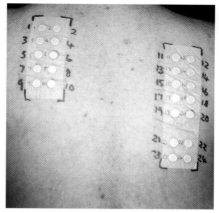

Fig. 2 **Patch test applied to the back.**

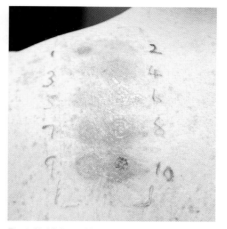

Fig. 3 **Multiple positive reactions at 48 h following application of patch test with a European Standard Battery.**

INTERPRETATION

The responses should be interpreted with the information available from the history and examination. Even a clearly positive reaction to an allergen may be due to irritation, or sensitization not relevant to current dermatitis, if there is no history of exposure. However, the history should be carefully checked in these circumstances. Once the relevance of a positive response is established, complete avoidance should lead to resolution. Occasionally, multiple positive responses are seen (angry-back syndrome). This may be due to a strongly positive reaction stimulating an irritant reaction by other allergens. If this is suspected, separate tests should be done for all the allergens producing a positive response.

If an allergen, which is strongly suspected from the history, gives a negative reaction, the test may be repeated with a higher concentration. However, the risk of an irritant reaction increases with a highly concentrated allergen. If the diagnosis of allergic contact dermatitis is strongly suspected on clinical grounds, a negative

result to the standard battery may simply mean that the causative allergen is not included. Some relatively common contact allergens such as corticosteroids are not included in the standard battery. Steroid sensitivity is relatively common in patients who use topical steroids frequently. Various factors such as hormones, drugs and ultraviolet radiation may influence patch-test reactions.

There is a small risk of sensitization during patch testing. If sensitization occurs, a reaction is seen after 10–14 days, which can be confirmed on retesting, when the reaction appears at the usual 48–96 h. Patients should be asked to report any reaction appearing after 1 week. Overall the benefits of patch test outweigh this small risk.

AVOIDANCE

The patient should be given detailed information as to where the allergen is likely to be found at home or work.

Written information should be provided about the characteristics of each allergen and the situations where the allergen may be encountered.

ATOPY PATCH TEST

In an atopy patch test, food or aeroallergens are applied to the skin (normal or abraded) of patients with atopic dermatitis. This leads to an eczematous reaction on the site of application with erythema, oedema and infiltration. The reaction is specific for patients with atopic dermatitis sensitized to the allergen, and is not observed in sensitized patients with asthma or rhinitis. The methodology is not standardized. In studies, allergens are used in various different forms and concentrations, and read at 20 min–72 h. A positive reaction may prove the relevance of an allergen in the pathogenesis of atopic eczema and the need for avoidance. However, its clinical usefulness has not been evaluated.

Patch tests

- The patch test is a useful diagnostic tool for the confirmation of allergic contact dermatitis and the identification of the offending allergen.
- A standard battery is used with optional addition of other allergens suspected from the history.
- The test should be read both at 48 and 96 h to minimize false-negative responses.
- The test should be interpreted with the information available from the history and examination.
- Irritant reaction should be differentiated from the true-positive reactions.
- There is a small risk of sensitization to one or more allergen being tested.
- Avoidance of the offending allergen should result in significant improvement in the condition.
- Atopy patch test has been devised for identification of the relevant allergens in patients with atopic dermatitis.

LABORATORY TESTS

The most commonly used laboratory tests for the diagnosis of allergic disorders are measurements of total and specific IgE antibodies. Blood eosinophils may be high in asthma but this has limited diagnostic value. A number of other tests may be useful occasionally in certain allergic disorders. Several cytokines and mediators and their metabolites can be measured in the serum and urine but their diagnostic value is still being evaluated.

TOTAL IgE

Immunoglobulin E or IgE is produced by B lymphocytes and plasma cells in the respiratory and gastrointestinal mucous membrane. In the tissues it is largely bound to the mast cells. However, it diffuses into the circulation and free IgE is present in the blood in small quantities. The foetus begins to make IgE from the 11th week of gestation. At birth the level of IgE is usually less than 1 ng/ml (0.4 IU/ml). The level of IgE rises throughout childhood to adult levels by early teens, and declines in older age. The normal adult range is 0–100 IU/ml.

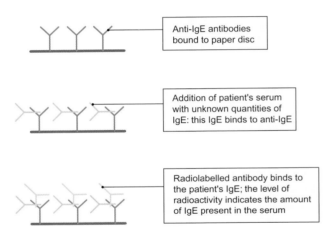

Anti-IgE antibodies bound to paper disc

Addition of patient's serum with unknown quantities of IgE: this IgE binds to anti-IgE

Radiolabelled antibody binds to the patient's IgE; the level of radioactivity indicates the amount of IgE present in the serum

Fig. 1 **Steps in the measurement of total IgE with paper radio-immunosorbent test (PRIST).**

Measurement

Immunoassay, using solid phase such as tube, sponges, beads or microtitre plate, are commonly used. Anti-IgE antibodies are coupled to the solid surface. The patient's serum, containing unknown quantities of IgE is added, and the IgE binds to the anti-IgE antibodies. In radioimmunoassay (RIA), a radiolabelled antibody is then added and the radioactivity is counted with a gamma scintillator (Fig. 1). Alternatively, a fluorochrome can be attached to the second antibody and the fluorescence measured in a fluorometer (fluorescence immunoassay or FEIA). In enzyme-immunoassay (EIA), an enzyme is attached to the second antibody. A substrate is added, which is hydrolyzed by the enzyme, and colour develops, which is quantitated in a spectrophotometer. The intensity of radioactivity, fluorescence or colour is directly related to the concentration of IgE present in the patient's serum. A standard curve is built in a parallel test with known quantities of the IgE antibodies to compare and quantify IgE present in the patient's serum.

Significance

Total IgE is elevated in patients with allergic conditions such as atopic asthma, eczema and rhinitis. High levels are seen in atopic eczema and patients with multiple organ involvement. However, there is a considerable overlap, and nearly half of the individuals with asthma or rhinitis sensitized to one or a few allergens have normal total IgE. Total serum IgE is high in other conditions, such as parasitic infestations and hyper-IgE syndrome. For these reasons, the value of total IgE as a diagnostic test is limited. Moreover, a high total IgE indicates an atopic status but it does not identify the causative allergen. High IgE at birth may predispose to the development of atopy later in life. However, its value as a screening test is limited because of poor sensitivity. Total IgE is high in bronchopulmonary aspergillosis and may be useful in the diagnosis and monitoring of disease activity. Measurement of total IgE is extremely useful in epidemiological and research studies, for improved understanding of the natural history and pathological associations of atopic diseases (Fig. 2).

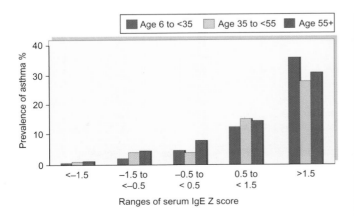

Fig. 2 **Total serum IgE is a valuable tool to investigate the cause of allergic diseases in epidemiological studies.** This graph shows a direct relationship between total IgE and asthma in all ages. (From Burrows B, Martinez F, Halonen M, Barbee RA, Cline MG 1989, N Engl J Med 320: 271–7.)

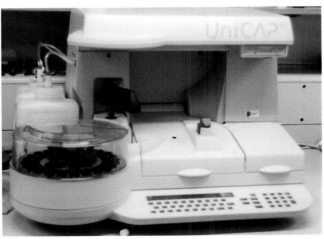

Fig. 3 **UniCAP is used to measure specific IgE in the serum with enzyme base immunoassay.**

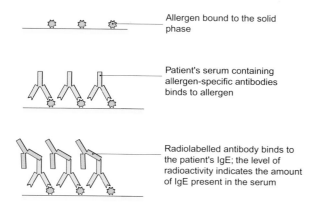

Allergen bound to the solid phase

Patient's serum containing allergen-specific antibodies binds to allergen

Radiolabelled antibody binds to the patient's IgE; the level of radioactivity indicates the amount of IgE present in the serum

Fig. 4 **Steps in the measurement of specific IgE with radioallergosorbent test (RAST).**

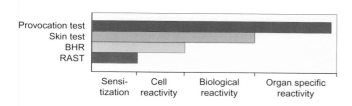

	Sensi-tization	Cell reactivity	Biological reactivity	Organ specific reactivity
Provocation test				
Skin test				
BHR				
RAST				

Fig. 5 **The relevance of various tests for the diagnosis of allergy.**

ALLERGEN-SPECIFIC IgE

Specific IgE to one or more allergen is commonly used in the diagnosis and management of allergic disorders (Fig. 3).

Measurement

The most commonly used technique is radioallergosorbent test (RAST) (Fig. 4). The serum to be tested for specific IgE is added to the solid phase allergen immunosorbent. After wash, this is incubated with radiolabelled purified or monoclonal anti-IgE. The amount of radioactivity reflects the quantities of allergen-specific antibodies in the patient's serum. Alternatively, enzyme or fluorescence conjugated antibodies may be used. This avoids the use of radioactive material. Specific IgE to all the common allergens can be measured with commercially available kits (allergen bound to the solid phase). The accuracy of the test depends on the quality of the allergen extract used. The results are given as scores (0–4). An improved version of RAST is the immunoCAP system with improved sensitivity and the results are quantified in kU/l. Multi-allergen tests (Phadiatop, MAST) have been developed where several allergens (common aero- or food) are bound to the solid phase. This is useful as a first stage screening test.

Significance

The sensitivity of the RAST is somewhat low (60–80%), i.e. a negative test does not exclude mild degrees of sensitization to the tested allergen. The specificity of the test is high (90%), i.e. a positive test definitely indicates sensitization. The presence of specific IgE to an allergen indicates sensitization, not clinical reactivity (Fig. 5). There is, however, good correlation with skin test and organ-specific responses (bronchial or nasal challenge). A detailed case history, in conjunction with specific IgE and/or

Table 1 **Indication for specific IgE measurement**

When skin test cannot be done	Supplementary to skin test
Patient is taking antihistamines Widespread skin disease Dermographism Skin test solution not available History of anaphylaxis (e.g. bee or wasp venom or peanut)	Skin test result is equivocal History is strongly suggestive but skin test is negative

Table 2 **Some other laboratory tests and their indications**

Test	Indications
Serum immunoglobulins and IgG subclasses	Immune deficiency states
Complement components	Urticaria/angioedema
C1 esterase inhibitor	Angioedema
IgG antibodies to fungal and avian proteins	Extrinsic allergic alveolitis
Plasma histamine/tryptase	Anaphylaxis
Specific IgG and subclasses	Monitoring of immunotherapy
RAST inhibition	Allergen extract standardization

skin-test results, gives a reliable diagnosis, and obviates the need for provocation tests in most patients. Skin prick-tests are generally preferred, as they are quick and inexpensive. However, measurement of specific IgE is useful in certain situations (Table 1).

BASOPHIL HISTAMINE RELEASE (BHR) TEST

This test gives an estimation of the allergen-specific IgE. Peripheral blood basophils are isolated and incubated with allergen. Histamine secreted from the basophils as a result of interaction of allergen with cell-bound IgE is measured. Its clinical applications are limited because of the need for fresh blood cells, the limited number of allergens that can be tested and the interlaboratory variability of the assay.

BLOOD EOSINOPHILS AND MEDIATORS

Eosinophils are predominantly present in the tissues and only 1% of the total eosinophils is in the circulation. Normal range is 100–400 cell/mm^3. Eosinophils are activated during allergic inflammation with the release of cytotoxic proteins such as major basic proteins and eosinophilic cationic protein. Kits are available commercially to measure these proteins. Eosinophilic cationic protein correlates with severity of asthma and possibly atopic dermatitis. However, its clinical usefulness remains uncertain. Other tests may be indicated in specific clinical situations (Table 2).

Laboratory tests

- The discovery of immunoglobulin E in 1966 has helped to improve our understanding of allergic diseases.
- IgE is present in very small quantities in the blood. However, it can be measured in the serum with sensitive immunoassays.
- High total IgE indicates atopic status but does not help the clinician in identifying the causative allergen.
- Specific IgE can be measured in the blood using radio-allergosorbent test (RAST) or its analogues.
- Measurement of specific IgE is highly specific and safe, and correlates well with provocation tests.
- The disadvantages of RAST are low sensitivity and cost.
- Eosinophils may be high in allergic and nonallergic asthma.
- Serum eosinophilic cationic protein correlates with the severity of asthma and atopic dermatitis.

SPIROMETRY

Pulmonary function tests are an objective measure of lung function in health and disease. There are several kinds of pulmonary function tests but spirometric examination is the most useful. Spirometry is the measurement of dynamic lung volumes (the amount of air coming in and out of lungs during various breathing manoeuvres). It is helpful in the diagnosis and monitoring of pulmonary diseases, particularly asthma (Table 1).

EQUIPMENT

There are several kinds of spirometers. A water-seal spirometer uses a rotating kymograph to record the displacement of a bell into water by the subject's breathing movements. The other common type is the dry rolling-seal where the piston moves into a cylinder. Pneumotachographs are the flow-sensing devices which employ flow signals to measure flow and volumes. These are often computerized, with facility for printouts (Fig. 1). The American Thoracic Society recommendations for diagnostic spiromtery equipment in terms of accuracy, precision, validation and quality control should be followed. Daily calibration with a precision syringe is essential.

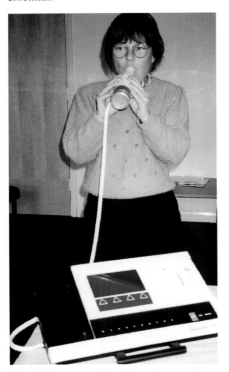

Fig. 1 **Spirometry can be performed as an out-patient procedure using portable pneumotachographs.**

METHOD

Spirometry is an effort-dependent manoeuvre that requires understanding and cooperation by the subject, and a clear explanation of the procedure should be given. The subject should be asked to avoid smoking, exercise, caffeine and bronchodilators for at least 6 h prior to testing. A number of parameters can be calculated from these breathing manoeuvres (Table 2). These should be corrected to BTPS (body temperature, pressure, saturated with water vapour).

PROCEDURE

Vital Capacity (VC)

The subject inhales maximally and then blows into the mouthpiece at a sustained and comfortable speed and continues to exhale fully.

Forced Vital Capacity (FVC)

The subject inhales maximally and then blows out in the mouthpiece as hard and as fast as possible and continues to exhale fully. Table 3 describes requirements for spirometry of good quality as recommended by the American Thoracic Society.

Peak Expiratory Flow (PEF)

PEF can be calculated from the FVC manoeuvre but this can be measured sep-

arately with a portable peak-flow meter. The FVC manoeuvre is performed as detailed above, but there is no need for maximal exhalation (1 or 2 s is adequate). At least three manoeuvres should be performed with variability of less than 5%. The best value is recorded.

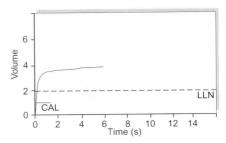
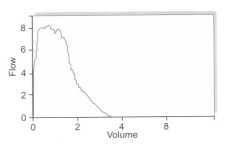

Fig. 2 **Spirometry in a normal subject.**
(a) Volume/time curve. Spirogram plotting volume changes against time in the FVC manoeuvre. (b) Flow/volume curve. The expiratory flow/volume curve plotting flow against volume.

Table 1 **Indications for spirometry**

Diagnostic	Monitoring	Public health/research
To evaluate: Symptoms, e.g. cough, dyspnoea and wheezing Signs, e.g. wheezing and cyanosis Abnormal results, e.g. hypoxia	*Monitoring progress:* Diseases: e.g. COPD, sarcoidosis, neuromuscular disease Occupational diseases Patients on certain drugs	*To screen people at risk of developing disease:* Smokers Workers in some occupations
To assess: Reversibility (bronchodilators, steroids) Disease severity Pre-operative risk Prognosis		Epidemiological surveys Healthy subjects Patients with a disease, e.g. asthma

Table 2 **Commonly used parameters from the relaxed and forced expiratory manoeuvres**

Measure	Definition
Vital Capacity (VC) (relaxed)	The maximal volume of air that can be expired during a relaxed expiration from full inspiration
Forced Vital Capacity (FVC)	The maximal volume of air that can be expired during a forced expiration from full inspiration
Forced Expiratory Volume in 1 s (FEV_1)	The maximal volume of air that can be expired in the first second of an FVC manoeuvre
Peak Expiratory Flow (PEF)	The maximal flow achieved during an FVC manoeuvre
Forced Expiratory Flow $_{25-75}$ (FEF_{25-75})	The flow achieved during the middle half of the FVC manoeuvre

```
Vitalograph compact 11

Date      : 23-04-00
Name      :
Ref. No.  : 1
Age       : 32
Sex       : female
Height    : 165cm
Race      : caucasian
Normals   : I.T.S.
Pre       : 6 tests  -0.3%
Values at B.T.P.S. : :-

A.T.S.     Best.
            Pred   Meas    %
FV          3.76   3.69    98
FEV1        3.17   3.11    98
FEV1/VC%    79      -      -
FEV1/FUC%   84     84      0
PEF         389    544    140
FEF25-75%   3.61   3.55    98
```

Fig. 3 **Most electronic spirometers calculate useful parameters (such as FEV$_1$ and FVC) from the FVC manoeuvre and the normal predicted range.**

INTERPRETATION

A graphic output is essential to ensure quality requirements. When measured with the old spirometers (e.g. dry bellows), a volume/time graph is displayed. FEV$_1$ and FVC can be measured from this graph. With the use of computerized pneumotachographs, both volume/time and flow/volume curves can be displayed and the computer calculates FVC and its subdivisions (FEV$_1$, PEF and FEF$_{25-75}$). There is usually an option to observe and print one or both graphs, and selected parameters (Figs 2 & 3).

A comment should be made on test quality and effort made by the subject.

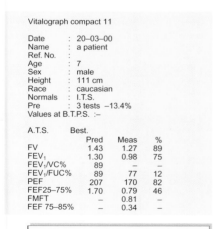

```
Vitalograph compact 11

Date      : 20-03-00
Name      : a patient
Ref. No.  :
Age       : 7
Sex       : male
Height    : 111 cm
Race      : caucasian
Normals   : I.T.S.
Pre       : 3 tests  -13.4%
Values at B.T.P.S. :-

A.T.S.     Best.
            Pred   Meas    %
FV          1.43   1.27    89
FEV1        1.30   0.98    75
FEV1/VC%    89      -      -
FEV1/FUC%   89     77      12
PEF         207    170     82
FEF25-75%   1.70   0.79     46
FMFT        -      0.81    -
FEF 75-85%  -      0.34    -
```

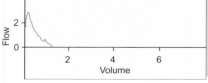

Fig. 4 **Airflow obstruction in a child with asthma.** Spirometry shows up reduction in FEV$_1$ and FVC and most prominently mid-flow obstruction (FEF$_{25-75}$) on expiratory flow/volume curve.

Spirometric values depend on age, height, sex and race of the patient. The interpretation involves comparing values measured in the patient, with reference values determined in population studies of healthy non-smokers. For a given age, height and sex there is a normal predicted value for each measurement. The subject's value is compared with this value to calculate the percent predicted (Fig. 3). Less than 80% predicted is generally considered abnormal.

VC and FVC

FVC is normally equal to VC, but it may be reduced in airway obstruction. Decreased VC and FVC are common in restrictive lung diseases such as pulmonary fibrosis.

FEV$_1$

This is the most widely used parameter for assessment of airway obstruction. It is reduced in both airway obstruction and parenchymal and chest-wall diseases.

Reversibility

Repeated measurement of FEV$_1$ following treatment with bronchodilator or steroids can be used to assess response to treatment. A 15% or more improvement in FEV$_1$, following a standard dose of short-acting bronchodilator, is characteristic of asthma.

Ratio of FEV$_1$ and FVC

In asthma, FEV$_1$ is reduced much more than FVC, thus causing a reduction in FEV$_1$:FVC ratio. This is the obstructive pattern of pulmonary function defect (Fig. 4). A restrictive pattern of pulmonary function defect means that the

lung volumes are small. Spirometry shows a reduction in both FEV$_1$ and FVC with a normal ratio.

FEF$_{25-75}$

This is indicative of the status of medium to small airways. Reduced values are common in early stages of obstructive airway disease such as asthma, when other measurements may be normal.

PEF

A single reading of PEF is less reliable than FEV$_1$ as a diagnostic tool. However, it is most useful for repeated observations, with small portable apparatus, to assess variability in airway obstruction (a characteristic of asthma) and response to treatment. Morning and evening peak-flow are measured (best of three blows), for a period of 4–6 weeks, before and after treatment. Regular home monitoring is recommended for moderate to severe asthma.

Table 3 **Performance criteria for spirometry** (adapted from the statement of the American Thoracic Society)

Procedure
Full inhalation before start of test
Satisfactory start of exhalation
Evidence of maximal effort
No hesitation, cough or glottal closure
Satisfactory duration of test: at least 6 seconds (up to 15 seconds in patients with airflow obstruction)
No evidence of leak
No evidence of obstruction of mouthpiece

Reproducibility
At least 3 manoeuvres are performed
For FVC and FEV$_1$, the two largest values should not vary more than 0.2 l
If these criteria are not met continue testing up to 8 trials
If criteria are still not met, proceed with interpretation, using 3 best tests
Select from tests of acceptable quality
Select the largest values for FVC and FEV$_1$

Spirometry

- Spirometry is an assessment of dynamic lung volume during specific breathing manoeuvres.
- It is extremely useful in the diagnosis and assessment of severity of asthma.
- Spirometric examination can be performed in the outpatient clinic and general practitioner's surgery.
- Accuracy of the equipment and correct performance of the procedure are important considerations.
- FEV$_1$ and a ratio of FEV$_1$:FVC are the best measures of assessing airway obstruction and reversibility.
- A reduction in FEF$_{25-75}$ is indicative of small airway disease and is highly sensitive for early airways obstruction in asthma and smokers.
- A single measurement of PEF is not useful in asthma. However, repeated measurements at home are used in the diagnosis, identification of the cause (e.g. occupation), monitoring of severity and response to therapy.

BRONCHIAL PROVOCATION TEST

The tendency of the bronchi to constrict in response to a variety of stimuli, i.e. bronchial hyperresponsiveness (BHR) is one of the main characteristics of bronchial asthma. Bronchial provocation test (BPT) or bronchial challenge to various physical, chemical and antigenic stimuli can demonstrate this hyperresponsiveness. The non-specific BHR is a measure of lability of the airways. The degree of non-specific BHR correlates with the severity of the disease. In allergic asthma, inhalation of a specific allergen to which the patient is sensitized not only causes immediate bronchoconstriction, but in most subjects also increases non-specific BHR.

METHODS

The protocol for a bronchial provocation test is similar whether assessing non-specific responsiveness with chemical agents, such as histamine or methacholine, or evaluating specific allergen sensitivity with an allergen extract (Fig. 1). FEV_1 is measured before the test (baseline) and after inhalation of normal saline through a nebulizer.

Two methods are commonly used. In the tidal breathing method, increasing concentrations of the aerosolized solution are inhaled for a fixed timed-period or number of breaths, and FEV_1 is measured twice after each inhalation. Alternatively, a dosimeter can be used which delivers a fixed dose with each breath. The number of breaths and the amount of dose delivered at each breath can be varied. The two methods are highly comparable. The inhalation continues with stepwise increase in concentration until a predetermined drop (usually 20%) in FEV_1 is attained or the maximum concentration is achieved. FEV_1 is plotted against log concentration of the solution and PC_{20} (provocative concentration causing 20% fall in FEV_1) is calculated. PD_{20} (provocative dose causing 20% fall in FEV_1) can also be calculated if a dosimeter has been used.

NON-SPECIFIC BHR

Non-specific BHR is measured with various physical and chemical stimuli (Fig. 2). These stimuli cause bronchospasm in most but not all asthmatics. Histamine and methacholine are

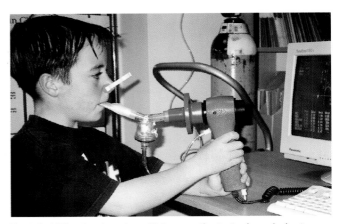

Fig. 1 **A child performing a bronchial provocation test using a dosimeter.**

used most commonly. In children, exercise may be a more physiological stimulus. Bronchial challenge with these agents can be used to diagnose asthma in difficult cases and they give a quantitative assessment of the severity of disease. In asthma, bronchial responsiveness varies from day to day. Treatment with steroids gradually reduces hyperresponsiveness. Patients with chronic bronchitis/emphysema (COPD) and rhinitis may also exhibit BHR.

ALLERGEN BRONCHIAL PROVOCATION TEST

Allergen bronchial provocation test (ABPT) or bronchial allergen challenge is used extensively in research to study the pathophysiological effect of exposure to allergen on airways, and to evaluate the effectiveness of pharmacological agents. Its clinical usefulness is limited except in occupational asthma. It represents a major undertaking with a predictable degree of patient discomfort and a significant risk of severe bronchospasm (Table 1).

Allergenic extracts are complicated mixtures of antigenic components with a number of detectable antigens. Ideally, standardized extracts should be used for allergen challenge. The type of diluent used to dilute lyophilized allergen extract, and storage conditions, may effect the allergenicity of the extract.

EARLY AND LATE ASTHMATIC RESPONSES

Airway response to an inhaled allergen is seen in only those asthmatics with specific sensitization to that allergen (Fig. 3). After inhalation of a sufficient dose of allergen, bronchoconstriction occurs immediately and gradually improves over the next 2 h, the early asthmatic response (EAR). This is a result of antigen/IgE antibody reaction on the surface of mast cells with the release of histamine, prostaglandins and leukotrienes causing smooth-muscle contraction. In nearly 50% of adults and 75% of children a second response is seen 2–3 h after challenge and may last up to 24 h, the late asthmatic response (LAR). Traditionally, a decrease in FEV_1 of > 15% between 2–12 h after challenge is considered diagnostic of LAR. The development of early and late asthmatic responses depends on the severity of asthma, the degree of allergen sensitization, non-specific bronchial hyperresponsiveness and the dose of allergen delivered.

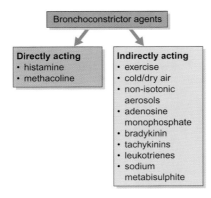

Fig. 2 **Bronchoconstrictor stimuli used to test non-specific bronchial hyperresponsiveness.** Some act directly on the smooth muscles whereas others act indirectly through cellular or neurogenic mechanisms.

During LAR, bronchoconstriction occurs as a result of inflammatory cellular (eosinophils, lymphocytes, basophils and neutrophils) influx, mucosal oedema and smooth-muscle contraction. An increase in eosinophil number and activation is observed (Fig. 4). Non-specific airway responsiveness, as assessed by histamine or methacholine challenge, is increased for a week or more after allergen challenge in those who develop LAR. β-2 agonists and sodium cromoglicate may inhibit EAR, whereas steroids and sodium cromoglicate may suppress LAR and ensuing non-specific bronchial hyperresponsiveness.

The doses used in bronchial provocation tests are not often encountered in daily life. Recently, some investigators have suggested that low-dose allergen inhalations repeated over several

Table 1 **Important points to remember**

- Patients should not have had a respiratory infection within the previous 6 weeks as this might increase BHR
- They are asked not to take their inhaled bronchodilator for 6 h, oral bronchodilator for 24 h and caffeine-containing foods for 12 h before the test, as these may suppress the response
- Baseline FEV_1 should be more than 70% predicted
- If FEV_1 drops more than 10% after normal saline, the test is aborted, as the subject is too reactive
- All subsequent values of FEV_1 are compared to the post-saline value
- Stimulants (such as histamine or methacholine) or allergen extracts are aerosolized through a nebulizer
- Inhaled bronchodilator is administered at the end of the procedure and spirometry repeated to make sure that FEV_1 has returned to baseline
- After histamine or methacholine challenge, a 2 h observation is recommended
- After allergen challenge, the patient should be monitored for 12–24 h as delayed bronchospasm may occur
- Bronchial challenge is highly reproducible (one doubling dose) within the same subject
- More than 100-fold variation in PD_{20} is seen between subjects

days or weeks may be a more appropriate form of bronchial allergen challenge (Fig. 5). In conclusion, BPT have many clinical and research indications. In clinical practice it is primarily used for the diagnosis of occupational asthma. In research, it has been used extensively to study the aetiology, mechanisms and treatment of asthma.

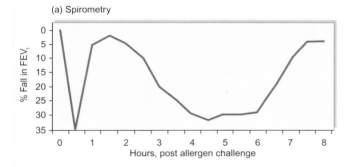

(a) Spirometry

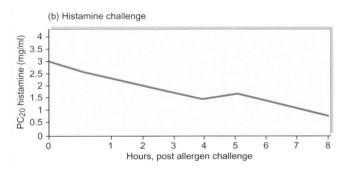

(b) Histamine challenge

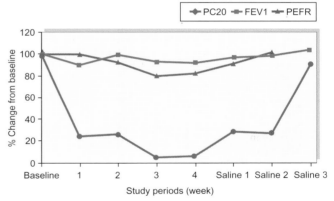

Fig. 3 **Bronchial provocation test with allergen.** FEV_1 falls within the first 2 h (early response) then recovers to fall again during 4–10 h post-challenge. The non-specific bronchial responsiveness, however, reduces gradually and remains low for several days following challenge.

Fig. 5 **Low-dose repeated allergen challenge.** Following repeated inhalation of low-dose of allergen over 4 weeks, the bronchial responsiveness increases (reduction in PC_{20}) and FEV_1 and PEFR decrease, but these measurements return to normal when normal saline is inhaled for the last 3 weeks. (Data from: Arshad SH, Adkinson NF, Hamilton RG 1998 Repeated exposure to small doses of allergen in sensitized individuals - a model for chronic allergic asthma. Am. J Respir Crit Care Med: 157, pp1900–1906).

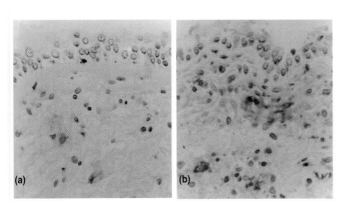

Fig. 4 **Eosinophils in bronchial mucosa (a) before and (b) 6 h after bronchial allergen challenge.** Eosinophitic infiltration is characteristic of late phase asthmatic response.(Immunohistochemical stain using antibody to EG2, ×550.)

Bronchial provocation test

- Non-specific bronchial responsiveness is one of the primary features of asthma.
- BPT measures specific and non-specific bronchial responsiveness.
- Different methods of BPT produce reliable and comparable data so far as standardized procedures are employed.
- Bronchial hyperreactivity correlates well with the severity of asthma.
- Allergen BPT measures target organ sensitivity in allergic asthma.
- Short-acting β-2 agonists inhibit early but not late response to allergen during allergen BPT.
- Steroids inhibit late asthmatic reaction following allergen BPT.
- Low-dose repeated allergen challenge might prove to be a useful method of allergen BPT.

FOOD CHALLENGE

Some physicians regard food allergy as a problem that is imagined by the patients. In contrast, a substantial section of the general population consider this to be the cause of a wide variety of ailments. Perhaps the truth lies somewhere in between these two extremes and double-blind placebo-controlled food challenge (DBPCFC) is the only way to uncover the truth in an individual complaining of food-related symptoms. Nearly a quarter of the adult population considers themselves to be allergic to one or more foods but only 5–10% of these can be proven on DBPCFC.

Performing a DBPCFC with masked foods in daily clinical practice can be a great challenge to the imagination and creativity of a dietitian. The development of recipes and the preparation of masked foods are time-consuming. However, it is possible, and indeed desirable, to perform DBPCFC as an outpatient/office procedure. Single-blind (SBPCFC) (patient unaware of the food given) and open food challenges are also useful in certain circumstances. A positive food challenge confirms an adverse reaction but does not indicate the mechanism (allergic or non-allergic).

RELATIONSHIP TO OTHER TESTS

Skin prick-tests (SPT) and radioallergosorbent test (RAST) are sensitive indicators of food-specific IgE antibodies. A negative test largely excludes IgE-mediated allergy, but a positive test does not necessarily indicate clinical reactivity. A positive test (SPT or RAST) and a positive challenge to the same food confirms the diagnosis of food allergy. Patients who are highly sensitized (≥ 8 mm reaction on SPT and/or RAST ≥ 3), to foods such as egg, milk, nuts and fish, have more than 95% likelihood of reacting on food challenge in the presence of a suggestive history. In these situations food challenge may not be needed (Fig. 1).

INDICATIONS

The history of adverse reaction to foods is commonly inaccurate and the relationship of symptoms to foods is often presumed, driven by the wish that symptoms will disappear when the responsible food is identified and excluded from the diet. The history is, therefore, primarily used to design the challenge, which will confirm or refute the food intolerance. Information needed from history includes type and amount of food required to produce symptoms, description of symptoms, and the time between ingestion and appearance of symptoms. If the history indicates immediate reaction with the development of objective signs, such as rash or bronchospsam, an open challenge may be sufficient. In all other cases single- or preferably double-blind challenges should be arranged (Fig. 1).

PROCEDURES

Before the challenge is arranged it is important that the suspected food has been eliminated from the diet. If no improvement occurs with the avoidance diet then the food is not responsible for the symptoms.

PREPARATIONS

For double- or single-blind challenges the taste, smell, colour and texture of the suspected food have to be hidden in such a way that the patient cannot tell which of the two foods (the active food or the placebo food) contains the suspected agent. Foods can be disguised in capsules. When the use of capsules as a vehicle is not feasible, recipes have to be developed for masking the suspected food with another food or drink that is tolerated. Once developed, the recipes have to be judged carefully to ensure that the foods do not contain ingredients other than the suspected agent that can possibly provoke complaints in the patient.

Dried food such as nuts and grain can be powdered using a blender and encapsulated or hidden in other foods. Powdered milk and dried egg or egg-white is also readily available. Preparation of fish, meat, vegetable or fruit can be a problem. These are sometimes available in freeze-dried form. Alternatively, they will have to be chopped or ground, to be hidden in other foods. For placebo, dextrose capsules or other foods that are tolerated can be used (Fig. 2).

LABIAL FOOD CHALLENGE

Labial food challenge is easy to perform and carries a low risk of systemic reaction (< 5%). Labial challenge is recom-

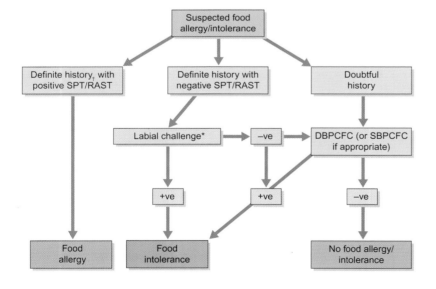

Fig. 1 **A proposed scheme to indicate the need for food challenges for the diagnosis of food allergy / intolerance.**
*An open challenge can be done instead where a negative test excludes the diagnosis, whereas a positive test should be confirmed with DBPCFC; †Definite history is where objective signs, such as rash, appear within 2 h of ingestion.

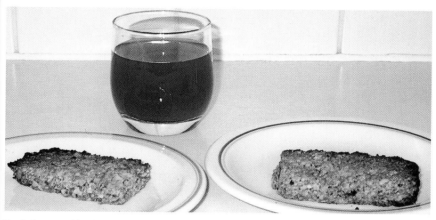

Fig. 2 **Suspected food can be mixed in a drink or other foods to disguise its taste, colour and smell.**

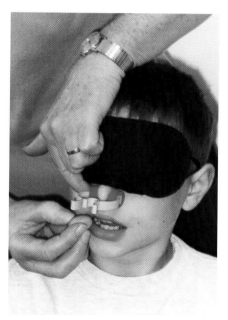

Fig. 3 **Labial food challenge with peanut.**

mended before the oral challenge if there is a risk of anaphylactic reaction. However, this is less sensitive than the oral food challenge. Positive results indicate the presence of food allergy, but negative results require further investigations preferably by DBPCFC.

Labial challenge is performed by placing a drop of the food in liquid solution, or rubbing the dry food, such as a peanut, on the outer edge of the lip (Fig. 3). Criteria for a positive reaction include the appearance within 15 min of labial erythema or oedema, perioral urticaria, or occasionally systemic reaction, e.g. generalized urticaria/angioedema. Initially an open labial challenge can be done but if subjective symptoms, such as localized numbness and itching, appear without the objective signs described above, the test should be repeated in a double-blind manner.

Table 1 **Reproducible symptoms on DBPCFC**

Gastrointestinal	Vomiting, diarrhoea, abdominal cramps, bloating
Cutaneous	Erythema, pruritis, eczema, urticaria, angioedema
Respiratory	Sneezing, rhinorrhoea, laryngeal oedema, cough and wheezing

Table 2 **Information from DBPCFC performed in clinical and research situations**

- Foods commonly causing reaction on DBPCFC include milk, egg, fish, nuts, wheat and soy. Chocolate, strawberries, orange and tomato are often incriminated but rarely proven
- Planning, preparation, administration and supervision of the procedure is time consuming
- Procedure is generally safe, but should only be performed under the supervision of a physician and where facilities for resuscitation are available
- Multiple food hypersensitivity is rare
- Behaviour changes, multiple-organ involvement, neurological or psychiatric symptoms are rarely proven on DBPCFC

ORAL FOOD CHALLENGE

The patient should have minimal allergy symptoms and no medication before the test. The first, and total cumulative, dose to be given depends on the severity of the anticipated reaction and the amount that has produced a reaction previously. Food or placebo is administered in gradually increasing quantities at 20–30 min intervals. Any signs or symptoms of a reaction are observed and recorded and if convincing, the test should be stopped (Table 1). Medication may be administered, if required. If a cumulative dose is given without a reaction, the patient should be observed for 1–2 h. Most reactions occur during this time, however late reactions, e.g. eczema, may occur and should be observed by a physician whenever possible.

In DBPCFC a series of tests is performed. The food, active or placebo, is prepared and coded by a person (usually a dietitian) not involved with the tests. Active or placebo food is administered, as described above, on separate days, in random order while both physician and patients are unaware of the nature of food. The exact number of tests required varies but usually five tests (two or three

each of placebo or active food) are needed. The codes are broken at the end of all tests. If the patient has reacted at least twice to the active food, the challenge is considered positive. Any reaction to placebo casts doubt on all other positive reactions (Table 2). A negative test should be followed by an open challenge in the amount usually consumed by the patient.

The procedure for single-blind challenge is the same except that the physician is aware of the food given. This is less desirable but has the advantage that the number of tests required can be reduced. For example, a negative result to the suspected food obviates the need for placebo test. Open challenge is least desirable as it is subject to bias, but is sometimes useful as a screening test. A negative test excludes the diagnosis whereas a positive test should be confirmed with DBPCFC.

Food challenge

- The history of an adverse reaction to foods is commonly inaccurate.
- DBPCFC is the gold standard for the diagnosis of food intolerance.
- Any new diagnostic test should be validated by the outcome of DBPCFC.
- Food challenge should not be performed if there is a history of anaphylactic reaction or an immediate reaction with a high level of sensitization.
- Most foods can be masked in capsules or other foods or drinks.
- Labial challenge is a useful screening test and carries a low risk of a systemic reaction.

ALLERGEN AVOIDANCE

Avoidance of an offending allergen is an integral part of the management of allergic disease. This is the only successful method available to prevent symptoms of food and occupational allergen-related disorders. In some children with infantile atopic eczema, avoidance of cow's milk and eggs may lead to significant improvement in the disease. Although the role of aeroallergens is established in the causation of allergic diseases (e.g. pollens in allergic rhinitis and dust mites in asthma), the effectiveness of allergen avoidance measures is still debated.

It is generally difficult to avoid aeroallergens completely. However, effective measures to reduce exposure to these allergens are available, although some of these may be expensive and may require considerable, and occasionally unacceptable, alteration to the patient's lifestyle. For example, many patients are unwilling to get rid of their pets. Despite these difficulties, advice on allergen avoidance should be considered in all patients. Measurement of allergen burden in the homes of patients is not of proven value. The extent of allergen avoidance measures should be in proportion to the disease severity. For example, it may not be appropriate to advise extensive changes in the house and lifestyle in a patient with mild allergic rhinitis caused by a sensitization to house-dust mite.

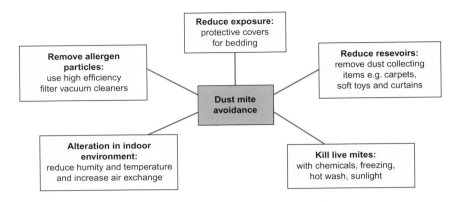

Fig. 2 **Methods available for the reduction in exposure to house-dust mite allergen.**

HOUSE-DUST MITE

Nearly 80% of atopic asthmatics are allergic to house-dust mites. Reduction in exposure to dust mite allergen improves symptoms, pulmonary function and non-specific bronchial responsiveness (Fig. 1). However, not all methods are of proven efficacy and improvement in some studies has been modest, at best. Most studies showing benefit have used some form of allergen-impermeable encasement of mattresses along with other strategies.

Mite control

The most important limiting factor for dust mite population is humidity. Although the mite growth and reproduction slows down in low humidity conditions, it is difficult to kill mites by reducing humidity alone. Mites can be killed by applying low or high temperatures or acaricides. Benzyl benzoate is the most widely used acaricide. The application of liquid nitrogen to mattresses, and placing soft toys in the freezers overnight, will also kill mites. Washable items (clothes, bed linen, some types of rugs, curtains and blankets) can be washed at high temperatures (> 55°). Steam-cleaning can kill mites in carpets, mattresses and upholstery. In warm climates, rugs and blankets can be laid in the sun. All these methods require repeated or regular application to be effective (Table 1). Killing mites does not remove the offending allergen, which may persist for months or even years in reservoirs of house-dust. The effect of vacuum cleaning is to remove the allergen, live mite and their food (human dander) but this is minimally effective, as mites tend to live in deep pores and cling to the fabric. Another method is to put a physical barrier between the allergen and the patient. This is suitable for bedding but not for other items such as carpet or upholstered furniture. A global strategy is therefore required (Fig. 2). It has been demonstrated in studies that people will adapt significant changes to their domestic environment and lifestyles, if the risks and benefits are explained.

ANIMALS

Animals frequently reported as the cause of allergic reactions are cats, dogs, horses, rats and birds. Domestic furred animals are important sources of allergen because of the risk of continuous

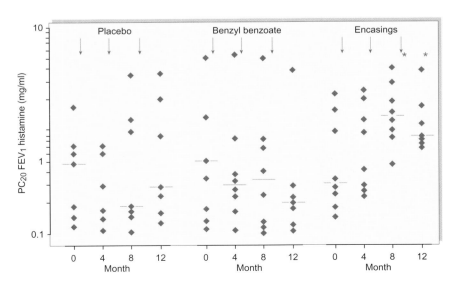

Fig. 1 **Effect of dust mite allergen avoidance on bronchial responsiveness.** The benefit was primarily seen in the mattress-encasing group (adapted from Ehnert B, et al. Journal of Allergy & Clinical Immunology 90(1): 135–38).

Table 1 **Dust mite allergen avoidance**

Varnished floors and washable rugs are preferable to fitted carpets – replace if possible
Vacuum carpets (if not removed) and upholstery, at least once a week
Allow adequate ventilation
Replace old mattresses
Use semi-permeable covers for mattresses, pillows and duvets
Use a damp cloth when dusting
Change and hot-wash (> 55°) pillow-cases, sheets, blankets and duvet covers every week
Replace woollen blankets with synthetic ones or washable duvets
Avoid using feather pillows or bedding
Have light washable curtains
Reduce the amount of upholstered furniture, especially old items
Expose mattress and bedding to the sunshine
Keep soft toys to a minimum, hot-wash or freeze regularly

Table 2 **Domestic animal allergen avoidance**

Never allow animals into the bedroom
Set aside areas in the home where pets are not allowed
Room where pets are allowed should have washable flooring, rather than carpets, to minimize accumulation of allergen particles
Pets should sleep outside the house, if possible
Vacuum clean regularly with a high-efficiency filter
Grooming or clipping should not be done in the house
Discourage animals from licking people
Do not allow visitors to bring animals into your home
Do not buy or replace pets in future
Allow adequate ventilation
Wash cat frequently, this reduces their surface allergen

exposure. Direct contact with an animal is not essential to experience allergic symptoms, since the whole environment of a household containing pets is contaminated. In homes with these animals, allergen can be detected in the carpet and upholstery dust, and in the air. The allergen is carried on clothes and hair to school and work-places. Avoidance of these allergens is an important measure in the treatment of sensitized patients with asthma and rhinitis.

The solution in the domestic environment is to remove the pet and thoroughly clean the home to remove the accumulated allergen. If this is not accepted by the patient, some sensible measures should be taken to minimize exposure

(Table 2). However, the value of these measures is not proven.

POLLENS

Pollens of grasses, trees and weeds are the most common cause of allergic disease. It is possible to reduce exposure to pollens to some extent but this is rarely sufficient to prevent symptoms of allergic rhinitis or conjunctivitis (Table 3). Pollens rise with the heat to high levels during the day. They come down to lower levels as the air begins to cool during the late afternoon, when the exposure is highest.

MOULDS

Moulds are microscopic living organisms, which usually grow on the surface of organic materials such as rotten foods. In the home, they are often found in damp basements, bathrooms, refrigerators and

upholstered furniture. They produce spores, which are found inside and outside the house and are present all year round. Measures should be taken to reduce the burden of this allergen by sensitized individuals with asthma or rhinitis (Table 4).

COCKROACH

If sensitivity to cockroach allergen is demonstrated, aggressive eradication of cockroaches, followed by thorough cleaning of the house, should be recommended. Re-infestation is common unless hygiene standards are improved.

FOODS

Food avoidance can be difficult, expensive and even harmful if appropriate replacement is not ensured. The help of a qualified dietitian is invaluable in these circumstances.

Table 3 **Pollen avoidance**

Avoid cutting the grass yourself
Avoid going out and keep windows closed in the late afternoon and early evening
Wear sun glasses when outdoors
If possible, keep the bedroom windows closed
Avoid picnic or camping holidays
Keep car windows closed when in the car

Table 4 **Mould allergen avoidance**

Avoid exposure to areas of high mould growth such as basements, compost piles, fallen leaves, cut grass, barns and wooded areas
Solve problems of dampness inside the house
Excess humidity produced by bathing and cooking should be reduced with an exhaust fan
Mould growing in the home can be killed with various products
Clean and disinfect air-conditioning conduits
Change and hot-wash pillow-cases, sheets, blankets and duvet covers every week
Allow adequate ventilation
Varnished floors and washables rugs are preferable to fitted carpets

Allergen avoidance

- Adequate explanation and written advice on allergen avoidance measures should always be made available to the allergic patient.
- For allergy to food and occupational allergens, avoidance is the only effective method available.
- Avoidance of aeroallergens is difficult and time consuming. Despite this, allergen avoidance should be part of the overall management of asthma and rhinitis
- The most effective dust mite avoidance measure is to use suitable covers for mattress and the bedding.
- Ideally cat or dog should be removed and the home vigorously cleaned to enhance allergen reduction.
- Cockroaches must be exterminated, followed by aggressive cleaning of the house to remove collected allergen.
- Some common sense measures to avoid exposure to high levels of pollen during the season are recommended.
- Reducing dampness and regular cleaning can reduce mould growth in the house.

ANTIHISTAMINES

Histamine H$_1$-receptor antagonists (or antihistamines) are the most frequently prescribed drugs for the treatment of allergic diseases. Antihistamines are used in the treatment of seasonal and perennial allergic rhinitis, urticaria and angioedema, and localized and systemic allergic reactions. They have been available since the 1930s. These first-generation antihistamines are effective, although they cause considerable sedation (sedative antihistamines, Table 1). Since the early 1980s, a second generation of antihistamines has been available, which do not cause significant sedation (non-sedative antihistamines, Table 2). These antihistamines are diverse in terms of chemical structure and clinical pharmacology, but have similar efficacy in the treatment of patients with allergic disorders.

MECHANISM OF ACTION

There are three types of histamine receptors (H$_1$, H$_2$ and H$_3$) distributed widely in many tissues including blood vessels, nerves and endothelium. H$_1$-receptors in the CNS and in peripheral tissues do not differ with regard to their affinity for H$_1$-blockers. The release of histamine during IgE-mediated allergic reactions, either locally or systemically, ensures the effectiveness of H$_1$ receptor antagonists in the treatment of allergic reactions (Fig. 1).

Antihistamines do possess some non-H$_1$-receptor effects. They inhibit histamine release from mast cells and basophils. In vitro studies have shown that antihistamines, particularly the second generation, can affect the function of most inflammatory cells. Larger doses of antihistamines can also inhibit allergic inflammation in vivo, including mediator release, accumulation and activation of leukocytes such as eosinophils, and adhesion molecule expression. However, at the recommended doses they cannot be regarded as anti-inflammatory drugs. The significance of these findings in the treatment of allergic disease is not certain. Tachyphylaxis, or loss of receptor blocking activity following regular use, has not been found for any of the second-generation antihistamines.

PHARMACOKINETICS

Second-generation antihistamines are well absorbed with the peak plasma concentration within 1–2 h and a duration of effects of 12–24 h. Most undergo metabolism in the liver prior to elimination from the body, except fexofenadine and cetirizine. The second-generation antihistamines do not accumulate in tissues during repeated administration and have a residual action of less than 3 days after a short course has been completed, the exception being astemizole, which takes 4 weeks to reach the steady state and residual effects may last for up to 8 weeks.

EFFECTS

Rhinitis

Antihistamines inhibit symptoms following nasal allergen challenge, (Fig. 2). The majority (75–80%) of patients with allergic rhinitis experience good symptomatic relief. They are particularly effective against rhinorrhoea, itching and sneezing but have little effect on nasal obstruction. There is little evidence that second-generation antihistamines are more effective than the first generation. However, with the reduction in adverse effects, especially drowsiness, the compliance is usually better with the second generation. They can be used as sole therapy in mild intermittent rhinitis or in combination with nasal steroids in moderate to severe disease.

Topical nasal and ocular administration of antihistamines, such as azelastine and levocabastine, is as effective as oral administration in allergic rhinoconjunctivitis. This may have a theoretical advantage of less systemic adverse effects.

Asthma

Airway hyperresponsiveness to histamine is a hallmark of asthma, and histamine inhalation reproduces asthma symptoms. The second-generation antihistamines demonstrate some bronchodilating effect. They may also protect against histamine and exercise-induced bronchospasm, and attenuate the first phase of the early asth-

Table 1 **Recommended dose schedule for some commonly used first-generation (sedative) antihistamines**

Antihistamines	Adult	Child (depending on age)
Promethazine	10–25 mg 6–8 hourly	5 mg once daily to 25 mg 6 hourly*
Chlorphenamine (Chlorpheniramine)	4 mg 4–6 hourly	1 mg 12 hourly to 2 mg 4–6 hourly**
Hydroxyzine	25 mg 6–8 hourly	5 mg once daily to 25 mg 6 hourly***
Trimeprazine	10 mg, 25 mg 6–8 hourly	2.5 to 5 mg 6–8 hourly*
Cyproheptadine	4–8 mg 6–8 hourly	2-8 mg 6–12 hourly*
*not recommended under 2 years ** not recommended under 1 years ***not recommended under 6 months		

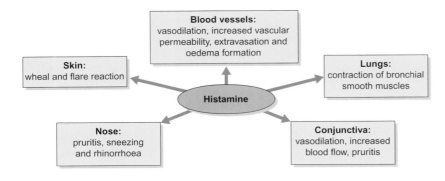

Fig. 1 **Actions of histamine.**

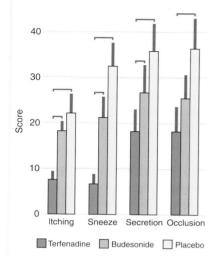

Fig. 2 Antihistamine on nasal allergen challenge. Symptom scores are least in the group treated with an anti-histamine. Adapted from Hillberg O. 1995 Effect of Terfenadine and budesonide on nasal symptoms olfaction and nasal airway potency following allergy challenge. Allergy 50 (8): 683-8.

Table 2 Recommended dose schedule for the second-generation (non-sedative) antihistamines

Antihistamines	Adult	Child (depending on age)
Acrivastine	8 mg 8-hourly*	
Astemizole	10 mg daily	5 mg daily**
Cetirizine	10 mg daily	5 mg daily (2–6 years)
Fexofenadine	120–180 mg daily*	
Loratadine	10 mg daily	5–10 mg daily (2–12 years)
Mizolastine	10 mg daily*	
Terfenadine	60 mg once or twice a day	1 mg/kg once or twice a day (2–12 years)
Azelastine (topical)	140 µg each nostril 12-hourly*	
Levocabastine (topical)	two sprays each nostril 12-hourly*	

*not recommended under 12 years
** not recommended under 6 years

Table 3 Adverse effects of antihistamines

Adverse effects	Details
Sedation	First generation, ketotifen, (occasionally cetirizine, loratadine and terfenadine)
Cardiac arrhythmias	Terfenadine, astemizole
Local irritation	Topical azelastine, levocabastine
Weight gain	Astemizole, mizolastine
Other adverse effects (rare)	Rashes, photosensitivity, sweating, myalgia, extrapyramidal effects, anticholinergic effects (first generation), hepatic dysfunction, depression, hypotension, hair-loss, blood disorders, convulsion, hypersensitivity reactions

matic response. In a recent study, a combination of cetirizine and leukotriene receptor antagonists, zafirlukast, reduced early and late asthmatic responses. However, these effects are generally seen at higher than recommended doses. At present, they cannot be recommended for the treatment of asthma, although they improve mild seasonal asthma symptoms in patients with seasonal allergic rhinitis. Cetirizine has also been shown to prevent the development of asthma in a subgroup of young children with atopic eczema.

Chronic urticaria

Antihistamines are usually very effective in chronic urticaria/angioedema. However, they may be less effective where wheals last longer than 24 h, and in urticaria vasculitis.

Acute allergic reactions

Antihistamines are used to treat symptoms of mild to moderate allergic reactions to food, drug or insect-bite. They are often administered intravenously as an adjuvant to adrenaline (epinephrine) in systemic anaphylaxis. Both first- and second-generation antihistamines are similarly effective.

Atopic dermatitis

Antihistamines are generally not effective in atopic dermatitis. However, the first-generation antihistamines are often used for their sedative effects, in children with moderate to severe atopic dermatitis.

ADVERSE EFFECTS

CNS

The first generation antihistamines slow neurotransmission and depress CNS function, causing somnolence, sedation, drowsiness, fatigue and psychomotor impairment (Table 3). In higher doses, they may also cause CNS stimulation (seizures, dyskinesia, dystonia and hallucination). Sedation can affect patients' daily activities, driving ability and performance at school and work. There may be an additive effect if alcohol or other sedative drugs are consumed. These effects are much less pronounced with the second-generation antihistamines, as they do not cross the blood–brain barrier. However, even the second-generation antihistamines (except fexofenadine), do produce some CNS depressant effects, which is variable in individuals.

Cardiac

Certain non-sedating antihistamines, mainly terfenadine and astemizole, may rarely cause cardiac effects including prolongation of the QTc interval and torsades de pointes. The risk is greater with a higher than recommended dosage, concomitant ingestion of imidazole or macrolide antibiotics, and in patients with underlying cardiac or liver diseases. This is a consequence of the blockade of one of the K^+ channels, IKr channels, by these drugs. Loratadine, cetirizine and fexofenadine do not show cardiac toxicity.

Antihistamines

- Histamine receptors are widely distributed in both central nervous system and peripheral tissues.
- Histamine is released by mast cells and basophils, following an allergic reaction.
- Stimulation of H_1-receptors causes allergic symptoms in the nose, eyes, skin and airways.
- Histamine H_1-receptor antagonists or antihistamines, block the effect of histamine, and are effective in relieving allergic symptoms.
- First-generation antihistamines cause sedation, and are now largely replaced by second-generation, non-sedative antihistamines.
- Second-generation antihistamines have some anti-inflammatory properties but the significance of this is not certain.
- Cardiotoxic effects of some antihistamines, such as terfenadine, are rare, but could be serious.
- Antihistamines are the first-line therapy in rhinoconjunctivitis.
- They are more effective in sneezing, itching and rhinorrheoa, but less effective in relieving nasal obstruction.
- They are not very effective in asthma or atopic dermatitis.

BRONCHODILATORS

Asthma is characterized by reversible airway obstruction. Bronchodilators are therefore an essential component of effective drug therapy for asthma. They are also used in other pulmonary disorders associated with bronchoconstriction, and occasionally during an allergic reaction to a drug, food, insect-venom or immunotherapy. β_2-adrenergic receptor agonists are the most commonly used bronchodilators. Other groups of bronchodilators include anticholinergic drugs and methylxanthines (Table 1).

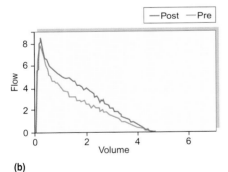

```
Date      :
Name      :
Ref. No.  : 1
Age       : 25
Sex       : male
Height    : 174cm
Race      : caucasian
Normals   : I.T.S.
Pre       : 3 tests −2.3%
Post      : 3 tests −1.0%
Values at B.T.P.S. : :−
```

A.T.S.	Best. Pred	Pre Meas	%	Post Meas	%	Change %
FVC	5.25	4.63	88	4.70	89	1
FEV₁	4.40	2.95	67	3.40	77	15
FEV₁/VC	80	–	–	–	–	–
FEV₁/FUC%	84	64	-20	72	-12	9
PEF	569	460	81	512	90	11
FEF25–75%	4.73	1.88	40	2.61	55	39
FMFT	0.61	1.23	50	0.90	68	37
FEF75–85%	1.52	0.64	42	0.87	57	35

(a)

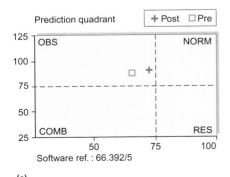

(b)

(c)

Fig. 1 **Reversibility to bronchodilator in a patient with asthma.** Spirometry, before and 20 min after the administration of salbutamol, 200 µg by inhalation. (a) parameters, (b) flow/volume curve, (c) prediction quadrants.

β_2-AGONISTS

The major effect of β_2-agonists on the airways is relaxation of airway smooth muscle (Fig. 1). They do have several other effects mediated through β_2-receptors expressed on other cell types. They may inhibit plasma exudation in the airways by acting on β_2-receptors on postcapillary venule cells. They may also inhibit the secretion of mediators from airway mast cells and other inflammatory cells. This anti-inflammatory effect may not be clinically significant, as they do not reduce the chronic inflammation of asthma. The selectivity for β_2-receptors is relative and in larger doses they may also stimulate β_1-receptors. Adverse effects are dose-related and include headache, tremor, tachycardia and palpitation.

Mechanism

β_2-adrenoceptors are located on the surface of many cells. Agonists bind in a pocket formed by transmembrane spanning domains where key contact points initiate receptor activation, inducing the generation of cyclic AMP. As with other pharmacological receptors, β_2-adrenoceptors in most tissues develop tolerance as a result of continuous β_2-stimulation. This tolerance is partial and an adequate residual protective effect remains. Several regions of the β_2-adrenergic receptor show genetic diversity, such that expression, coupling, and agonist regulation may be different in individuals with these polymorphisms.

SHORT-ACTING β_2-ADRENERGIC AGONISTS

Indications

Salbutamol and terbutalin are two commonly used short-acting β_2-agonists. They are highly effective in relieving symptoms of asthma. They are also useful for prevention of exercise-induced and nocturnal asthma symptoms. They should be used to relieve symptoms on an as-required basis, and regular use should be avoided. These are commonly used via an inhaler. Their bronchodilatation effect starts within 5 min, peaks at 30–90 min and lasts for 4–6 h. Administered via a nebulizer, they are very effective in relieving acute bronchospasm. Alternatively, in acute asthma, these drugs can also be given through an intravenous, intramuscular or subcutaneous route or using an inhaler in combination with a spacer device. Oral formulations are rarely used.

Short-acting β_2-agonists and asthma mortality

An increase in asthma mortality in the 1960s in the UK and in the 1970s in New Zealand has been related to the regular use of potent short-acting β_2-agonists. Regular and excessive use of these agents may increase airway responsiveness, and impair control of asthma, hence increasing the number of asthmatic patients at risk of death in an acute attack. However, a recent study did not confirm impairment in control of asthma with regular use of short-acting β_2-agonists.

LONG-ACTING β_2-ADRENERGIC AGONISTS

Salmeterol and eformoterol have prolonged bronchodilator activity (>12 h). Significant bronchodilatation is achieved more rapidly with eformoterol than salmeterol. Their long duration of action may depend upon a higher lipophilicity, affinity, selectivity, and potency than most short-acting agonists. They have

Table 1 **Commonly used bronchodilators**

Class	Common drugs	Usual dose range
Short-acting β_2-agonists (inhaled)	Salbutamol (aerosol) Salbutamol (nebulized) Terbutaline (aerosol) Terbutaline (nebulized)	100–200 µg qid and/or prn 2.5–5 mg qid 250–500 µg qid and/or prn 5–10 mg qid
Long-acting β_2-agonists (inhaled)	Formoterol (eformoterol) Salmeterol	12–24 µg bid 50–100 µg bid
Theophyllines	Theophylline oral (s.r.) Aminophylline i.v. (infusion)	175–500 mg bid 500 µg/kg/h
Anticholinergics	Ipratropium (aerosol) Oxitropium (aerosol) Ipratropium (nebulized)	20–80 µg qid 200 µg tid 100–500 µg qid

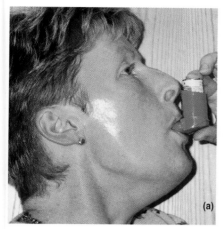 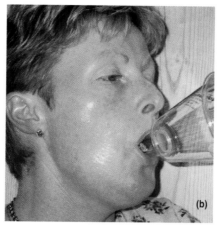

Table 2 **Theophylline has a narrow therapeutic range and side-effects appear commonly unless plasma levels are monitored and dose adjusted accordingly**

Theophylline plasma concentration	Effects
10–20 mg/ml	Therapeutic range
20–30 mg/ml	Nausea, vomiting, diarrhoea, headache, insomnia
30–40 mg/ml	Tremor, agitation, restlessness, sinus tachycardia, palpitation, arrhythmias, hypokalaemia, hyperglycaemia
> 40 mg/ml	Haematemesis, convulsions, death

Fig. 2 **An adult asthmatic using (a) metered-dose inhaler (MDI) and (b) a spacer device (volumatic).**

similar β_2 selectivity to salbutamol but are about ten times as potent. They protect against allergen, exercise and methacholine-induced bronchoconstriction and are said to have some anti-inflammatory properties, but should not be used as an alternative to steroids.

Given in twice-daily doses, they improve asthma control and pulmonary function and decrease the number of exacerbations with improvement in quality of life. These agents have shown particular benefit for patients who continue to have symptomatic asthma despite the regular use of inhaled corticosteroid therapy and require frequent short-acting β_2-agonist. They are effective in preventing nocturnal asthma and exercise-induced bronchoconstriction. Some studies have shown that their addition to low-dose inhaled steroids is more effective than increasing the dose of steroids. There is some tendency to develop tolerance with longer-acting β_2-agonists as a consequence of down-regulation of β_2-receptors. Despite this, there is no evidence of loss of bronchodilator effect after regular use. Long acting β_2-agonists should not be used for rescue bronchodilatation.

ANTICHOLINERGIC AGENTS

Anticholinergics inhibit acetylcholine-induced bronchoconstriction by competitive inhibition of muscarinic receptors. Ipratropium bromide and oxitropium bromide are effective bronchodilators though less potent than β_2-agonists. They cause bronchodilatation by the inhaled route for 6 h and need to be given four times a day. They are added to β_2-agonists to achieve maximum bronchodilatation, either as long-term therapy in severe

asthma, or in nebulized form for acute exacerbation. It has been shown that combining a nebulized β_2-agonist with an anticholinergic agent produces a greater improvement in pulmonary function than β_2-agonist alone.

METHYLXANTHINES

Theophylline, the commonly used methylxanthine, is an effective bronchodilator with some anti-inflammatory properties. It probably acts by inhibiting the breakdown of cyclic AMP by phosphodiesterase, thus increasing the level of intracellular cyclic AMP. It is used orally as maintenance therapy in slow-release formulations, when it is particularly effective in preventing nocturnal asthma symptoms. In acute asthma it can be given as slow intravenous infusion. It may be more cost-effective than long-acting β_2-agonists. However, it has a narrow therapeutic margin and in higher doses stimulates the heart and the nervous system (Table 2). It has a variable hepatic metabolism and higher doses require monitoring of plasma levels.

DELIVERY SYSTEMS

β_2-agonists and anticholinergic drugs are often given through the inhaled route as pressurized metered-dose inhalers (MDI) with or without spacers (Fig. 2), dry powder inhalers (DPI) or nebulizers. Due to direct delivery into the airways, the drug is effective in relatively small doses. The replacement of chlorofluorocarbon (CFC), with more ozone-friendly gases such as hydrofluoroalkanes (HFAs), for gas propellant metered-dose inhalers, is underway. Replacement formulations for almost all inhalant respiratory medications have been or are being produced and tested. It is anticipated that the transition to CFC-free MDIs will be complete in the next few years. DPI and nebulizers do not use a propellant gas and have no effect on the ozone layer.

Bronchodilators

- β_2-agonists cause relaxation of bronchial smooth muscles.
- Short-acting β_2-agonists are effective in relieving symptoms of asthma. For chronic asthma, they are recommended to be used as needed, by the inhaled route. For acute asthma, they can be administered regularly through nebulizer.
- Long-acting β_2-agonists are a useful adjuvant to anti-inflammatory therapy in chronic asthma. They are very effective in nocturnal and exercise-induced asthma.
- Anticholinergic drugs are effective through the inhaled route only, with a duration of effect of 4–6 h. In acute asthma, nebulized anticholinergic can be combined with short-acting β_2-agonists for added bronchodilatation.
- Theophylline is an effective bronchodilator but toxic effects are common at higher dose. Slow-release preparation can be combined with β_2-agonists for added effect.

CORTICOSTEROIDS

Corticosteroids are widely used for the suppression of inflammation in chronic inflammatory diseases, including most allergic disorders. Topical steroids are the first-line prophylactic therapy for asthma and allergic rhinitis. Short courses of systemic steroids are also useful in asthma exacerbation and systemic allergic reactions. Long-term treatment with systemic steroids should be avoided because of their adverse effects (Table 1).

Different corticosteroids vary in their glucocorticoid (anti-inflammatory and metabolic) and mineralocorticoid (water-retaining) effects. Hydrocortisone is less potent than others in its anti-inflammatory activity but is used as intravenous injection for acute systemic reactions in addition to adrenaline (epinephrine). Prednisolone has more potent glucocorticoid activity and is often used if oral therapy is required.

MECHANISM OF ACTION

Glucocorticoids (steroids) bind to their intracellular specific receptors and the complex is transported to the nucleus, resulting in increased transcription of genes coding for anti-inflammatory proteins. They also inhibit the production of proinflammatory cytokines and mediators by their inhibitory effect on activated transcription factors, such as nuclear factor-κB and activator protein-1, which regulate the inflammatory gene expression. Other effects of steroid include decreased capillary permeability and up-regulation of β-adrenoreceptors (Fig. 1).

A single dose of steroid has been shown to inhibit late-phase asthmatic reaction following allergen challenge. Long-term treatment is associated with suppression of both early and late-phase asthmatic responses and reduction in bronchial hyperresponsiveness. These

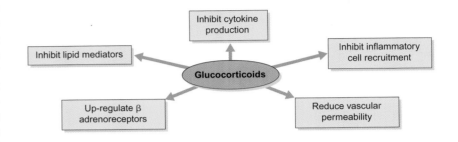

Fig. 1 **Anti-inflammatory effects of glucocorticoids in allergic inflammation.**

effects are seen with both systemic and inhaled steroids. Similarly, administration of topical nasal steroids in allergic rhinitis suppresses nasal mucosal inflammation and improves nasal patency.

SYSTEMIC STEROIDS

Used with care, systemic steroids can be extremely effective in the treatment of allergic diseases without undue toxicity (Fig. 2). Short courses of oral steroids are indicated in asthma exacerbation, and occasionally in severe rhinitis, ezcema and urticaria. There is no risk of adrenal suppression when oral steroids are used at standard doses (Prednisolone 40 mg daily or equivalent) for up to 2 weeks. A longer course requires gradual reduction in doses. Depot intramuscular steroids have been used for the management of severe allergic rhinitis. However, their advantage over a short course of oral steroids has been questioned.

INHALED CORTICOSTEROIDS

The introduction of inhaled steroid in the 1970s revolutionized the treatment of asthma. With increased awareness of the significance of mucosal inflammation in asthma, inhaled steroids are being used at an earlier stage of the disease. They are now recommended for all degrees of severity of asthma, except in those with very mild, intermittent disease. They provide the most potent and consistent long-term control of adult and childhood asthma, with improved lung function and quality of life (Fig. 3). Several inhaled steroids are in common use (Table 2). In terms of relative topical potency, mometasone and fluticasone are twice as potent as beclometasone.

Inhaled steroids owe their favourable safety profile to a high topical-to-systemic bioavailability ratio compared to oral steroids. The delivery device and the patient's inhaler technique determine the amount of drug reaching the airways. A spacer device attached to a metered dose inhaler reduces oropharyngeal deposition and increases lung deposition. Recently, an improved formulation of beclomethasone with smaller particle size (1.1 microns) has become available, which increases lung deposition. Budesonide is also available as respules to be given through a nebulizer.

Side-effects

Local side-effects include oropharyngeal complications such as thrush and dysphonia. Systemic toxicity is less likely

Table 1 **Adverse effects of corticosteroids**

Mineralocorticoid	Hypertension, sodium and water retention, potassium loss and adrenal suppression
Glucocorticoid	Diabetes, osteoporosis, psychosis, proximal myopathy, peptic ulceration, cataract, increased intraocular pressure, skin atrophy, hirsutism, reduction in ability to fight infection and retarded growth in children

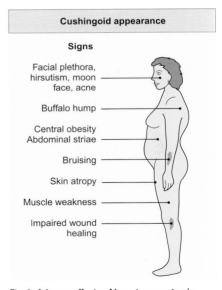

Fig. 2 **Adverse effects of long-term systemic therapy with corticosteroids.** (Adapted from Mygind N, Dahl R, Pedersen S, Thostrup-Pedresen K 1996 Essential Allergy 2nd edn, Blackwell Science.)

below a dose of beclometasone 1000 μg in adults and 400 μg in children. When laboratory assays of adrenal function or bone formation are measured, inhaled steroids can be shown to cause suppression of these markers, especially at high doses (beclometasone ≥ 2000 μg in adults and 800 μg in children). Growth monitoring (in children) and mineral bone density measurement may be indicated when high doses of inhaled steroids are prescribed.

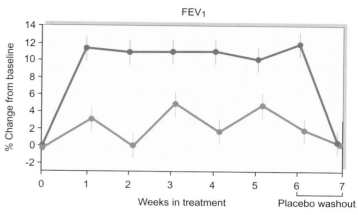

Fig. 3 **Inhaled steroid effect in asthma.**

TOPICAL NASAL STEROIDS

Chronic mucosal inflammation of allergic rhinitis responds to topical administration of steroids. Intranasal steroids are more effective than antihistamine in nasal obstruction. Intranasal preparations of beclometasone and budesonide have been available for more than two decades (Table 2). Newer drugs, such as mometasone furoate and fluticasone propionate appear to have substantially higher topical potency and lipid solubility, and lower systemic bioavailability. However, most nasal steroids are effective in controlling symptoms of seasonal and perennial allergic rhinitis. Local side-effects include dryness of nasal mucosa and epistaxis. Mometasone has been reported not to cause atrophy of the nasal mucosa.

TOPICAL SKIN PREPARATIONS

Topical steroids are used for the treatment of inflammatory skin conditions such as atopic and contact eczema. They are effective in the inflammatory exacerbation of eczema, but long-term regular treatment should be avoided. They are available in various potencies (Table 3). Potent steroids should be avoided in children, and on the face and neck. Very potent steroids should only be used for a short treatment course. Local side-effects include skin atrophy, spread of infection and contact sensitization. Regular use of potent topical steroids may cause systemic toxicity and adrenal suppression.

OTHER ANTI-INFLAMMATORY AGENTS

Sodium cromoglicate

Sodium cromoglicate, a sodium salt of chromone-2-caboxylic acid, is an anti-inflammatory agent used in the treatment of allergic asthma and rhinitis. It inhibits the release of mediators from mast cells and basophils although this does not fully explain its effectiveness. It is a less effective but a safer alternative to steroid and therefore often preferred as a first-line therapy in mild asthma, particularly in children. In asthma, it is administered through a dry powder inhaler or nebulizer and in rhinoconjunctivitis, as nasal spray and eye drops. It has to be given three to four times a day. Nedocromil sodium is a similar compound, which has been shown to be at least equally effective. It is available as inhaler and eye drops.

Immunosuppressive drugs

Methotrexate has proven efficacy in patients with steroid-insensitive asthma. Careful monitoring of adverse effects, especially for hepatic and haematological toxicity, is mandatory. Ciclosporin has also been used in difficult asthma and, rarely, in severe urticaria and angioedema.

Table 2 **Commonly used inhaled and intranasal steroids for asthma and allergic rhinitis**

Drugs	Inhaled steroids (Daily-dose range, μg)		Intranasal steroids (Daily-dose range, μg)	
	Adult	Child	Adult	Child*
Beclometasone dipropionate	200–1600	100–800	300–400	300–400
Budesonide	200–1600	100–800	200–400**	
Triamcinolone acetonide	200–1600	100–800	110–220	110
Flunisolide	200–2000	100–800	200–300	100–150
Fluticasone propionate	100–2000	50–400	200–400	100–200
Mometasone furoate			100–400**	

* 4–6 years or older
** 12 years or older

Table 3 **Topical corticosteroid preparations according to their potencies**

Potency	Examples
Mild	Hydrocortisone 0.1–1.0%
Moderately potent	Clobetasone butyrate, fluocortolone, fluroxycortide (flurandrenolone)
Potent	Hydrocortisone butyrate, beclometasone, betamethasone, diflucortolone, fluticasone, mometasone, triamcinolone, fluocinonide
Very potent	Clobetasol, halcinonide

Corticosteroids

- Glucocorticoids are powerful anti-inflammatory drugs. Long-term systemic administration is associated with a number of adverse effects.
- Short courses of oral prednisolone are indicated for asthma exacerbation, or to bring the disease under control.
- Prophylactic therapy with inhaled steroids is now considered an essential part of asthma therapy.
- Systemic adverse effects may occur at high doses of inhaled steroids.
- Intranasal steroids are the preferred form of treatment in perennial and seasonal allergic rhinitis.
- Topical steroids for eczema should be used intermittently for exacerbations.
- Sodium cromoglicate and nedocromil sodium have minimal adverse effects, and could be used in mild to moderate allergic asthma.
- In severe, steroid insensitive asthma, methotrexate has been found to be a useful anti-inflammatory agent.

NOVEL ANTI-INFLAMMATORY DRUGS

With increased awareness and understanding of the underlying inflammatory mechanisms in asthma and other allergic diseases, the indications for anti-inflammatory therapy are expanding. Steroids have been the mainstay of anti-inflammatory therapy in allergic diseases. However, there is concern about their adverse effects, especially with increased usage. Moreover, steroids do not possess disease-modifying potential. Recent advances in molecular and cell biology have paved the way for the discovery of novel therapeutic agents, that may be safer and effective, and may even alter the natural history of the disease (Fig. 1).

Extensive research is being carried out with a rational approach, to inhibit allergic inflammation. The success of the new therapies depends on their effectiveness and the absence of adverse effects. Some of the most promising new therapies are discussed.

MEDIATOR ANTAGONISTS

Inhibition of synthesis of mediators, or receptor antagonism, may reduce inflammation in allergic diseases. Several such mediator antagonists have been studied. Apart from antihistamines, only anti-leukotrienes have so far been used in clinical practice. The platelet activating factor seems to be an important mediator in asthma. However, potent PAF inhibitors failed to show efficacy in clinical trials. Some other mediator antagonists are being studied.

Anti-leukotrienes

Anti-leukotriene agents are the first new class of asthma medication to be approved in the last 20 years. Leukotrienes C4, D4 and E4, are released by numerous inflammatory cells, and are potent mediators of inflammation (Table 1). Leukotriene antagonists can inhibit the effect of leukotrienes either via receptor antagonism or inhibition of synthesis.

Table 1 **The pro-inflammatory effects of leukotrienes C4, D4 and E4**

- Bronchoconstriction
- Chemoattraction
- Eosinophil recruitment
- Increase vascular permeability
- Plasma extravasation
- Mucus hypersecretion
- Mucosal oedema
- Bronchial hyperreactivity

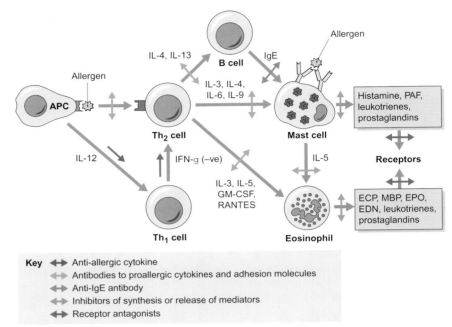

Fig. 1 **Rational approach to novel treatments for allergic diseases, based on the knowledge of cellular immune mechanisms.**

Receptor antagonists

The receptor antagonists demonstrate a significant effect and are generally well tolerated (Table 2). Oral administration and relatively few adverse effects improves compliance. Montelukast, zafirlukast and pranlukast are the currently available leukotriene-receptor antagonists. Their overall effect is nearly equal to the inhaled beclometasone at a dose of 400 μg daily. They are recommended for mild to moderate asthma, usually as an additional treatment to inhaled steroids. Whether they can be used as sole anti-inflammatory therapy in mild persistent asthma, remains to be seen. Their effectiveness in allergic rhinitis is currently being studied and preliminary results are promising.

Inhibition of synthesis

The 5-lipoxygenase inhibitors have shown an anti-inflammatory effect in experimental asthma models and clinical studies.

Antitryptase

Tryptase has been implicated, as a mediator, in allergic conditions including asthma and rhinoconjunctivitis. In animal studies, tryptase inhibitors have been effective in inhibiting the late-phase bronchoconstriction and airway hyperresponsiveness following allergen challenge. Moreover, the intradermal injection of tryptase inhibitor blocks the cutaneous

response to allergen. Further studies are needed before the usefulness of this mediator antagonist becomes clear.

Phosphodiesterase inhibitors

Theophylline exerts its bronchodilator and anti-inflammatory effects by inhibiting phosphodiesterase (PDE) enzyme activities (Fig. 2). Several isoenzymes have been identified in airway smooth muscles. By selective inhibition of these isoenzymes, it may be possible to retain bronchodilator and anti-inflammatory properties without adverse effects of theophylline. Several PDE inhibitors have been studied. A selective phosphodiesterase IV inhibitor shows both anti-inflammatory and bronchodilator characteristics in animal studies. Clinical trials are currently being carried out.

CYTOKINES AND ADHESION MOLECULES

Adhesion molecules are important in inflammatory cellular activation, and transportation from circulation to the site of inflammation. Monoclonal antibodies to several adhesion molecules have been investigated and show some promise in animal studies. Results of human studies with these antibodies are not yet available.

Cytokines modulate immune responses in both a pro- and an anti-allergic manner.

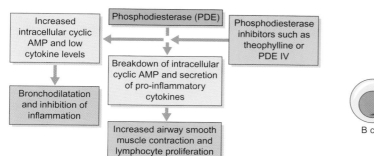

Fig. 2 **Mechanism of action of phosphodiesterase inhibitors such as theophylline and PDE IV inhibitor.**

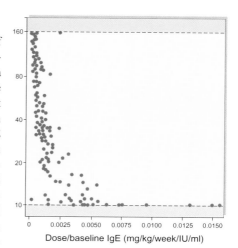

Fig. 3 **Anti-IgE molecule binds to the free IgE in the circulation and those expressed on B cells. IgE is therefore not available to bind to its high- and low-affinity receptors on mast cells and other inflammatory cells. The initiation of allergic reaction can thus be inhibited.**

Anti-allergic cytokines, such as IL-12 and interferon-γ promote Th1, and inhibit Th2, response to allergen. These can therefore be used to inhibit allergic inflammation. However, recent trials with these cytokines have shown marginal efficacy with considerable toxicity. Monoclonal antibodies to pro-allergic cytokines such as IL-4, IL-5 and IL-13 can be used to suppress allergic inflammation.

Anti-interleukin-5 (anti-IL-5)

IL-5 is important for the differentiation, activation and survival of eosinophils. Monoclonal antibody to IL-5 has been shown to suppress allergen-induced late-phase asthmatic responses in animal studies. A recent study in mild asthmatics, however, failed to show any effect on allergen-induced asthmatic responses, or non-specific bronchial hyperresponsiveness, despite being effective in reducing sputum eosinophilia.

ANTI-IMMUNOGLOBULIN E (ANTI-IgE)

IgE plays a critical role in the initiation of allergic inflammation. Monoclonal antibody to IgE has been developed with a high affinity for the IgE molecule. The antibody has been humanized so that it does not provoke an immune reaction (non-anaphylactogenic). The anti-IgE binds to the circulating IgE to form an IgE/anti-IgE complex (Fig. 3). The half-life of anti-IgE is 2–4 weeks. Repeated administration ensures that no IgE is available for binding to mast cells and other inflammatory cells (Fig. 4). In experimental studies in asthma and rhinitis, it has been successful in inhibiting allergen-induced responses, and improves symptoms. Clinical studies are underway to determine its usefulness in clinical practice. The advantage of anti-IgE antibody is that it may prove to be useful in all IgE-mediated allergic diseases, irrespective of causative allergen, or the organ involved.

Dose/baseline IgE (mg/kg/week/IU/ml)

Fig. 4 **Serum IgE in patient treated with humanized monoclonal antibody to IgE (E-25).** The reduction in IgE is dose-related, though beyond 0.005 mg/kg/week/IU/ml very little IgE can be detected in blood. (From Casale TB, Bernstein IL, Busse WW, et al. 1997 J Allergy Clin Immunol, 100:110–21.)

Table 2 **Effects of leukotriene antagonists**

Experimental models of asthma
Decrease in the number of inflammatory cells: • eosinophils • lymphocytes
Inhibition of bronchial hyperresponsiveness induced by: • cold dry air • exercise • allergen • hyperventilation • aspirin Bronchodilator effects Additive to β-agonists and antihistamine
Clinical asthma
Improvement of: • asthma symptoms • quality of life • air flow obstruction • lung function
Reduction in: • β 2-agonist- use • corticosteroid-use • asthma exacerbations

Novel anti-inflammatory drugs

- There is need for new anti-inflammatory drugs in allergic diseases which do not possess adverse effects associated with steroids.
- With better understanding of immune regulation and inflammatory mechanisms, it is possible to devise novel therapies.
- Leukotrienes are important mediators of inflammation.
- Anti-leukotrienes have proved successful in improving symptoms and lung function, and reducing the need for bronchodilators and steroids.
- Anti-leukotrienes are the first new mediator antagonists to be approved for clinical use.
- Extensive research is being carried out in modifying immune responses through the use of anti-allergic cytokines or monoclonal antibodies to pro-allergic cytokines and adhesion molecules.
- Anti-IL5 antibody has not been found to be effective in inhibiting asthmatic responses to allergen challenge.
- Humanized monoclonal antibody to IgE has proved useful in clinical trials of allergic asthma and rhinitis.

ALLERGEN IMMUNOTHERAPY 1 – INTRODUCTION

Specific allergen immunotherapy (IT) or hyposensitization was introduced in 1911 for the treatment of asthma and allergic diseases and remains the only treatment modality with disease-modifying potential. However, its efficacy, indications and risk–benefit ratio has been extensively debated over the years with extreme views prevailing in the medical community. Some recommend allergen IT as the first-line treatment for all or most allergic diseases, whereas others believe it has no role to play in the modern medical practice.

IT aims to induce tolerance to the allergen and thus improve symptoms related to exposure to that specific allergen. In conventional IT, periodic injections of allergen extract is administered in gradually increasing quantities, until maintenance dose is reached. Thereafter, the injections are given at longer intervals for 3–5 years.

MECHANISM

The exact mechanism of how IT works is not known. Both antibody-mediated and cell-mediated mechanisms have been proposed.

Antibody-mediated

It was suggested that IT stimulates the production of allergen-specific blocking IgG antibodies which intercept the allergen before it can bind to the IgE on the cell surface (Fig. 1). Blocking IgE antibodies may provide protection in venom IT but their relevance in respiratory allergy has been questioned, as clinical improvement may precede a rise in their titre. Moreover, the level of blocking IgG antibody generally does not correlate with the degree of improvement. It was also suggested that the increase of specific IgG subclass 1 (IgG1) in relation to IgG4 (ratio of IgG1–IgG4) might influence the induction of tolerance, but this has not been proven. IT initially causes a rise in allergen-specific IgE, with gradual decline over years. However, changes in the level of allergen-specific IgE or in the size of skin-test reaction also do not correlate with the efficacy of IT.

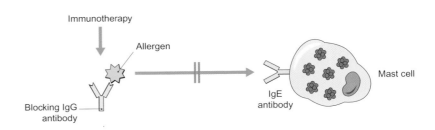

Fig. 1 **Proposed mechanism for immunotherapy:** Allergen-specific IgG antibodies bind to the allergen preventing antigen binding to IgE antibody and thus inhibiting allergic reaction.

Cell-mediated

A number of studies have shown reduction in target organ allergen sensitivity with suppression of early and late phase skin and bronchial responsiveness, due to decrease in mediator release from inflammatory cells. A reduction in the number of mast cells and eosinophils has also been observed following prolonged IT. Recent work has suggested that this might be due to a switch from a Th2 into a Th1 reaction pattern in the T cell regulation (Fig. 2). In atopic individuals, allergen exposure causes naïve lymphocytes to preferentially differentiate into Th2 type cells, with its specific cytokine profile (IL-4, IL-5, IL-13). IT induces Th1 cellular activity with increased production of IL-2 and IFN-γ, with the concomitant inhibition of Th2 cell proliferation. This results in a decrease in eosinophilic infiltration, IgE production and mediator release.

EFFECTIVENESS
Rhinitis

The clinical efficacy of IT in seasonal allergic rhinitis has been convincingly documented in double-blind, placebo-controlled trials. This includes grass (e.g. rye, timothy), tree (e.g. birch) and weed (e.g. ragweed) pollen allergy. IT with a single pollen species, such as rye grass, is as effective as treatment with four or five species. The evidence for autumn rhinitis due to mould (e.g. *Cladosporium, Alternaria*) allergy is less forthcoming. This is possibly due to the unavailability of standardized extracts to moulds. About 20–30% of patients with pollen-induced allergic rhinitis develop asthma. Some studies have shown a prophylactic effect of immunotherapy in reducing the development of asthma in these patients. IT is also effective in house-dust mite and cat-sensitive perennial allergic rhinitis. However, the outcome may be diffi-

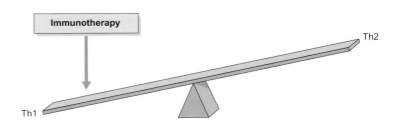

Fig. 2 **The balance of T cell regulation is tilted in favour of Th1 responses, thus inhibiting allergic inflammation mediated by Th2 cytokines.**

cult to assess because of the complicating features of perennial rhinitis such as nasal polyposis and sinusitis. Therefore, the effectiveness of immunotherapy, compared to standard pharmacotherapy, is not known.

Asthma

The evidence supporting its effectiveness in the treatment of asthma is much more limited. However, a number of controlled studies published during the last decade show a clear tendency towards a beneficial effect, especially in children. Studies of pollen-sensitive asthma have demonstrated beneficial effects of specific immunotherapy for grass, birch, and ragweed pollen-induced asthma. House-dust mite IT has benefited asthmatic children more than adults. Controlled trials have shown a benefit of IT in asthma due to cat allergy, but evidence for allergy to other animals (dog, horse) and mould is insufficient.

In asthma, reduction in allergen responsiveness is more convincingly demonstrated but improvement in non-specific responsiveness, symptoms, medication usage and pulmonary function is modest. Some recent studies have shown improvement in respiratory function, bronchial hyperreactivity, and quality of life with sub-lingual IT in house-dust mite-related asthma. Whether immunotherapy has any long-term prophylactic effects on airway remodelling and subepithelial fibrosis is not convincingly demonstrated.

Other diseases

IT has been shown to prevent anaphylaxis to insect (wasp, honeybee, hornet) venom in patients with a history of systemic reactions to their stings. IT is not effective in non-allergic rhinitis, atopic or contact dermatitis, urticaria and food allergy or intolerance (Table 1).

Single vs. multiple allergens. Clinical trials with IT for single allergens such as house-dust mite, cats, pollen, and mould are convincing in showing benefit. There is no convincing evidence that multiple allergen therapy in a patient sensitized to

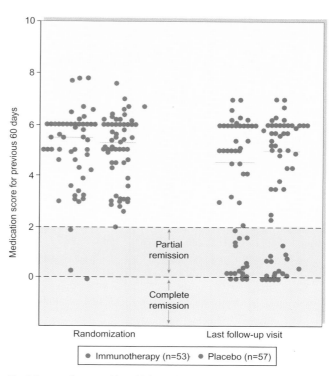

Fig. 3 **Immunotherapy with multiple unrelated allergen extracts in a randomized controlled trial failed to show any benefit over and above placebo.** The reduction in medication requirement was similar in the two groups (Adkinson et al. 1997 N Engl J Med 336: 324–331).

several unrelated allergens is beneficial (Fig. 3). IT with a low-dose regime is generally not effective, although it may have fewer side-effects (Table 2).

Clinical vs. statistical benefit. Although the effectiveness of immunotherapy has been shown in a number of well designed studies, the statistical improvement is not equal to clinically relevant benefit. For optimal effectiveness, IT should be restricted to appropriately selected patients with proven IgE-mediated disease. Immunotherapy rarely cures the disease. However, a considerable reduction in symptoms and drug consumption may be achieved.

Table 1 **Efficacy of allergen-specific immunotherapy in IgE-mediated allergic diseases**

Efficacy	Diseases
Definite	Seasonal allergic rhinitis and asthma (pollen allergy), insect allergy
Probable	Perennial rhinitis and asthma (dust mite and animal dander), IgE-mediated drug allergy
Possible	Perennial rhinitis and asthma (mould allergy)
None	Atopic eczema, acute and chronic urticaria, food allergy

Table 2 **Some issues regarding the efficacy of immunotherapy**

Issues	Comments
Seasonal versus perennial	More effective in seasonal than perennial disease
Single versus multiple allergens	Less effective in patients with multiple allergy
Mild versus severe disease	Mild disease can be controlled with simple drug treatment but risk of reaction is high in severe asthma
Asthma versus rhinitis	Efficacy better proven in rhinitis
Low-dose versus high-dose	Low-dose regimens, although safer, are of unproven efficacy
Early versus late in the disease process	Possible advantage in early treatment, of disease-modifying effect

Allergen immunotherapy – Introduction

- Immunotherapy induces tolerance to the allergen.
- Several immunological changes are observed following immunotherapy.
- Allergen-specific blocking IgG antibodies are produced.
- T cell regulation is influenced towards a Th1 response to allergen exposure.
- Bronchial, nasal and skin sensitivity to the allergen is reduced.
- Inflammatory cell recruitment and mediator release is inhibited.
- Efficacy in pollen allergic rhinitis and asthma and insect allergy is proven beyond doubt.
- Efficacy in allergy to dust mite, mould and animal dander is convincing but the benefit is marginal.
- Children and young adults benefit more than older patients.
- Statistical improvement does not necessarily means clinically relevant benefit.

ALLERGEN IMMUNOTHERAPY 2 – RISKS AND BENEFITS

INDICATIONS

There is ample evidence of the effectiveness of immunotherapy (IT) in allergic rhinitis, insect venom allergy and asthma. However, proven efficacy does not necessarily mean IT is indicated in all or most patients with these diseases, as effective and safe pharmacological treatment is available. IT should be considered in patients with:

- significant disease not adequately controlled with allergen avoidance and standard pharmacotherapy, or the requirement for systemic steroids
- allergen exposure clearly related to symptoms
- a single or group of allergens (e.g. grass pollen) responsible for most symptoms.

IT is recommended for the treatment of seasonal allergic rhinitis due to grass, tree or weed pollen allergy. It may also be used for pollen-induced asthma. It is strongly recommended for patients with insect (wasp, honeybee) venom allergy with a history of anaphylaxis and demonstrable venom-specific IgE. However, its value in those with a mild or local reaction to insect sting is not clear. It may be used in perennial allergic rhinitis, where allergen avoidance is difficult.

IT may be indicated in a few highly selected patients with perennial asthma, although it should be avoided in those with severe unstable asthma because of an increased risk of anaphylaxis. Some investigators have suggested its use early in the disease process in asthma, to prevent airway remodelling due to chronic persistent inflammation. More evidence is needed before this can be recommended. IT should generally be used in conjunction with pharmacotherapy, which remains the first line of management. However, the requirement for medication may be reduced with successful IT.

Allergens used for immunotherapy include pollen, dust mites, mould and some animal dander such as cat, dog and horse. The allergen should be well characterized. For example, IT should not be done with house-dust, which is a mixture of allergenic and non-allergenic substances, but specifically to house-dust mites. Similarly, patients with allergy to insect sting should be treated with venom and not whole-body extract. The availability of purified and standardized extract also determines the use of IT. Standardized allergen extracts are not available for all common mould or animal dander. IT should not be done with extracts prepared from foods, feathers, synthetic material, bacterial extract, enzymes and occupational allergens. Allergen immunotherapy is not recommended for patients with atopic or contact dermatitis, food allergy and urticaria. IT should be avoided in certain situations, which increase the risk of side-effects (Table 1).

SELECTION OF PATIENTS

When selecting patients for IT, a careful evaluation should be made for each individual, considering the severity of disease for the kind of treatment, balancing the relative benefits, risks, cost and inconvenience (Table 2). Avoidance of the offending allergen should be preferred, however this is not always possible. Effective pharmacotherapy is available for most allergic diseases. IT should be used in addition to pharmacotherapy in a selected group of patients who will benefit most (Fig. 1). The benefit of IT should be additional to what can be obtained from standard pharmacotherapy (Table 3), such as an improved control of disease or reduced need for systemic steroids.

Table 1 **Some relative and absolute contraindications for immunotherapy**

- Pregnancy
- Significant cardiovascular diseases
- Presence of other serious diseases
- Treatment with β-blocker
- Pulmonary function below 70% predicted

Table 2 **Arguments for and against immunotherapy**

Advantages
• the only treatment with disease-modifying potential
• reduces sensitivity to allergens such as pollen, cat and dust mite
• clinical efficacy documented in allergic rhinitis, insect allergy and in selected patients with asthma
• benefit may continue after discontinuation of IT

Disadvantages
• requires compliance with the treatment for long periods and therefore highly motivated and cooperative patients
• can cause serious side-effects including anaphylaxis
• standardized allergen extracts are not available for all common allergens
• the mechanisms of action are not yet understood
• many protocols have been devised empirically

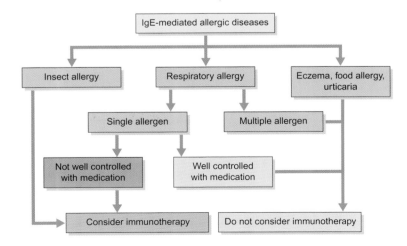

Fig. 1 **Protocol for selecting patients for consideration of immunotherapy.**

Table 3 **Comparison of specific allergen immunotherapy and standard pahrmacotherapy**

	Immunotherapy	Pharmacotherapy
Mechanism	Intervene early in allergy cascade	Intervene later in allergy cascade
Duration of therapy	Discontinue after 3–5 years	Usually for life
Efficacy	Less proven	Better proven
Immediate relief	No	Yes
Disease modifying capacity	Possible but not proven	Not proven
Life threatening side-effects	Yes	Rare
Cost	Less expensive	More expensive
Convenience of therapy	Less convenient	More convenient

Table 4 **Type of reaction encountered during the course of immunotherapy**

Type of reaction	Time	Signs
Local	Immediate (<30 min.)	Localized erythema and swelling
	Delayed (4–24 hours)	Diffuse swelling
Large local	Anytime	Diffuse swelling and erythema (> 20 cm)
Systemic	Commence < 30 min	Itching, urticaria / angioedema, throat tightness, bronchospasm, hypotension

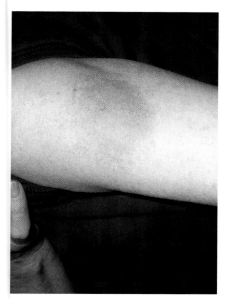

Fig. 2 **A localized reaction to specific immunotherapy to grass pollen in a patient with severe hayfever.**

Before initiating IT the following questions must be answered:

- Is there evidence of a close relationship between symptoms and allergen exposure? (e.g. seasonal allergic rhinitis)
- Is it possible to achieve efficient allergen avoidance? (e.g. allergy to cat)
- Is simple drug-treatment not sufficient? (e.g. inhaled corticosteroids or oral antihistamines)
- Is there evidence in the literature of effectiveness of IT for this allergen? (e.g. pollen)
- Is the patient able to comply with a long and constraining treatment?

RISKS

IT carries certain risks, including the possibility of life-threatening anaphylaxis (Table 4). Local reactions at the site of injection are common, but systemic reactions are fortunately rare, if appropriate precautions are taken. Patients with severe asthma, and those who are highly sensitized, are at a higher risk of having systemic reactions to IT (Table 5).

A localized reaction consists of a pruritic, erythematous induration at the site of injection (Fig. 2). This usually responds to oral antihistamine. Systemic reactions occur, on average, one in every 1000–2000 injections (approximately 5–10% of patients). They usually occur within 30 min of the injection. Adverse reactions commencing after 60 min are almost never life-threatening. Symptoms include generalized urticaria, bronchospasm, breathing difficulty and rarely hypotension and shock. Most reactions are mild and respond quickly to adrenaline (epinephrine) 0.3–0.5 ml of 1:1000 solution and parenteral antihistamine. Oral corticosteroids may help to reduce the intensity of any late reaction. Reactions to IT can rarely be fatal.

Nineteen deaths were reported due to IT in the USA between 1987 and 1991. Systemic reactions are more common in the dose-escalation phase and may be related to the rate of escalation.

Table 5 **Risk factors for systemic reactions to IT**

- Symptomatic asthma
- Highly sensitized patients
- New vaccine vial
- Dosing errors
- Concomitant high allergen exposure
- Short period of observation
- Use of β-blocker

Allergen immunotherapy – Risks and benefits

- Immunotherapy is recommended for the treatment of allergic rhinitis, insect allergy and in some highly selected patients with asthma.
- It is indicated where simple pharmacotherapy does not adequately control symptoms.
- It should be used in conjunction with pharmacotherapy for optimal control with minimal side-effects.
- Evidence of a causative relationship of allergen exposure to symptoms is essential
- Each individual should be carefully assessed, regarding the benefit, risks, cost and inconvenience.
- A detailed explanation should be given to the patient of the procedure, expected benefits and risks.
- It is not recommended in patients with atopic or contact dermatitis, urticaria and food allergy.
- Localized reactions at the site of injections are common.
- Systemic reactions are rare and usually start within 20 min of injection.
- A life-threatening reaction should be treated immediately with adrenaline (epinephrine) and parentral antihistamine.

ALLERGEN IMMUNOTHERAPY 3 – PROCEDURES

ALLERGEN EXTRACTS

Aqueous extracts

Only purified and standardized extracts should be used, containing all important antigens of the specific allergen. Aqueous extracts were originally introduced in 1911 and these are still commonly used. Lyophilized (frozen, dried) extracts can be stored for long periods before reconstitution. Aqueous extracts tend to lose potency as the proteins adhere to the surface of the glass. The addition of albumin to an aqueous solution helps to preserve potency. Highly concentrated extracts retain potency for longer periods than more diluted solutions, which should be used for short periods only. Manufacturers supply extracts in various dilutions (Fig. 1). These extracts should be kept refrigerated to reduce loss of potency.

Modified extracts

A number of modified extracts have been developed to delay absorption and thus reduce the risk of anaphylaxis. Another advantage of depot preparation is that less frequent injections are needed. Depot extracts with allergen adsorbed to aluminium hydroxide are in clinical use. The modified extracts have similar efficacy to the aqueous extract.

Units of potency

Previously, the potency of the extract was measured in protein nitrogen units (PNU) or the amount of allergenic material present in the solution, weight-to-volume (w/v). For example, 1 g of pollen extracted in 10 ml of water is 1:10 w/v solution. The potency in these solutions was difficult to predict and varied widely, depending on the source of material and method of extraction. More recently, the potency has been assessed by in vitro tests such as RAST inhibition (IgE-binding capacity of the allergen in the extract indicates potency), measurement of major antigens, and in-vivo assays (skin testing with end-point titration). The potency is expressed in allergy units (AU), in biological units (BU) or standardized quality (SQ) units. Unfortunately, these units are not interchangeable. It is therefore important not to make changes in the supplier during the course of treatment.

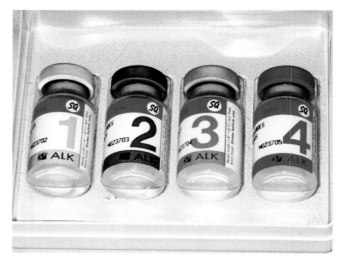

Fig. 1   **Allergen extracts for immunotherapy are available in 10-fold dilutions.**

ROUTE OF ADMINISTRATION

The principal and most effective route of allergen administration is the subcutaneous injection. The intramuscular route is not appropriate, as rapid absorption of the allergen will be associated with higher risk of anaphylaxis. The efficacy and safety of topical administration of allergen extracts have been investigated. This includes nasal, bronchial, oral and sublingual IT. Their effectiveness is not proven and these cannot yet be recommended for clinical practice except in the context of research.

SCHEDULES

Conventional

The most concentrated solution has the same potency as used for skin-prick tests. Manufacturers often provide serially (usually 10-fold) diluted solutions in colour-coded vials. The initial dose which would be tolerated by all patients is low, such as 0.1 ml of 1:1000 or 1:10 000 dilution of the most concentrated solution containing 100 000 units/ml. Some prefer to do skin end-point titration to find an appropriate starting-dose for each patient. The dose is gradually increased at weekly or twice weekly intervals (Table 1), the maximum possible dose being 1 ml of the concentrated solution. The maintenance dose is the maximum dose tolerated by the patients. Variations in the dose escalation regimen are common in different centres. The regimen needs to be tailored to the individual, according to their sensitivity and clinical condition. It generally takes 12–20 weeks to achieve the maintenance dose. The dose interval is then increased to 2, 3 and then 4 weeks (6 weeks if using the modified extract). Injections are given at 4–6 weeks interval for a period of 3–5 years. The optimal duration of IT is not known. Some continue to give IT for longer than 5 years if the benefit continues, whereas others may stop after 2 years. The benefit generally lasts for several years after a 3-year course.

Preseasonal therapy for pollen is started 3–4 months before the season until the maintenance dose is achieved. The therapy is discontinued during the season and restarted before the next season. In perennial therapy, maintenance dose is administered

Table 1   **A sample schedule for conventional immunotherapy***

Dilution	Concentration	Volume (ml)	Dosage (SQ-U)
1:1000	100 SQ-U/ml	0.2	20
		0.4	40
		0.8	80
1:100	1000 SQ-U/ml	0.2	200
		0.4	400
		0.8	800
1:10	10 000 SQ-U/ml	0.2	2000
		0.4	4000
		0.8	8000
1:1	100 000 SQ-U/ml	0.1	10 000
		0.2	20 000
		0.4	40 000
		0.6	60 000
		0.8	80 000
		1.0	100 000

*This regimen is for guidance only when using SQ units. It should be altered according to the allergen sensitivity and other factors, such as allergen exposure

Table 2 **Some practical issues in the use of immunotherapy**

Issues	Comments
Preseasonal versus perennial administration	Perennial regimen is safer and more convenient
Aqueous or modified extract	Modified extracts are more convenient as fewer injections are needed
Parenteral versus oral/sublingual	Effectiveness better established for parenteral therapy
Conventional versus rush or cluster protocols	Conventional protocols are safer
Standard extract versus peptides and DNA vaccines	Peptide extract and DNA vaccines are experimental at present

Table 3 **Adverse effects of IT can be minimized if care is taken in the selection of patients and administration of extracts**

- IT should only be administered under direct supervision of a trained allergist, and where facilities for resuscitation are available
- Adrenaline(epinephrine), parenteral antihistamines and bronchodilators should be at hand
- Only standardized extracts from a reputable laboratory should be used
- Avoid IT in patients with severe asthma and those on β-blockers
- IT should not be administered to asthmatic patients with $FEV_1 < 70\%$ predicted
- Patient should wait at least 30 min in the department after each injection. A longer waiting period may be necessary for high-risk subjects
- A close cooperation between patients, their family practitioner and allergist is important for the success of this treatment

all year round. The efficacy of the two treatment protocols is similar. Perennial therapy is preferred as fewer injections are required and the overall risk of reaction is less during maintenance therapy (Table 2).

Modified schedules

Cluster or rush immunotherapy refers to a shortened schedule of immunotherapy. Patients receive rapidly increasing doses of allergen to reach the maintenance dose within a period of days or weeks. This schedule has been used most frequently for immunotherapy to insect venom. Although IT has been shown to be successful in several studies with the shorter schedules, the risk of adverse reactions is greater. It is not generally recommended for the treatment of respiratory allergy.

Precautions

Appropriate care should be taken in the selection of patients and the administration of extracts to avoid systemic reactions (Table 3). Most reactions occur in the dose-escalation phase, and general rules should be followed (Table 4). Care should also be taken when a new vial is opened as the allergen often degrades with storage. The new vial may be more potent compared to the old, despite having the same designation. Every precaution should be taken to avoid errors in the calculation and administration of the appropriate dose. IT should only be done where facilities for resuscitation are available.

FUTURE TRENDS

The characterization of IgE-binding sites on antigen opens the possibility of using recombinant allergens in various immunotherapeutical approaches, for example, the administration of allergen peptides, allergen fragments, allergen isoforms or mutated allergens. Th2 lymphocytes play a central role in the regulation of allergic inflammation. For stimulation, T cells require the presentation of allergen epitope (the part of the antigen molecule which recognizes and combines with the T cell receptor), by antigen-presenting cells. Injection of allergen epitope can occupy the T cell receptor without stimulating the cell, thus blocking allergic reaction.

A novel concept is the use of plasmid DNA for IT. pDNA immunization induces a Th1 response by causing antigen-presenting cells (e.g. macrophage) to secrete INF-α, INF-β and IL-12, cytokines, that induce naïve T cells to differentiate into $CD4^+$ Th1 cells and $CD8^+$ Tc1 cells. Immunization with pDNA, encoding for allergen, has been shown to cause a shift in T cell response from Th2 to Th1 in preliminary studies. Allergen-pDNA immunotherapy is unlikely to carry the risk of the anaphylactic reactions associated with conventional IT. This approach promises to be safe and effective.

Table 4 **Guidelines for the administration of IT**

- Carefully check dose and concentration before administration
- Increase the dose slowly in patients:
  - with moderate asthma
  - who are highly sensitized
- Reduce the rate of escalation or repeat the same dose:
  - if moderate size local reaction occurs
  - with concurrent high allergen exposure
- Repeat the same dose or scale down:
  - if large local reaction occurs
  - if the interval between injections is 2 weeks or more
- Scale down
  - when a new vial is opened
  - if systemic reaction occurs
- Source (manufacturer of allergen extract) should not be changed during therapy

Allergen immunotherapy – Procedures

- Only purified and standardized extracts should be used for IT.
- Modified extracts have similar efficacy to the aqueous extract and may be safer.
- The principal and most effective route of allergen administration is the subcutaneous injection.
- Topical (nasal, bronchial, oral and sublingual) IT is not yet recommended for clinical use.
- Conventional immunotherapy is given in gradually escalating doses until maximum tolerable (maintenance) dose is achieved.
- Maintenance therapy continues for 3–5 years, although ideal duration is not known.
- In cluster or rush immunotherapy, rapidly escalating doses are given to achieve maintenance dose within days or weeks.
- Every precaution should be taken to avoid excessive risk to the patient.
- IT should only be done where facilities for resuscitation are available.
- Manipulation of immune regulation with specific molecules such as T cell epitopes or plasmid DNA may prove to be effective and safer forms of IT.

ASTHMA 1 – DEFINITION AND CHARACTERISTICS

DEFINITION

It has been difficult to achieve a consensus on definition. The difficulty arises as none of the proposed definitions encompass all the features of asthma. Recently *The National Asthma Education Program Expert Panel Report* has produced a comprehensive definition:

'Asthma is a lung disease with the following characteristics:

- Airway obstruction (or airway narrowing) that is reversible (but not completely so in some patients) either spontaneously or with treatment
- Airway inflammation
- Airway hyperresponsiveness to a variety of stimuli.'

CHARACTERISTICS

Asthma can present in many different ways. The aetiology is known in some forms of asthma such as occupational asthma, whereas there may be no clues to the cause in other forms, for example, non-atopic or intrinsic asthma (Table 1).

Clinical syndrome

Asthma is a syndrome with many overlapping features (Figs 1 & 2). Bronchial obstruction is a cardinal feature and is reversible, at least to a degree, in most asthmatics (Table 2). Bronchial hyperresponsiveness is present in most but not all patients with asthma, as is atopy. Eosinophilic airway inflammation is probably the most consistent feature.

Atopy

The relationship of asthma and atopy is complex. Both are inherited and it is possible that some common genetic loci are involved. The vast majority of asthma in children and young adults is atopic. In adults, late onset asthma is often non-atopic. In an individual, atopy can be confirmed by positive skin test, the presence of specific IgE to common allergens, or a high total serum IgE.

Bronchial hyperresponsiveness

Bronchial responsiveness is the ease with which the airway narrows in response to external stimuli. In asthma, airways contract too much and too easily (hyperresponsiveness), which is one of the

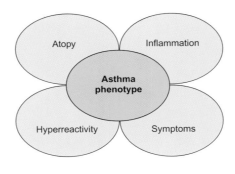

Fig. 1 **Features of asthma: relationship of atopy, bronchial hyperreactivity, symptoms and bronchial inflammation.**

main characteristic of asthma. However, bronchial hyperresponsiveness may not be present in some subjects who clearly have asthma, whereas others may bronchoconstrict easily without any symptoms of asthma. The measurement of the degree of bronchoconstriction provides an objective tool to assess the severity of asthma.

Airway inflammation

Asthma is a chronic inflammatory disorder. This inflammation results in mucosal oedema, accumulation of leukocytes, especially eosinophils, in the mucosal surface and lumen, and thickness of the basement membrane. These changes cause narrowing of the airway lumen and bronchial hyperresponsiveness. Allergenic and non-allergenic triggers and neurogenic stimuli then cause further narrowing by bronchial smooth muscle contraction.

MORBIDITY AND MORTALITY

Asthma is one of the most common chronic conditions. Overall, 10–15% of children and 5–10% adults suffer from asthma in the Western world. Boys are twice as likely to have asthma as girls. In adults, women may have a slightly higher prevalence, but severe or life-threatening asthma is almost twice as common in women.

It is now generally agreed that the prevalence of asthma is rising. At least a

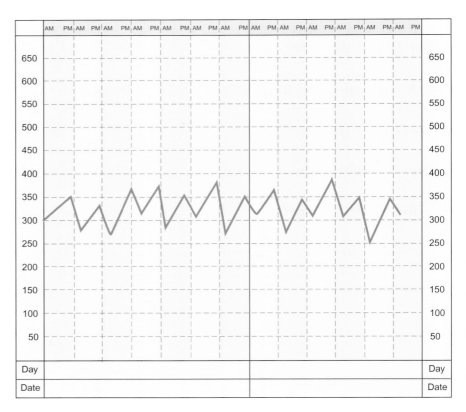

Fig. 2 **Diurnal and day-to-day variability is a characteristic of asthma indicating airway lability.** Morning peak flows are usually lower than evening readings.

Table 1 **Types of asthma**

Type of asthma	Features
Atopic	High serum IgE, sensitization to common allergens, presence of other allergic diseases
Early-onset, non-atopic	Often severe persistent asthma
Late-onset, non-atopic	Often associated with eosinophilia, sinusitis and nasal polyps
Associated with other lung disease	'Asthmatic component' of chronic obstructive pulmonary disease, bronchiectasis
Associated with arteritis	Churg–Strauss syndrome, polyarteritis nodosa
Exercise induced asthma	Symptoms on exercise, often in children
'Cough variant'	Chronic dry cough, bronchial hyperreactivity
Aspirin-sensitive asthma	Aspirin intolerance, rhinitis, nasal polyposis
Occupational asthma	Occupational exposure to gases, vapours and fumes at work

Table 2 **Clinical features of asthma**

Type of asthma	Features
Episodic	Episodes of cough, wheezing and shortness of breath
Symptom variability	Symptom severity varies from day to day, often worse at night and early morning (morning tightness)
Peak flow variability	Day to day variability and low morning readings (morning dip) are characteristic. A 20% or more variability is diagnostic of asthma
Lack of symptoms	In mild asthma, there may be days or weeks of symptom-free periods. However, patients may adopt their lifestyle to avoid symptoms (such as lack of physical activity)
Reversibility	The obstruction to airflow is reversible in the majority of patients. A 15% improvement following bronchodilator or steroid treatment is regarded as evidence of reversibility.

two-fold increase in the prevalence of asthma has been seen during the last two decades. Hospital admission rates for asthma increased during the 1970s and 1980s but seems now to have stabilized. In several countries there was an increase in asthma mortality in the 1960s. Since then, despite an increase in the prevalence of asthma, the mortality rates have remained around 10–15 per million population in the Western world (Fig. 3).

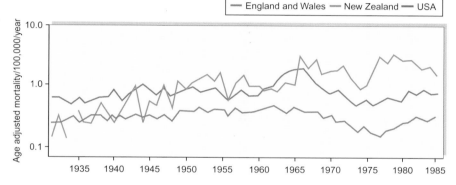

Fig 3 **Asthma mortality in England and Wales, New Zealand and the USA.** There was a decline in mortality in the USA but a rise was observed in New Zealand in the 1980s. (From: Holgate ST, Church MK 1993 Allergy, London: Gower Medical Publishing.)

DEVELOPMENT AND NATURAL HISTORY

Genetics of asthma

It has been known for some time that genetic factors are important in the causation of asthma. The exact mode of inheritance is not known but seems likely to be multifactorial. A history of asthma and atopy in the parents remains the most reliable indication of this genetic susceptibility. The search for genes for asthma, atopy and related clinical characteristics continues.

Environmental risk factors

Environmental factors that may influence the development of asthma include allergens (food and inhalant), viral infections, pollutants such as cigarette smoke, SO_2, NO_2, ozone and particulate matter and occupational allergens. The evidence is strongest for exposure to inhalant allergens, such as dust mites, to facilitate the development of asthma in those with genetic susceptibility. The effect of these environmental factors may be strongest during the first few months of life.

Natural history of asthma

Wheezing is very common in early childhood. The majority of these children are non-atopic and symptoms are related to respiratory viral infections. Most of these children do not continue to wheeze. Most of the asthmatic children are atopic, and allergens, viral infections and exercise are the main triggers for their symptoms. In 30–50% of children, symptomatic asthma disappears during adolescence, but in a proportion may reappear in adult life. Even among those who become asymptomatic, lung function abnormalities and bronchial hyperresponsiveness may persist.

Asthma may develop for the first time during adult life (late-onset asthma), may persist from childhood or recur after a period of remission. Late-onset asthma is often non-atopic and in some may be related to occupational exposure to allergens. Viral infections remain a common trigger of symptoms, in addition to allergens and pollutants. Mild intermittent asthma may improve in late adult life, but severe asthma often results in declining lung function and irreversibility of airways obstruction.

Asthma – Definition and characteristics

- Asthma is one of the most common chronic conditions.
- Prevalence of asthma is rising.
- Symptomatic asthma may disappear during adolescence, but sometimes reappears in adult life.
- Reversible airway obstruction is a cardinal feature of asthma.
- Bronchial hyperresponsiveness is present in most but not all asthmatics.
- Most children have atopic asthma with evidence of other allergic diseases.
- Eosinophilic airway inflammation is probably the most consistent feature.

ASTHMA 2 – PATHOPHYSIOLOGY

The clinical features of asthma are due to the airway narrowing causing obstruction to airflow. This airways obstruction has three elements:

- Bronchial smooth muscle contraction
- Thickening of bronchial wall
- Excessive secretions in the lumen.

BRONCHIAL SMOOTH MUSCLE CONTRACTION

Airway smooth muscles are innervated by adrenergic, cholinergic and NANC (non-adrenergic, non-cholinergic) nerves (Fig. 1). Normally, adrenergic ($\beta2$)-receptors are stimulated by adrenaline, causing bronchodilatation. Cholinergic (muscarinic) receptors, through vagus, cause bronchoconstriction. The physiological role of the NANC system is unclear. In addition, several inflammatory mediators of asthma, such as histamine, bradykinin, prostaglandins and leukotrienes act directly on their specific receptors to cause bronchoconstriction. In asthma, the smooth muscles contract easily and excessively following exposure to these mediators, perhaps due to heightened sensitivity of their receptors. On the other hand, $\beta2$-receptors may have a diminished response.

Bronchial hyperresponsiveness

Bronchial hyperresponsiveness is a major feature of asthma, which can be defined as the ease with which the airway narrows in response to external stimuli. The measurement of the degree and ease of bronchoconstriction, in response to these stimuli, provides an objective tool to assess the severity of asthma. Although, the degree of hyperreactivity reflects the severity of asthma, this is not so in every asthmatic subject.

THICKENING OF BRONCHIAL WALL

Thickening of the bronchial wall is due to inflammatory and fibrotic changes (Fig. 2). Increased capillary permeability allows plasma exudation into the mucosa causing oedema and infiltration of the epithelium and submucosa with activated eosinophils, mast cells and Th2 lymphocytes. Thickening of the basement membrane with deposition of collagen is a prominent feature (Fig. 3). This fibrotic process may lead to irreversible obstruction in chronic severe asthma. Hypertrophy of the bronchial smooth muscle may also contribute.

EXCESSIVE SECRETIONS IN THE LUMEN

Bronchial biopsy in asthmatic patients shows that the epithelium is fragile and damaged epithelial cells are found in the sputum (Fig. 4). Impaired ciliary function encourages retention of thick mucus in the lumen. During severe exacerbation, the lumen of the airway is blocked by thick mucus, plasma proteins and cell debris (Fig. 5).

All the three features described above, i.e. bronchial wall thickening, excessive secretions and bronchial hyperresponsiveness, are due to the underlying airway inflammation.

AIRWAY INFLAMMATION

In most patients, especially children, this inflammation is initiated by IgE antibodies (allergic asthma) but in others this may be IgE-independent (non-allergic asthma). In either case, the process is orchestrated by T lymphocytes and regulated by a network of cytokines. This results in recruitment and activation of inflammatory cells in the respiratory mucosa following up-regulation of endothelial adhesion molecules.

Allergic asthma

Sensitization

In atopic individuals, initial exposure to the antigen results in sensitization. The antigen-presenting cells, such as macrophages, engulf the antigens, and after processing, present these to the naïve T cells (Th0) which differentiate into Th2-type cells. Th2 cells secrete cytokines, IL-4 and IL-13, among others. These cytokines cause switching of B cells to IgE-producing B and plasma cells, specific to the antigen. The IgE is mostly bound to high-affinity receptors ($Fc\varepsilon R1$) on the surface of mast cells and low affinity receptors ($Fc\varepsilon R2$) on eosinophils, macrophages and platelets.

Early response

On subsequent exposure, antigen–antibody reaction occurs on the surface of the mast cell. Cross-linking of two adjacent Fab fragments results in the activation of the cell and release of preformed (histamine, heparin) and newly synthesized (prostaglandins, leukotrienes, platelet activating factor and

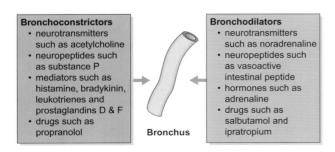

Fig. 1 **Neurotransmitters, mediators and drugs causing bronchoconstriction and bronchodilatation.**

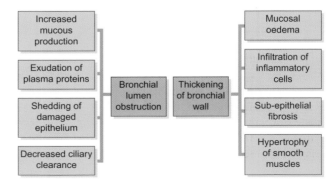

Fig. 2 **Causes of bronchial lumen obstruction and thickening of the bronchial wall.**

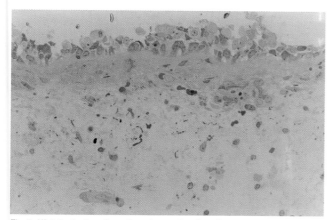

Fig. 3 **Histological section of an airway showing disruption and damage to the epithelial layer and thickening of the basement membrane** (immunohistochemical stain × 550).

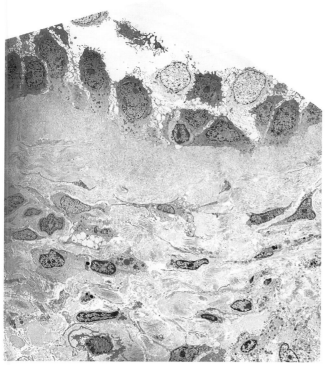

Fig. 4 **Electron micrograph showing epithelial damage and excessive shedding of the superficial layers, characteristic of asthma** (× 1600).

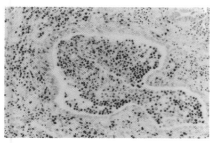

Fig. 5 **Histological section of an airway from a case of fatal asthma.** The lumen is infiltrated heavily with inflammatory exudates, fibrin and cellular debris. Immunohistochemical staining with monoclonal antibody against EG2 indicates that the majority of the cells are eosinophils (× 275).

bradykinin) mediators. The immediate effects on the bronchi include bronchoconstriction and increased bronchial responsiveness. Release of cytokines such as IL-3, IL-4, IL-5 and IL-6 activate T and B lymphocytes, stimulate mast cells and attract eosinophils, further augmenting the inflammatory process.

Late response

A few hours after the allergen exposure, events initiated during the early response result in vascular dilatation and increased permeability, oedema formation and the accumulation of cells. Upon activation, eosinophils release mediators such as eosinophilic cationic protein (ECP), major basic protein (MBP), leukotrienes and prostaglandins. Clinically this results in bronchoconstriction 4–12 h later (late-phase response) and prolonged bronchial hyperresponsiveness. Further secretion of a host of cytokines, including IL-3, IL-4 and IL-5, contribute to an on-going inflammation.

Chronic inflammation

With continued or repeated exposure to allergen, a state of chronic inflammation develops with increased numbers of activated Th2 cells, expressing mRNA for the secretion of IL-3, IL-4, IL-5 and GM-CSF. These cytokines are important in the continuation of inflammation and the attraction of mast cells and eosinophils. These cells cause further increase in histamine, prostaglandins and eosinophilic toxic products. Under the influence of IL-4 from mast cells, more B cells are switched to the production of IgE antibodies, thus maintaining allergic reaction.

Even in patients with mild intermittent asthma, a state of low-grade inflammation persists, in the absence of symptoms. It is hypothesized that almost continuous exposure to very small amounts of allergens, such as house-dust mite, or pollen during summer, contribute to this ongoing allergic reaction without causing symptoms. Bronchoscopy studies reveal increased numbers of activated inflammatory cells and cytokines in the respiratory mucosa and secretions.

Non-allergic asthma

T lymphocytes (Th2 type) release cytokines, particularly IL-5, which attract, proliferate and activate eosinophils. Upon degranulation, eosinophils release toxic products and a host of cytokines including IL-4 and IL-5. This causes inflammatory changes very similar to allergic asthma through an IgE-independent mechanism. Bronchial hyperresponsiveness can be demonstrated, and non-specific triggers such as histamine and methacholine cause bronchoconstriction as in allergic asthma. To some extent IgE-independent mechanisms also operate in allergic asthma, especially when it is chronic.

Asthma – Pathophysiology

- In asthma, airflow obstruction is due to bronchial muscle contraction, thickening of wall and excessive secretions in the lumen.
- Bronchial wall thickening is due to mucosal oedema, sub-epithelial fibrosis and smooth muscle hypertrophy.
- Bronchial hyperresponsiveness is a major feature and indicates severity.
- After allergen exposure, an early and late response is seen.
- Inflammatory changes are present in all grades of severity.

ASTHMA 3 – DIAGNOSIS

In a clinical setting, asthma is not usually difficult to diagnose. Typically, a child or young adult presents with a history of intermittent cough and wheeze. Other common symptoms are chest tightness and difficulty in breathing (Table 1). Once patients have narrated their story, it is important to ask specific questions with options for responses, to make an accurate assessment of the severity. Details of the triggers for their asthma should also be noted (Table 2).

DIFFERENTIAL DIAGNOSIS

Cough is a common symptom of many chest diseases (Fig. 1). Wheezing is common in cystic fibrosis and bronchiectasis as chronic infection induces a state of hyperresponsiveness in the airways (Table 3). However, copious infected sputum should point to the correct diagnosis. Wheezing may also occur in left ventricular failure (cardiac asthma). In some non-asthmatic individuals, cough and wheeze may develop for a limited period after a viral infection. Asthma may present in many different forms (Table 4).

PHYSICAL EXAMINATION

Between exacerbations

In mild asthma, physical examination may be normal. However, in more severe forms, breathlessness may be apparent. Chest auscultation may reveal prolonged expiration and inspiratory and/or expiratory wheezing. In chronic asthma of long duration, hyperinflation with increased anteroposterior diameter of the chest may be present. Signs of other atopic diseases such as eczema and rhinoconjunctivitis should be looked for.

During an exacerbation

During an exacerbation the patient is breathless, apprehensive and restless. Clinical cyanosis and the use of accessory muscles of respiration may be seen. Walking and even talking may be difficult. Tachycardia and tachypnoea (increased respiratory

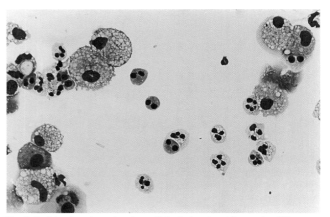

Fig. 1 A slide of sputum showing cellularity (eosinophils, neutrophils, macrophages), typical of asthma. Sputum induction is an increasingly used research tool in asthma. Nebulized hypertonic saline is used to induce sputum, examined for differential count. Inflammatory mediators and cytokines can be measured in the supernatant.

rate) is almost always present and a paradoxical pulse may develop. Wheezing may be pronounced, but in severe cases the chest may be silent due to reduced air entry.

INVESTIGATIONS

Peak expiratory flow

Peak expiratory flow (PEF) is the maximum flow achieved during forced expiration starting at full inspiration. A single reading of peak flow is not very helpful. However, a peak-flow measurement twice a day for several weeks may reveal diurnal and day to day variation characteristic of asthma. This is helpful in diagnosis, as well as monitoring the response to treatment. Patients should also make a record of the best peak flow achieved following optimal treatment. Any deterioration can be detected early as not only the average peak flow declines, but there is also an increase in variability.

Spirometry

Spirometry is essential in the diagnosis and management of asthma as both patient and physicians often have an inaccurate perception of the severity. The procedure is simple. Following maximum inspiration, the patient expires forcefully and completely into the spirometer. Forced expiratory volume in one second, or FEV_1, is the volume of air expired in the first second. Forced vital capacity or FVC, is the maximal volume of air expired during the procedure.

FEV_1 is reproducible and it is a sensitive indicator of the severity of asthma. FEV_1 values should be compared to those pre-

---

Table 1 **Symptoms of asthma**

Type of asthma	Features
Cough	Dry or productive of mucoid sputum
Wheezing	Whistley sounds from the chest during inspiration and expiration occurs frequently in asthma. In mild asthma wheezing occurs on exposure to certain triggers, but in more severe forms this could occur spontaneously or even continuously
Dyspnoea	Difficulty in breathing is a subjective symptom and its perception is variable. Many patients do not complain of dyspnoea even at considerably reduced lung function
Chest tightness	Subjective feeling of heaviness in the chest, which is variable from patient-to-patient.

Table 2 **Asthma triggers**

Stimuli which provoke symptoms and make asthma worse	Allergens: dust mite, pollen, animals, moulds Occupational sensitizers Respiratory infections
Stimuli which provoke symptoms of short duration	Osmotic stimuli: exercise, cold air, hyperventilation Psychomotor: stress, emotion Irritant: smoke, air pollutants

---

Table 3 **Difficulties in the diagnosis of asthma**

- Cough may be the only presenting symptom of asthma but is common to many respiratory diseases
- Some patients have symptoms only after exercise (exercise-induced asthma)
- Wheeze is not always due to asthma
- Recurrent wheeze is common in early childhood (wheezy bronchitis), but the majority of these children do not develop asthma
- Physical examination and lung function may be normal
- There is no diagnostic biomarker for asthma

Table 4 **Some of the many different forms of asthma**

In chronic obstructive pulmonary disease (COPD)	Middle-aged and elderly smokers with COPD may have significant reversibility to bronchodilator and/or steroids (asthmatic or reversible component). Cough is usually productive, symptoms are persistent and dyspnoea on exertion is prominent. Peak-flow reading does not show significant variability.
Occupational	Occupational asthma is caused by the inhalation of an agent at work. It accounts for 2–5% of all cases of asthma. More than 200 chemicals have been incriminated. These include airborne dusts, gases, vapours and fumes in the working environment. It is important to obtain a full medical history and the precise occupational exposures, including the relationship of symptoms to periods of exposure. Peak-flow monitoring at work and at home might be diagnostic. Specific inhalation challenges may need to be performed to confirm the diagnosis.
Aspirin-induced	Approximately 20% of adults with non-allergic asthma have sensitivity to aspirin and other non-steroidal anti-inflammatory drugs (NSAIDs). Other manifestations of aspirin intolerance such as non-allergic rhinitis, nasal polyposis, urticaria and angio-oedema may be present. Diagnosis is suggested by history and confirmed, if necessary, by oral provocation tests. Avoidance should be strictly adhered to. Treatment is with steroids, bronchodilators and leukotriene antagonists.
Exercise-induced	Exercise induces bronchoconstriction in most asthmatics due to its cooling and drying effect on airway mucosa. However, in some patients, especially children, this may be the only symptom. An exercise test such as free running for 6 min is diagnostic. The bronchoconstriction can be prevented by the inhaled β2-agonists or sodium cromoglicate.
Cough-variant	Chronic dry cough may be the only symptom of asthma, without wheezing or breathlessness. Pulmonary function is usually normal, but bronchial hyperresponsiveness can be demonstrated by bronchial provocation tests. Treatment with bronchodilators and steroids is effective. Other causes of chronic cough such as chronic rhinitis/sinusitis, gastro-oesophageal reflux and angiotensin-converting enzyme inhibitors should be considered.

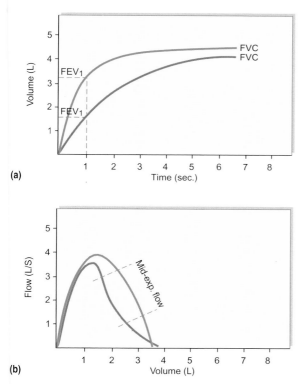

(a)

(b)

Fig. 2 **Spirometry (a) volume/time and (b) flow/volume curves in normal subject (blue) and asthma (red).** In graph (a), the reduction in FEV_1 is more pronounced than FVC. In graph (b), the reduction in mid-expiratory flow can be easily seen.

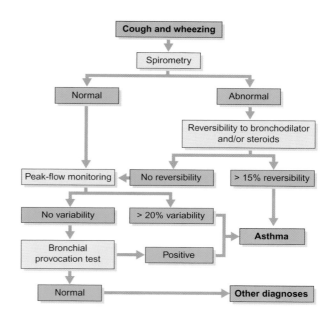

Fig. 3 **Diagnostic approach to asthma.**

Allergy tests

Skin-prick tests are often used to identify causative allergens. Usually about 6–8 common allergens are selected, with additional allergens added if suspected. Alternatively, IgE antibodies to suspected allergens can be measured in the blood using immunoassays such as radioallergosorbent test.

dicted according to the age, height, sex and race of the patients. A value less than 80% of predicted is considered abnormal. A 15% improvement in FEV_1, following bronchodilator, demonstrates reversibility. In asthma both FVC and FEV_1 are reduced, but the reduction in FEV_1 is proportionately greater, thus causing a reduction in FEV_1/FVC ratio (obstructive pattern) (Fig. 2).

Bronchial provocation tests

Bronchial provocation tests are employed to assess bronchial hyperresponsiveness objectively. Chemicals, such as methacholine or histamine, cause bronchoconstriction in most asthmatics. Other stimuli used are exercise, cold air and hypertonic saline. The test is only occasionally required for the diagnosis of asthma when other tests are inconclusive (Fig. 3).

Asthma – Diagnosis

- A history of intermittent cough and wheeze is characteristic of asthma.
- Other common symptoms are chest tightness and difficulty in breathing.
- These symptoms may also occur in chronic bronchitis, left ventricular failure and bronchiectasis.
- Home peak-flow monitoring is useful in the diagnosis, assessment of severity and response to treatment.
- >15% improvement in FEV_1 following bronchodilator demonstrates reversibility.
- Bronchial provocation tests to methacholine or histamine assess non-specific bronchial responsiveness.

ASTHMA 4 – TREATMENT OF CHRONIC ASTHMA

ASSESSMENT OF SEVERITY

To evaluate severity, it is important to consider frequency of symptoms, level of pulmonary function, frequency and severity of exacerbation, and if already on treatment, the requirement for medication (Table 1). A history of previous admission to hospital and need for ventilation should also alert the physician.

PHARMACOTHERAPY

Asthma therapy is aimed at treating underlying inflammation and controlling symptoms (Table 2). Topical treatment of asthma through the inhaled route is preferable, as the dose can be kept small and side-effects are minimal.

Anti-inflammatory therapy

Sodium cromoglicate and nedocromil have anti-inflammatory effects but are less effective than steroids. In adults, steroids by inhalation are given as the first-line therapy (Fig. 1). Systemic adverse effects are rare. Asthma exacerbations are treated with a short course of oral steroids, but severe asthmatics may need regular oral steroids. The dose of oral steroids should be kept to a minimum with the addition of high-dose inhaled steroids and other supplementary therapy. The patient should be warned of the possible adverse effects.

Montelukast and zafirlukast are recently introduced leukotriene receptor antagonists. They are orally effective and useful as additional anti-inflammatory therapy (Fig. 2). They

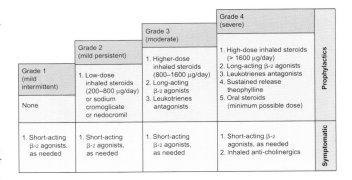

Fig. 1 **Stepwise approach to asthma treatment.** An appropriate level of treatment is chosen according to the grade of severity. During follow-up, step up or down in the treatment depends on the response to treatment, residual symptoms and lung function. The sequence of additional treatment within each grade may be altered.

Table 2 **Aims of treatment**

• Keep patients free of symptoms
• Minimize risk of exacerbation
• No restriction to daily activities including exercise
• Pulmonary function as near to normal as possible
• Minimal requirement for as-required bronchodilator
• Minimal possible side-effects from the medications

may prove to be very useful in aspirin-sensitive and exercise-induced asthma. Theophylline is an effective bronchodilator with some anti-inflammatory properties.

Symptomatic therapy

Salbutamol and terbutalin are commonly used short-acting β-2 receptor stimulants. They are used, as required, for intermittent symptoms, except in severe persistent asthma when regular use may be indicated. Salmeterol and formoterol have prolonged bronchodilator activity. Given in twice-daily doses, they improve asthma control and prevent nocturnal asthma symptoms. Ipratropium bromide, an anti-cholinergic drug, causes bronchodilatation by the inhaled route.

CHOICE OF INHALERS

Metered-dose inhalers (MDI)

The drug is suspended in a vaporizable gas such as chlorofluorocarbon (CFC) within a pressurized container. CFC has undesirable effects on the ozone layer and is being replaced by ozone-friendly gases. Normally, only about 10–15% of the drug is deposited in the lung and the rest is swallowed. Correct tech-

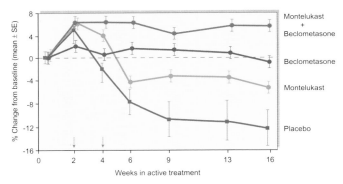

Fig. 2 **The addition of the leukotriene antagonist montelukast to beclomethasone has an additive effect on FEV$_1$.** (From: Laviolette M, Malmstrom K, Lu S, et al. 1999 Am J Respir Crit Care Med 160: 1862–68.)

Table 1 **Grades of asthma severity**

	Grade 1 Mild intermittent	Grade 2 Mild persistent	Grade 3 Moderate	Grade 4 Severe
Day symptoms	< 1/week	>1/week	>1/day	Continuous
Nocturnal symptoms	< 2/month	> 2/month	>1/week	most nights
FEV$_1$	Normal	Normal	> 60% – < 80% predicted	≤ 60%
Peak-flow variability	< 20%	20–30%	> 30%	> 30%
Bronchodilator requirement	Occasional	< 1/day	Daily use	Several times/day
Exacerbation	Often self-limiting, may not require oral steroids	Affects activity, may require oral steroids	Affects activity and sleep, requires oral steroids	Frequent and may be severe

Presence of one of the features of severity puts the patients in the higher grade (adopted from 'Global Initiative for Asthma, NHLBI/WHO Report')

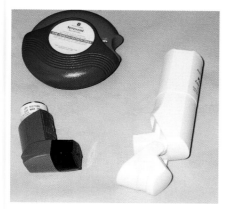

Fig. 3 **Commonly used inhaler devices: (a) Acuhalor, (b) Easibreathe, (c) metered-dose inhaler (MDI).**

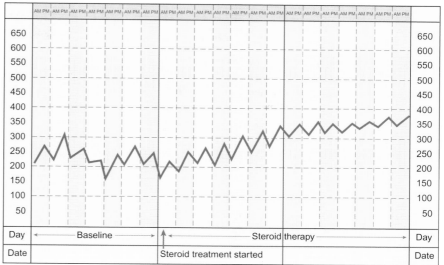

Fig. 4 **Labile peak flow and response to therapy.** During the base period, peak flow shows greater variability. With steroid therapy, peak flow improves over a 2-week period with reduction in day-to-day and diurnal variability.

nique, to coordinate the inspiration with actuation of the inhaler, is crucial for proper use of the MDIs. A modification of the MDI is a breath-actuated inhaler, where actuation is triggered by the inspiratory effort, thus avoiding the need for coordination (Fig. 3). An alternative is to use large volume spacer devices where the drug is released into the plastic chamber before being inhaled by the patient. Use of spacer devices is preferable as coordination is not needed, delivery to the lung is greater and deposition in the pharynx is reduced.

Dry-powder inhalers (DPI)
These inhalers contain powdered drug. A certain inspiratory effort is required to move the small particles from the inhaler to the airways. DPI do not require vaporizable gas and are not affected by the new rules banning the use of CFC.

Nebulizers
In a nebulizer, air passes through the drug solution at high pressure, creating a mist, which the patient inhales through a mask. Nebulizers can be electrically driven, or oxygen at high pressure can be used to form the mist. These are extremely useful in the treatment of acute severe asthma, and in young children, as patients do not have to make inspiratory efforts.

ENVIRONMENTAL CONTROL
Reduction in exposure to allergen and irritants may reduce symptoms, bronchial reactivity and medication requirement. Dust mite avoidance measures are aimed at removal of dust reservoirs and containment and killing of mites. In pet-allergic patients, removal

of the pet from the household should be strongly advised. Mould growth can be reduced by cleaning and by keeping the indoor humidity at a low level. Cockroaches can be killed by pesticide and regular cleaning will avoid their re-infestation. For pollen-sensitive asthmatics, simple measures such as staying indoors on high pollen days help to a certain degree.

Asthmatic patients should never smoke and should avoid a smoking environment. They have a much higher risk of developing fixed airways obstruction.

SELF-MANAGEMENT PLAN
It is important for patients to understand their disease and take control of management once the disease is under control (Table 3). It is helpful to define the best peak flow achieved by the patient (personal best). They should be able to increase or decrease the level of treatment depending on symptoms, need for rescue bronchodilator and peak-flow variability (Fig. 4). A written management plan for each individual patient, highlighting the need for monitoring, indications for step up or down in the treatment and when to seek medical help, is essential.

Table 3 **Steps in asthma management**

Confirm the diagnosis and assess the grade of asthma severity	History, examination, peak-flow monitoring and spirometry
Decide on appropriate pharmacotherapy Allergen avoidance	Stepwise treatments Instructions for avoidance measures
Follow-up treatment	Adjust the level of medication
Education	Ensure that the patient understands the disease and its implications.
Management plan	Self-adjustment of treatment

Treatment of chronic asthma
- A short course of oral steroids may be required at the outset to control the disease and achieve maximum lung function.
- Regular use of β-2 agonists indicates a need to increase prophylactic therapy.
- Monitoring of symptoms and home peak flow indicates if the treatment needs to be increased or reduced.
- Regular follow-up is recommended initially until asthma control is achieved.
- Review inhaler technique at each visit.
- Before stepping up treatment, make sure of the compliance to treatment and environmental control of allergens and adjuvants.
- Asthma control must be satisfactory for 3 months before treatment is scaled down.

ASTHMA 5 – TREATMENT OF ACUTE ASTHMA

Intermittent exacerbations (asthma attack, status asthmaticus, acute severe asthma) are a feature of asthma. Frequency depends on the adequacy of treatment and avoidance of triggers. Although an exacerbation can occur within minutes or hours, there is usually a history of progressive worsening of symptoms over days. Regular peak-flow monitoring is useful in moderate to severe asthmatics as deterioration can be detected early. The aim of management is to restore the patient's clinical condition and lung function to their best possible level, maintain optimal function and prevent early relapse.

ASSESSMENT OF SEVERITY

Initial assessment should be with a brief history (Table 1), physical examination and relevant investigations, including functional assessment (Table 2), for evaluating the severity of the current exacerbation (Table 3).

DRUGS USED FOR ASTHMA EXACERBATION

Bronchodilators

Nebulized bronchodilators are used frequently as the first-line therapy in the treatment of asthma exacerbation. This method of delivery is preferable for bronchodilators, as the onset of effect is rapid and high doses can be administered. Oxygen can be given at the same time and patients are not required to make inspiratory efforts, which many find difficult during an asthma attack. β-2 agonists are given alone or in combination with anti-cholinergics. Some investigators have suggested that a metered-dose inhaler with a large volume spacer may be equally effective.

Both β-2 agonists and aminophylline achieve bronchodilatation through the intravenous route, but toxic effects may appear. Therefore these are used as a second-line bronchodilator therapy.

Corticosteroids

Systemic corticosteroids should be given for most, if not all, asthma attacks. Mild to moderate exacerbation can be treated with a course of oral steroids

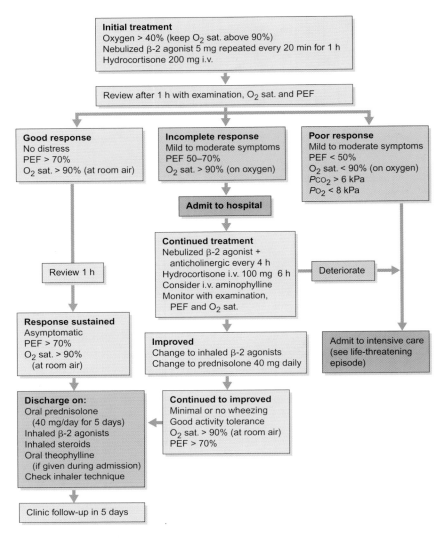

Fig. 1 **Management of moderate to severe asthma attack.**

such as prednisolone 40 mg/day. Intravenous hydrocortisone is given for moderate to severe exacerbation but the onset of effect is in hours and the maximal effect may not be achieved for days. There is generally no need to taper the dose of systemic steroids if given as a short course for less than 2 weeks, and inhaled steroids are concomitantly prescribed.

MANAGEMENT OF ASTHMA EXACERBATION

Mild exacerbation

Mild exacerbation can be managed in the community. β-2 agonists are administered through a nebulizer and repeated at 15-min intervals (up to three times) with peak-flow monitoring. If there is little or no improvement, the severity should be considered as moderate and immediate

Table 1 **History**

- Confirm the diagnosis
- Time of onset and cause of present exacerbation
- Severity of symptoms including exercise limitation and sleep disturbance
- All current medications
- Sgnificant prior cardiopulmonary disease
- Prior hospitalization and emergency visits
- Prior history of respiratory failure and mechanical ventilation due to asthma

Table 2 **Functional assessment**

- Evaluate alertness, posture, breathlessness, breathing pattern, presence of cyanosis, and ability to talk
- Pulse rate
- Respiratory rate
- Paradoxical pulse (> 10 mmHg)
- Chest auscultation (wheezing, silent chest)
- Peak flow (% predicted or personal best)
- Oxygen saturation (O_2 sat.)
- Arterial blood gases (in severe exacerbation)

Table 3 **Assessment of the severity of exacerbation**

	Mild	Moderate	Severe	Life-threatening
Breathless	on walking	on talking	at rest	at rest
Posture	can lie down	prefers sitting	hunched forward	hunched forward
Speech	sentences	short phrases	words	words or none
Alertness	normal	may be agitated	usually agitated	drowsy
Respiratory rate	increased	increased	> 30 (adults)	> 30 (adults)
Use of accessory muscles	no	yes	yes	yes
Wheeze	moderate	prominent	prominent	absent
Pulse rate (adults)	< 100	100–120	> 120	≤ 80
Pulsus paradoxus	absent	may be present (10–25 mmHg)	often present (> 25 mmHg)	may be absent due to fatigue
PEF (% predicted)	> 70%	50–70%	< 50%	may not be able to perform
O_2 saturation	> 95%	91–95%	< 90%	< 85%
Pao_2	> 12 kPa	> 8 kPa	< 8 kPa	< 8 kPa
$Paco_2$	< 6 kPa	≤ 6 kPa	≥ 6 kPa	> 6 kPa

(adopted from 'Global Initiative for Asthma, NHLBI/WHO Report')
Presence of two or more characteristics put them in the higher degree of severity

Table 4 **Hospital management – things to keep in mind**

- Avoid sedation
- High doses of β-2 agonists may cause hypokalaemia
- Omit bolus dose before an intravenous infusion of aminophylline, if the patient has been on oral theophylline
- Check theophylline levels if the patient is treated with aminophylline
- Check arterial blood gases in severe asthmatics who are not improving, and in all patients with life-threatening exacerbation
- Request a chest X-ray if pneumonia or pneumothorax is suspected
- Request total and differential white cell count in patients with fever or purulent sputum
- Consider antibiotics if there is neutrophilia, purulent sputum or consolidation on chest X-ray
- Make sure that follow-up care is organized before discharging the patient

Table 5 **Criteria for admission to intensive care**

- Poor response to initial therapy in emergency room
- Rapidly deteriorating condition despite treatment
- Signs of exhaustion (tiredness, bradycardia, normal or low respiratory rate)
- Confusion, drowsiness or loss of consciousness
- Po_2 < 8 kPa (despite supplemental oxygen)
- Pco_2 > 6 kPa

hospital referral is indicated. If symptoms disappear and peak expiratory flow (PEF) improves to > 80% predicted or personal best, subsequent management can be at home with regular inhaled β-2 agonists and peak-flow monitoring. A short course of oral steroids may be required, or doubling the dose of inhaled steroids may suffice. If symptoms recur, the patient should be admitted to hospital.

Hospital management (moderate, severe and life-threatening exacerbation)

Figures 1 and 2 outline the management of moderate to severe, and life-threatening exacerbation. Initial management in the emergency or admission room is followed by subsequent management as an in-patient (Table 4), or admission to Intensive care (Table 5).

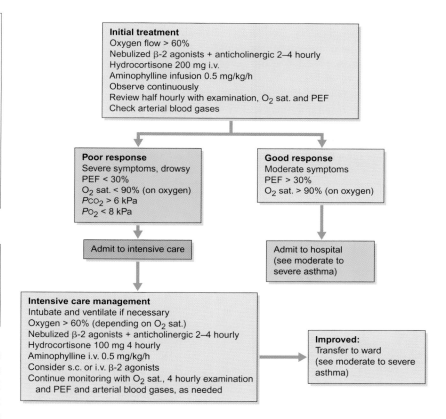

Initial treatment
Oxygen flow > 60%
Nebulized β-2 agonists + anticholinergic 2–4 hourly
Hydrocortisone 200 mg i.v.
Aminophylline infusion 0.5 mg/kg/h
Observe continuously
Review half hourly with examination, O_2 sat. and PEF
Check arterial blood gases

Poor response
Severe symptoms, drowsy
PEF < 30%
O_2 sat. < 90% (on oxygen)
Pco_2 > 6 kPa
Po_2 < 8 kPa

Good response
Moderate symptoms
PEF > 30%
O_2 sat. > 90% (on oxygen)

Admit to intensive care

Admit to hospital (see moderate to severe asthma)

Intensive care management
Intubate and ventilate if necessary
Oxygen > 60% (depending on O_2 sat.)
Nebulized β-2 agonists + anticholinergic 2–4 hourly
Hydrocortisone 100 mg 4 hourly
Aminophylline i.v. 0.5 mg/kg/h
Consider s.c. or i.v. β-2 agonists
Continue monitoring with O_2 sat., 4 hourly examination and PEF and arterial blood gases, as needed

Improved:
Transfer to ward (see moderate to severe asthma)

Fig. 2 **Management of life-threatening episode.**

Treatment of acute asthma – Remember!

- Acute asthma is a potentially fatal condition
- A decline in lung function (FEV_1, PEF) is a more reliable indication of severity than symptoms
- Morbidity and mortality in asthma is associated with under-assessment of the severity and under-treatment
- Regular follow-up is the best way to avoid recurrent exacerbation

ASTHMA IN CHILDREN 1 – EPIDEMIOLOGY AND DIAGNOSIS

Asthma is the most common chronic disease of childhood (Fig. 1) and ranks as the top reason for acute paediatric hospital admissions. Although the underlying airway inflammatory processes are similar in adult and childhood asthma, there are significant differences specific to this age-group that merit separate discussion. Growth of the child modifies the disease process; for example, asthma may become less severe during the teenage years (Fig. 2). In addition, asthma may slow the growth of the child. More than 80% of asthma in children is atopic and heredity plays a major role in its causation.

WHEEZING IN INFANCY

Wheezing is extremely common in infancy and early childhood. The cumulative prevalence of wheezing in children under 3 years is thought to be around 25%. Not all of this is regarded as true asthma as most of these children will cease to wheeze between the ages of 3–6 years. Several factors account for the prevalence of this symptom in children under 3 years (Fig. 3). Wheezing is often associated with respiratory infections, in particular, respiratory syncitial virus, which is common in young children. The bronchi are small and have a reduced cross-sectional area. This increases the likelihood of wheezing in the presence of mucosal swelling and inflamma-

tory exudates associated with infection. Non-specific irritants, such as cigarette smoke, also contribute. However, about a third of these children are atopic with positive skin test to egg and aeroallergens, such as house-dust mite, and show other signs of atopy, e.g. eczema. Most of these children have a family history of asthma, especially maternal asthma, and are likely to continue to wheeze.

DIAGNOSIS
History taking

There are problems in history taking from children of any age. In younger children, parental observations have to be relied upon. Parents often under- or over-state the symptoms depending upon their own perception of the disease. An attempt should be made to gain a more objective assessment of the child's disease by asking specific questions (Table 1).

Wheezing is not always due to asthma, and asthma is not always associated with wheezing and other diagnoses should be considered. Acute onset of wheezing could be due to a foreign body in the respiratory tract. More persistent wheezing may be due to the recurrent infections associated with cystic fibrosis. A chronic and recurrent cough, especially nocturnal, may be the only symptom of asthma in some children. Exercise-induced asthma is also very common and symptoms may be present only

Table 1 **Specific questions asked during history-taking of a child**

- Do you get any of these symptoms:
      Coughing, wheezing, shortness of breath, chest tightness?
- How often do you get these symptoms on average:
      Occasionally, once per week, once per day, several times a day or continuously?
- How often do you use your rescue bronchodilator (if prescribed):
      Never, occasionally, once per week, once per day or several times a day?
- How often do you wake up in the night because of your asthma:
      Never, occasionally, once a week or most nights?
- How often do you feel tightness in your chest in the mornings:
      Never, occasionally, once a week or most mornings?
- Have you ever been hospitalized because of your asthma?

Fig. 1 **Worldwide variation in the prevalence of self-reported asthma symptoms using a standardized questionnaire.** (From ISAAC Study Group 1998 The Lancet 351: 1225–32.)

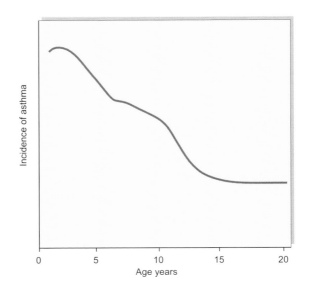

Fig. 2 **Incidence of asthma with age.** Incidence declines during the teen years.

after sports at school. As these children find it difficult to participate competitively they start to dislike the sports and avoid the situations which precipitate their symptoms. Often, children can adjust to their disability so well that their restricted lifestyle appears to be quite normal to them.

Physical examination may be completely normal. However, it may show signs of chronic lung disease or wheezing on auscultation. There may be evidence of other atopic diseases such as eczema and rhinitis.

Pulmonary function tests

Valid and reproducible spirometric manoeuvres can be performed by a child of 5 years or older, with explanation and encouragement. FEV_1, FVC and PEF readings are useful in assessing baseline lung function and degree of airflow obstruction. If FEV_1 is lower than expected, or FEV_1/FVC ratio is less than 80%, repeat spirometry after 2–4 puffs of inhaled bronchodilator is useful to assess the degree of reversibility. This is traditionally considered to be significant at >15%. Some children with chronic asthma do not reverse completely. A period of intensive treatment may be required to achieve the best possible values of FEV_1, and PEF (steroid reversibility). These values should be recorded and reference made to them in future visits. However, the values may change as the child grows.

Normal pulmonary function test results do not exclude the diagnosis of asthma and in the absence of infection, or other precipitating factors, are in fact the norm in mild-to-moderate asthma. In these situations, variability could be assessed by twice-daily peak flow readings performed at home for several weeks. A diurnal or day-to-day variability of >20% is generally considered sufficient for the diagnosis (Fig. 4). In children with a history of exercise-induced asthma, spirometry after exercise is useful to demonstrate bronchoconstriction. Only rarely are tests for bronchial reactivity, such as methacholine challenge, required for the diagnosis.

Skin-prick tests

These can be done from the age of 3 months. However, skin reactivity may not fully develop and thus reactions are usually smaller until children reach the age of 1–2 years. Skin tests are performed using a battery of common allergens pertinent to the geographical location. Common aeroallergens include house-

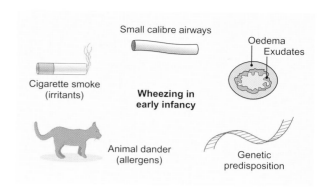

Fig. 3 **Causes of wheezing in children under 3.**

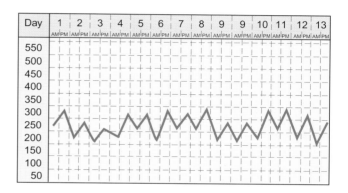

Fig. 4 **Diurnal and day-to-day variability in peak flow in a child with uncontrolled asthma.**

dust mite, grass pollen, tree pollen, cat and dog. In younger children, egg, milk and peanut are often included in the test battery to look for evidence of atopy. Skin tests provide information about the atopic status of the child and help with specific advice on avoidance measures (Fig. 5). Specific IgE levels could be measured with a radioallergosorbant test (RAST), if skin tests cannot be done.

A chest X-ray is not required for the diagnosis of asthma but may be needed to exclude other diagnoses. A sweat-test should be performed if cystic fibrosis is suspected.

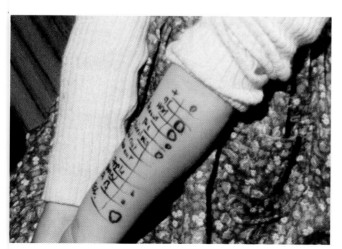

Fig. 5 **Asthma is usually allergic in childhood.** Multiple allergen sensitivities tested on an asthmatic child.

Asthma in children – Epidemiology and diagnosis

- Asthma is the most common chronic disease of childhood.
- Heredity plays an important role in the causation of asthma, but environmental factors, especially in the first months of life, are also important.
- More than 80% of asthma in children is atopic.
- In children under 3 years, wheezing is common and only caused by asthma in around 25% of cases.
- Passive smoking is an important risk factor for early childhood wheezing.
- Normal results of examination and pulmonary function tests do not exclude asthma.
- Variable peak flow is a useful indicator of the presence of asthma.

ASTHMA IN CHILDREN 2 – TREATMENT

Treatment should be aimed at achieving a normal and unrestricted life for the child and minimizing the risk of exacerbation. This can only be achieved through an understanding of the causal factors and a positive approach towards preventive treatment. Parents are often reluctant to let children take regular medication, in particular steroids, for fear of side-effects. Older children may not like taking inhalers at school because it reminds them of their illness. Time spent on discussing the problem and explaining the rationale behind the suggested measures usually results in improved compliance.

General measures include avoidance of allergens detected by skin tests and irritants such as cigarette smoke. In addition to written recommendations, which parents can read in their own time, verbal explanations are often very helpful.

Drug treatment remains the mainstay of asthma therapy. The choice of drug and route of delivery depends on the age of the child and severity of their asthma. Inhaler therapy is preferable as the dose can be kept small and side-effects minimized. Children aged 5 years or more should be able to use an inhaler. Traditional inhalers (metered dose inhalers, MDI) may not be suitable for many children as good technique is mandatory. A range of devices is available to counter this problem. The use of a spacer device attached to the inhaler increases pulmonary deposition while reducing the occurrence of local and systemic side-effects (Fig. 1). However, these devices are cumbersome. Breath-actuated inhalers also avoid the need for coordination, as do some dry powder inhalers.

Children less than 5 years will need a spacer or a nebulizer for effective delivery of a drug. For children aged over 5 years, nebulizers should be reserved for the emergency treatment of acute asthma.

ANTI-INFLAMMATORY THERAPY

Anti-inflammatory therapy should be given to most children with more than occasional symptoms. The choice of anti-inflammatory therapy depends on the severity of the disease and the likelihood of patient compliance with frequent doses. Inhaled sodium cromoglicate or nedocromil sodium is a safe and effective treatment in atopic asthma. However, it has a short half-life, requiring at least 4 daily doses, and it is less effective than inhaled steroids. There are several inhaled steroids that can be taken in twice-daily doses, thus increasing compliance.

The dose should be adjusted to achieve optimum symptom control. Some of the newer inhaled steroids claim reduced systemic bioavailability. Although there is concern about side-effects of steroids, in particular their effect on growth and the adrenal axis, inhaled steroids have been proven to be safe below a dose of 1 mg/day. The effect of asthma on growth may be greater than the side-effects of any treatment. A common local side-effect is oropharyngeal candidiasis which can be avoided by using a spacer device and rinsing the mouth after taking a dose.

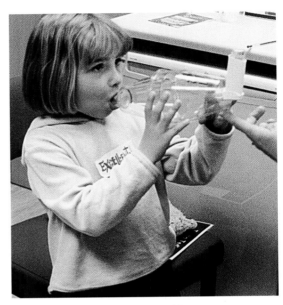

Fig. 1 **A child using a spacer device (volumatic).**

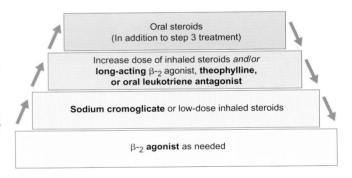

Fig. 2 **Step treatment strategy for treating children with asthma.**

Oral steroids
(In addition to step 3 treatment)

Increase dose of inhaled steroids *and/or* **long-acting β-2 agonist, theophylline, or oral leukotriene antagonist**

Sodium cromoglicate or low-dose inhaled steroids

β-2 **agonist** as needed

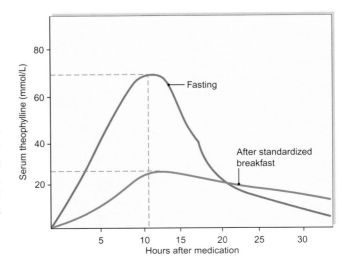

Fig. 3 **Variable absorption of theophylline in children due to food intake**

BRONCHODILATOR THERAPY

Bronchodilator therapy should primarily be used as a rescue treatment for breakthrough symptoms. It can also be used prophylactically before exercise. Short acting ß-2 agonists such as salbutamol or terbutalin by inhaler are most appropriate. Children younger than 2 years respond better to anticholinergics such as ipratropium. In moderate to severe asthma, longer-acting ß-2 agonists, such as salmeterol or eformoterol, are added to inhaled steroids in a twice-daily regime (Fig. 2), or if troublesome nocturnal cough is a prominant symptom.

Oral theophyllines have been used effectively for many years in the treatment of childhood asthma. Slow-release preparations in a twice-daily regime may be useful for more severe asthma. The dose of theophyllines should be carefully monitored and plasma theophylline determinations may be required (Fig. 3).

TREATMENT PLAN

A written treatment plan that includes peak-flow measurements should be given to all except those with very mild asthma (Fig. 4). Children and their parents should be encouraged to make necessary changes in the treatment depending on the frequency of symptoms and variability in peak flow (Fig. 5).

PROGNOSIS

It is often presumed that most children with asthma will grow out of their disease. Long-term follow-up studies indicate that this may not be entirely true. Around 50% of children with asthma sufficiently improve during their teenage years to not require further treatment. However, many can be shown to have persistent bronchial hyperreactivity on performance of a stress-test. In some, there is a recurrence of symptoms in adult life. More severe and chronic asthma, if under-treated, may lead to permanent abnormalities in lung function. The onset of puberty and growth may be delayed but eventual height-gain is often normal.

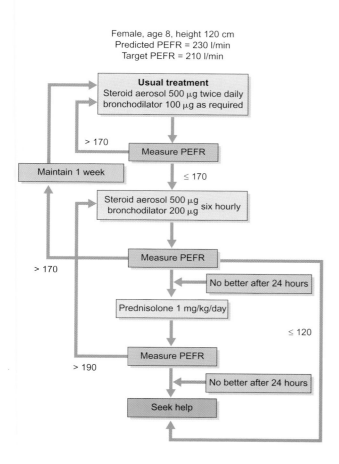

Fig. 4 **A typical management plan in the treatment of asthma.** A written plan to deal with exacerbation should be provided to all patients with asthma. (Adapted from: Holgate ST, Church M 1996 Allergy, Gower Publishing.)

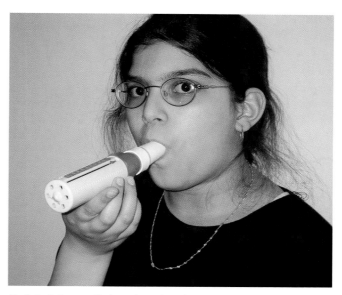

Fig.5 **Peak-flow monitoring at home is an integral part of the management of asthma in children.**

Asthma in children – Treatment

- Asthma is generally under-diagnosed and under-treated.
- Treatment should be aimed at achieving an unrestricted lifestyle.
- Avoidance of allergens is crucial.
- Inhaler therapy is preferable because of minimal side-effects.
- Spacer is essential in children under 5 years when using an MDI.
- Anti-inflammatory therapy with sodium cromoglicate or inhaled steroids should be given to all children with more than occasional symptoms.
- Under-treated asthma may lead to permanent abnormalities in lung function.

RHINITIS 1 – CLASSIFICATION AND PATHOGENESIS

The symptoms of rhinitis include sneezing, rhinorrhoea, nasal blockage and itching. Typical symptoms on most days, lasting for at least 1 h, are considered sufficient for clinical diagnosis. As there is no universally agreed definition, and the difference between normal and abnormal is indistinct, it is difficult to estimate the exact prevalence. Various studies suggest that the cumulative prevalence of rhinitis is about 10–20% of the population. Allergic rhinitis usually starts in late childhood, the median age of onset being around 10 years. The condition most commonly occurs at 10–25 years. Like other allergic diseases, the prevalence of rhinitis is increasing.

PATHOPHYSIOLOGY

The nose is designed to deliver air to the lungs at constant temperature and humidity, and to remove noxious substances as the air passes through its tortuous passages. Particulate matter settles on the epithelial surface or gets entangled in the mucous secretions. Ciliary activity then removes these particles anteriorly towards the nostrils or posteriorly towards the nasopharynx. Sneezing also helps to get rid of the particles and other noxious material. The nasal mucosal blood supply and ciliary movements are primarily under the control of sympathetic nerves, which drive the nasal cycle with increased airflow through one side, alternating every 2–4 h.

The nasal mucosa responds to exogenous stimuli by the mucosal swelling and increased secretions responsible for the nasal obstruction observed early in rhinitis. There is increased blood flow through the nasal mucosa, and increased vascular permeability leads to excess nasal secretions. Nasal secretions consist of albumin, immunoglobulins, enzymes, inflammatory cells and mediators. The mucosa become hyperreactive and stimulation of the nerve-endings causes sneezing. Nasal responsiveness is measured in terms of symptoms and nasal airway resistance after histamine challenge. Rhinitis is classified into allergic and non-allergic rhinitis, and further divided into seasonal and perennial (Fig. 1).

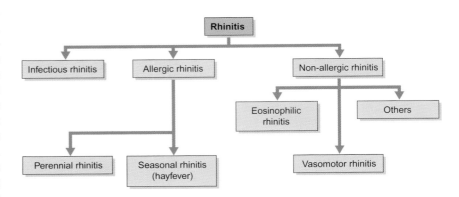

Fig. 1 **Classification of rhinitis.**

ALLERGIC RHINITIS

Allergic rhinitis often develops in children who already have some evidence of atopy. Some may have asthma and others may have had eczema in early childhood. Severely atopic children tend to develop eczema in infancy, asthma at 5–10 years and rhinitis at 10–15 years-of-age. This is often termed 'the allergy march'. Seasonal allergic rhinitis often improves in adult life and it is uncommon in old age. Perennial rhinitis, however, does not have such a favourable prognosis.

In line with other allergic diseases, atopic inheritance plays a major role in the causation of allergic rhinitis. The exact mode of inheritance, however, is not yet known. In children who are genetically susceptible, environmental influences, especially in the first year of life, may contribute to the development of the disease. Environmental influences may include exposure to allergens, ciga-

Table 1 **Environmental factors in the development of rhinitis**

- Exposure to allergens:
  –Pollen; higher incidence in children born in spring or summer
  –House-dust mites and moulds; damp houses with high humidity
  –Cigarette smoke may induce allergic sensitization
- Viral infections
- Family size (children of smaller families are at higher risk) and position in the family (the oldest child at a higher risk)
- Pollutants such as ozone, SO_2, NO_2
- Occupational allergens such as isocyanates, wood dust, etc.

rette smoke and other pollutants (Table 1). Most of these factors continue to be important in later life.

Seasonal allergic rhinitis (hayfever)

Seasonal allergic rhinitis is caused by airborne pollens of trees, grasses and weeds. Tree pollens are most common in spring, grass pollen in summer and weed pollen in autumn. Symptoms of allergic rhinitis may therefore occur in different seasons, depending on the type of allergic sensitization. Different geographical locations may have a higher prevalence of different allergens. For example, grass pollen allergy is common in the UK with a prevalence of 10–15%. The condition was termed hayfever during the last century with the observation that exposure to flowering grass (from which hay is obtained) caused an illness with predom-

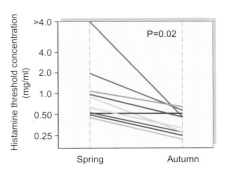

Fig. 2 **Nasal responsiveness to histamine is increased with increased exposure to dust mites in autumn, in patients with allergic rhinitis.** Each colour represents a different patient. (From Gerth van Wijk R, Dieges PH, Van Toorenebergen AW 1987 Rhinology 25: 41–48.)

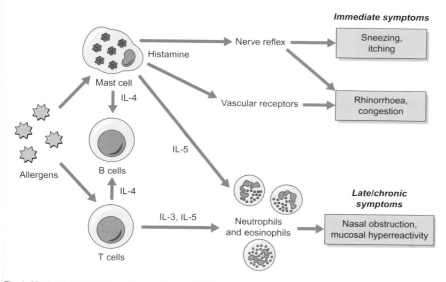

Fig. 3 **Mechanism of inflammation in allergic rhinitis.**

inant symptoms of rhinoconjunctivitis. In Scandinavian countries birch pollen allergy is very common, and in some parts of the USA, allergy to ragweed is the commonest cause of allergic rhinitis.

Pollens are large particles of 20–25 microns in diameter and they therefore settle on the superficial mucosal surfaces such as nasal or conjunctival mucosa. However, the antigen protein from the pollen may dissolve in the nasal secretions and trickle back to the respiratory mucosa, to cause pollen asthma. The symptoms vary during the season according to the concentration of pollen in the air.

Perennial allergic rhinitis

Allergy to house-dust mite is the commonest cause of perennial allergic rhinitis and symptoms are usually present on most days (Fig. 2). Allergy to the skin, fur or saliva particles of animals such as cat, dog and horses is also common, but symptoms may be intermittent. Mould allergy less often causes significant rhinitis, as the mould spores are smaller than 5 microns in diameter and generally bypass nasal passages to end up in lower airways. Many patients are allergic to both house-dust mites and pollen, and have perennial symptoms with worsening of symptoms during the pollen season.

Symptoms of perennial allergic rhinitis are similar to seasonal allergic rhinitis except that conjunctival symptoms are minimal and nasal obstruction is more prominent. The nasal mucosa is hyperreactive due to the continuous low-grade inflammation. Therefore, apart from the known allergens, these patients also react

to a range of non-specific triggers such as cold air, dust, smoke, chemicals and cosmetics.

PATHOGENESIS OF ALLERGIC RHINITIS

Mast cells and basophils are found in increased numbers in the nasal mucosa of patients with allergic rhinitits. Antigens react with the specific IgE bound to mast cells and basophils, and immediately release preformed mediators, such as histamine, tryptase and heparin. Thereafter, these cells slowly release newly synthesized mediators, such as prostaglandins and leukotrienes (Fig. 3). Histamine acts directly on the vascular receptors, increasing vascular permeability and causing mucosal oedema. It also stimulates the sensory nerves to cause sneezing, pruritis and reflex vasodilatation.

Just like asthma, early- and late-phase responses to allergens may be demon-

strated in the nose of patients with rhinitis. The late phase is initiated by mediators such as IL-4, IL-5, IL-3 and GM-CSF released from the mast cells, and Th2 type lymphocytes causing cellular recruitment. The cellular infiltration of eosinophils, basophils and neutrophils thus perpetuates an inflammatory reaction and causes a nasal obstruction that is less responsive to treatment with antihistamine. IL-4 further stimulates B-lymphocytes to produce specific IgE antibodies against the allergen that initiated the initial response.

NON-ALLERGIC RHINITIS

When symptoms of perennial rhinitis exist without any identifiable allergen (either from history or from tests such as skin-prick test or RAST), the condition is called 'non-allergic rhinitis'. This condition is more common in the older age group. Aetiology is varied and unclear. In some cases there may be an imbalance of autonomic nervous supply and peptidergic nervous mechanisms may also be involved. This sub-group is called 'vasomotor rhinitis', as the prominent abnormality is engorged blood vessels leading to increased nasal secretions and consequent nasal obstruction. In other cases, excessive eosinophilia can be demonstrated in the nasal secretions, and mucosal inflammation is similar to allergic rhinitis. In this sub-group non-allergic asthma (or 'intrinsic asthma') often coexists, and inflammatory changes can be shown in the nasal mucosa. Non-immunologic stimuli, such as cold air, can degranulate mast cells with mediator release and this may be another mechanism in non-allergic rhinitis.

Rhinitis – Classification and pathogenesis

- The nose is designed to deliver air to the lungs at a constant temperature and humidity and remove noxious substances.
- Nasal mucosa responds to exogenous stimuli by mucosal swelling and increased secretions.
- Rhinitis is a clinical diagnosis and typical symptoms on most days, lasting for at least 1 h, are considered sufficient for the diagnosis.
- Symptoms of rhinitis include sneezing, rhinorrhoea, nasal blockage and itching.
- Allergic rhinitis can be classified into seasonal and perennial. Non-allergic rhinitis is always perennial.
- The most common cause of seasonal rhinitis is pollen. The most common cause of perennial allergic rhinitis is allergy to dust mites.
- Mast cells and eosinophils play an important role in the pathogenesis of allergic rhinitis.
- The aetiology and pathogenesis of non-allergic rhinitis is varied and unclear.

RHINITIS 2 – DIAGNOSIS

PATIENT HISTORY

Rhinitis is a clinical diagnosis and the importance of a careful history cannot be overstated. The objective is to differentiate rhinitis from other causes of nasal blockage and determine the type and severity of disease (Fig. 1). When taking the history, the following points should be considered:

- Determine the type and relative importance of nasal symptoms such as sneezing, rhinorrhoea, blockage and itching (Table 1).
- Look for the presence of associated eye symptoms such as itching, congestion and redness, which favour allergic, especially seasonal, rhinitis.
- Determine the severity of symptoms by evaluating interference with daily activities. A more objective assessment can be achieved by using symptom scores (this is mandatory in research but may not be essential in routine clinical practice).
- Headaches or pain over nasal sinuses may indicate chronic sinusitis.
- The presence of diseases such as asthma and eczema, or a family history of allergy, supports allergic rhinitis.
- Allergens such as pollens, household pets, dust mites or moulds may cause symptoms in allergic rhinitis, whereas non-specific irritants such as dust, smoke, pollutants or chemicals may precipitate symptoms in both types of rhinitis (Table 2).
- Determine any seasonal variation in symptoms.
- Questions about the nature of patient's work and working environment may reveal precipitating factors.
- The presence of household pets and cigarette smoking inside the house should be established.

PHYSICAL EXAMINATION

Face

Long-standing rhinitis can manifest itself with bagginess and dark circles around the eyes (allergic shiners) due to engorged veins. The patient may also have a transversal nasal crease resulting from upward rubbing of the nose (allergic salute), and open-mouth breathing (allergic gape) as a result of nasal blockage (Fig. 2).

Rhinoscopy

Superficial examination of the nostrils may reveal the condition of the nasal mucosa and any external nasal deformity. Anterior rhinoscopic examination with the help of a light source and nasal speculum is more satisfactory. Posterior rhinoscopy and endoscopic examination of the nasal passages are required for a detailed examination.

Mucous membrane – In chronic rhinitis, the mucosa may look pale with a bluish tint but in acute states it is usually erythematous and swollen.

Secretions – The presence and type of secretion should be noted to differentiate between infective (thick, yellow) and other causes of rhinitis (whitish, mucoid).

Turbinates – Middle and inferior turbinates may hypertrophy in long-standing rhinitis and cause mechanical obstruction.

Polyps – In chronic rhinitis, polyps may develop contributing to the nasal obstruction (Table 3).

Septum – Septal deviation is usually asymptomatic but may augment nasal blockage in the presence of rhinitis.

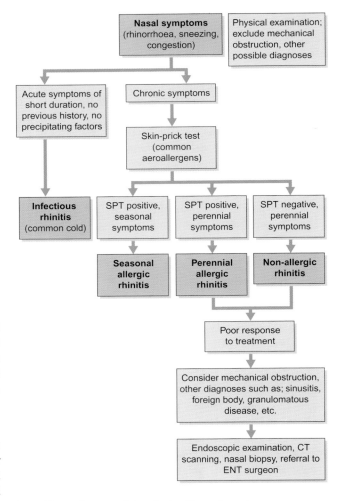

Fig. 1 **Diagnostic approach to patients with nasal symptoms.**

Table 1 **Diagnostic features of non-infectious rhinitis**

	Seasonal allergic	Perennial allergic	Perennial non-allergic
Time of year	Seasonal	Perennial	Perennial
Age of onset (median)	10–20 years	10–20 years	Adult
Prominent nasal symptoms	Rhinorrhoea, sneezing, itching	Rhinorrhoea, blockage, sneezing	Blockage, rhinorrhoea
Eye symptoms	Common	Uncommon	Not present
Nasal cytology	Eosinophils	Eosinophils	Eosinophils / neutrophils
Skin tests / RAST	Pollens	Dust mite / animal / moulds	Negative
Nasal polyps	Uncommon	Uncommon	Frequent

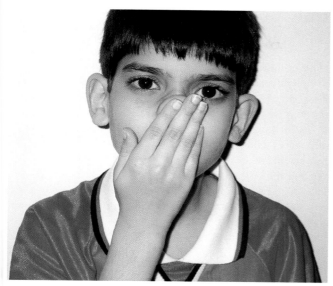

Fig. 2 'Allergy salute' is a characteristic sign of children with chronic allergic rhinitis.

Table 2 Triggers in rhinitis

- Pollens (tree, grass, weed, flower)
- Dust mites (symptoms on dusting, vacuum cleaning and making beds)
- Exposure to animals (cat, dog, horse)
- Occupational allergens (symptoms worse at work)
- Weather changes
- Cigarette smoke
- Chemicals/perfumes
- Exercise
- Pollutants such as CO, NO_2, SO_2, ozone, exhaust fumes/particles, etc.
- Stress/emotions
- Spicy foods
- Medications

Table 3 Differential diagnosis of nasal obstruction

• Deviated nasal septum	• Nasopharyngeal tumours
• Nasal polyps	• Foreign body
• Sinusitis	• Wegener's granulomatosis
• Adenoiditis	• Congenital choanal atresia

General

The eyes should be examined for the presence of conjunctivitis, which is often associated with allergic rhinitis (rhino-conjunctivitis). Ears should be examined for the condition of the tympanic membrane and middle-ear pathology, as middle-ear problems are common in association with rhinitis, especially in children. Signs of other atopic diseases such as eczema or asthma may also be present.

INVESTIGATIONS

Skin testing

Skin testing is done routinely to differentiate between allergic and non-allergic rhinitis, and to determine the specific allergen sensitivity (Table 4). Skin testing is sensitive, specific and provides useful information within 15 min. Prick-testing is a semi-quantitative method of detecting the presence of specific IgE to the antigen used and is the method of choice. The size of the reaction (mean diameter) indicates the amount of antibodies present.

The standard battery of allergens tested should include pollens, dust mites, animal proteins and moulds. The exact choice of allergen depends on the geographical location. A grass-pollen mix, using the most common grass species in the local area, is essential. Common varieties of moulds and dust mites should be included. One or two types of tree-pollen mixes are required. Sensitivity to common pets such as cats and dogs is usually tested, and other animals may be included depending on the exposure.

Blood test for IgE

Total IgE is not very useful as normal value does not exclude specific allergy and the causative agent is not identified. Measurement of specific IgE with methods such as RAST or

PRIST may be useful in certain circumstances where skin tests are not possible. These may include extensive eczema or inability to withdraw antihistamine. The disadvantage is that the result is not available at the time of initial consultation. In addition the test may be less sensitive than prick-testing.

Other tests

Nasal smear – A nasal smear-test for differential cells count can occasionally be useful to differentiate between infective (neutrophils) and non-infective (eosinophils) causes of rhinitis.

Rhinomanometry – Objective assessment of nasal airways resistance after the use of a decongestant may be used to evaluate the mechanical component of nasal obstruction, to predict the response to surgery.

CT scan – CT scan of the paranasal sinuses is indicated if chronic sinusitis is suspected from the history and examination. Plain radiographs of the sinuses are not helpful.

Nasal challenges – Nasal mucosa can be challenged with a non-specific stimulant such as histamine, methacholine or cold air, to assess airway hyperreactivity. The response can be measured as a symptom score or an estimation of nasal secretions. The normal range is wide and this test is not very useful clinically. Specific challenges to an allergen or occupational allergen may occasionally be indicated when history is not reliable (Table 4).

Rhinitis – Diagnosis

- When taking the history, determine the type and severity of nasal symptoms.
- The presence of diseases such as asthma and eczema, or a family history of allergy, indicates allergic rhinitis.
- Rhinoscopy should reveal the condition of the mucosa, the nature of secretions and any bony abnormalities.
- Endoscopic and CT examination is sometimes necessary to exclude other causes of nasal obstruction.
- Skin tests should be done to a range of common aeroallergens.
- Measurement of specific IgE can be substituted for skin tests
- Nasal provocation challenges are rarely required.

Table 4 Diagnostic tests in rhinitis

• Skin-prick tests	• Rhinomanometry
• Specific IgE measurements	• Acoustic rhinometry
• Nasal cytology	• Nasal peak-flow measurements
• Nasal challenges	• CT scanning
–Histamine/methacholine	• Nasal biopsy
–Allergen provocation	

RHINITIS 3 – TREATMENT

Rhinitis is not a fatal disease. Nonetheless, it can cause serious illness and suffering. An explanation of the causes and natural history of the disease goes a long way to reassure patients that symptoms can be effectively controlled and, at least in seasonal allergic rhinitis, the long-term prognosis is excellent.

ALLERGEN AVOIDANCE

Sometimes patients are aware of their allergic triggers. Others can be revealed on skin tests. Avoidance of allergens in all forms of allergic rhinitis reduces symptoms and medication requirements, and is the first priority in patients with moderate to severe symptoms. Details of avoidance measures can be found on p. 40.

Reducing humidity inside the house prevents growth of both moulds and dust mites. Animals should be easier to avoid, but often allergy sufferers prefer to tolerate symptoms than to remove their pets. Allergens from furry pets, especially cats, can be found in high concentrations in carpet-dust and indoor air samples from houses containing these animals. Therefore, it is not enough just to avoid close proximity; animals should be kept outside the house. In seasonal allergic rhinitis, however, avoidance is less practical. Even then taking simple steps, such as keeping the windows closed and using pollen filters in the car ventilation system, can help.

DRUG THERAPY

Antihistamines

Most of the symptoms of rhinitis can be reproduced by the instillation of histamine in the nose. This reflects the impor-

tance of this mediator in the causation of the disease and hence the effectiveness of blockage of its receptor in relieving symptoms (Fig. 1). Antihistamines are the drugs used most frequently for the treatment of rhinitis. Antihistamines block H_1-receptors, and some second-generation antihistamines may also have mild anti-inflammatory properties. Antihistamines prevent and relieve symptoms of rhinitis such as sneezing, itching and rhinorrhoea. They are less effective in relieving nasal blockage (Table 1). Oral absorption of antihistamines is excellent and they reach a peak concentration within 2 h of administration. Second-generation antihistamines have a prolonged half-life and need be given only once daily. Antihistamines such as azelastine, are effective topically as a nasal spray and have a rapid onset of action. For chronic symptoms, second-generation antihistamines, such as loratadine or cetirizine, should be given orally, whereas topical use may be indicated for intermittent symptoms.

First-generation antihistamines such as chlorpheniramine easily cross the blood–brain barrier and cause drowsiness, fatigue and confusion (Table 2). They may also cause urinary retention and tachyarrythmias. Second-generation antihistamines are better but some such as terfenadine can cause torsades de pointes and should be used with caution.

Anticholinergics

Rhinorrhoea is due to cholinergic stimulation. An anticholinergic drug, ipratropium bromide, used topically in the nose, is effective when watery discharge is a prominent symptom in perennial rhinitis. It should be used as required, the effect lasting for 8–12 h.

Sodium cromoglicate

Sodium cromoglicate and nedocromil sodium inhibits IgE mediate allergic reaction. They are effective in allergic rhinitis

Severe persistent symptoms
- Allergen avoidance
- Intra-nasal steroids
- Regular use of non-sedating oral antihistamine
- Occasional use of topical decongestant
- Immunotherapy, if appropriate
- Systemic steroids (short courses of oral prednisolone or longer acting depot injections)

Moderate persistent symptoms
- Allergen avoidance
- Intra-nasal steroids
- Regular use of non-sedating oral antihistamine
- Occasional use of topical antihistamine or decongestant

Mild persistent symptoms
- Allergen avoidance
- Adults: low-dose intra-nasal steroids
- Children: intra-nasal cromoglicate or nedocromil
- Non-sedating topical or oral antihistamine as needed

Mild intermittent symptoms
- Allergen avoidance
- Non-sedating topical or oral antihistamine as needed

Fig. 1 **Stepwise approach to the treatment of allergic rhinitis.** Patient should start treatment appropriate to the severity and move up or down depending on the response. ENT referral may be considered if significant mechanical obstruction is suspected. Associated eye symptoms may need additional topical treatment with cromoglicate.

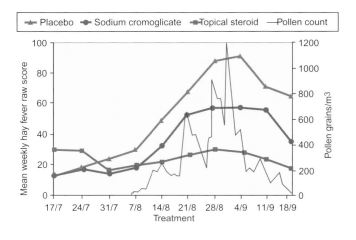

Fig. 2 **Topical steroids are more effective than sodium cromoglicate in reducing the symptoms of seasonal allergic rhinitis, in this case due to ragweed pollen** (from: Welsh PW, Stricker WE, Chei CP, et al. 1987 Mayo Clin Proc 62: 125–34).

Table 1 **The effect of different classes of drugs on various symptoms of rhinitis**

	Discharge	Blockage	Sneezing	Itching
Antihistamine (topical or oral)	++	+	+++	+++
Sodium cromoglicate (topical)	+	+	++	++
Steroids (topical)	+++	+++	++	++
Steroids (systemic)	+++	+++	++	++
Anticholinergic (topical)	+++	–	–	–
Sympathomimetic (topical or oral)	++	+++	–	–

Table 2 **Side-effects of first-generation antihistamine**

Antiserotonin effects	Anticholinergic effects
• Drowsiness, fatigue, confusion	• Urinary retention
• Slowed reaction time	• Dry mouth
• Learning impairments	• Impotence
• Dizziness	• Tachycardia
• Appetite stimulation	

when used topically. They are well tolerated with minimal side effects. They are not as effective as nasal steroids and need to be administered three to four times a day, which reduces compliance (Fig. 2). However, in children sodium cromoglicate is often preferred over steroids in mild to moderate disease.

Intranasal corticosteroids

Intranasal corticosteroids are the mainstay of therapy in allergic and non-allergic rhinitis. They suppress the inflammatory process by decreasing vascular permeability, reduce cytokine secretion and inhibit cell migration. They reduce nasal congestion, sneezing, rhinorrhoea and itching. They are effective locally with minimal systemic side-effects, which makes long-term therapy acceptable. Local side-effects occur occasionally, including nasal bleeding. Intranasal corticosteroids are effective a few days after commencing the treatment, but their peak effect may not be reached for several weeks. Therefore, these drugs should always be given regularly rather than as needed. In seasonal rhinitis, the drugs should be started before the pollen season. The dose should be adjusted to the minimum required. Beclometasone, budesonide and triamcinolone have been available in nasal spray formulation for several years. Recently fluticasone and mometasone have been introduced which are slightly more potent and may be given in a once daily regimen.

Systemic corticosteroids

Systemic steroids are sometimes used to treat severe rhinitis that is not responding adequately to other medications. For a non-fatal condition it is obviously not appropriate to give long-term systemic steroids. However, oral steroids such as prednisolone, can be used as a short course (1–3 weeks) to bring the disease under control before changing to intranasal therapy. Depot preparations of methylprednisolone and triamcinolone can be used in severe seasonal allergic rhinitis. From one to three injections are often needed to cover the pollen season.

Sympathomimetic drugs

Drugs that stimulate α-adrenergic receptors are commonly used as decongestants. These include pseudoephedrine, phenylephrine and xylometazoline. Most 'cold' and hayfever remedies available over-the-counter contain one of these agents. These drugs act as vasoconstrictive agents and reduce nasal congestion. They have a rapid onset of action when used topically.

Their regular use leads to rebound congestion and tachyphylaxis. Prolonged topical use can cause rhinitis medicamentosa in which the mucosa becomes red and swollen and unresponsive to therapy. Oral administration may cause tachyarrhythmias, hypertension and bladder dysfunction. These drugs should not be given to patients with ischaemic heart disease, hypertension or glaucoma.

Allergen immunotherapy

Before the discovery of antihistamines, the management of allergic rhinitis consisted of avoidance of allergen where practical, and immunotherapy. Immunotherapy involves subcutaneous administration of standardized and purified allergen extract. The extract is diluted to 1:100 000 w/v concentration, and weekly injections are given, increasing the dose and concentration until a maintenance dose is achieved. This dose is then continued monthly for 3–5 years. Short-term therapy can be given for seasonal rhinitis. Local reactions are common and potentially life-threatening anaphylaxis does occasionally occur. Local nasal immunotherapy in which freeze-dried extract is applied to the nasal mucosa, has been shown to be effective and safe in recent studies.

Most authorities agree that immunotherapy is effective in allergic rhinitis caused by pollen, dust mites and animal dander. However, the treatment is expensive, requires frequent visits and there is a potential for serious side-effects. For these reasons, immunotherapy is indicated only when allergen avoidance and pharmacotherapy have failed to suppress symptoms adequately and/or systemic steroids are needed to control symptoms. Moreover, immunotherapy should always be prescribed by a trained allergist and should be administered where facilities for resuscitation are available.

SURGERY

Surgery may be required for the treatment of mechanical obstruction contributing to nasal symptoms. Correction of deviated nasal septum with sub-mucus resection may be helpful. Polypectomy or ethmoidectomy may be required for nasal polyposis.

Rhinitis – Treatment

- Reduction in allergen exposure should be attempted in all patients.
- Antihistamines can be used intermittently for mild disease and regularly for more severe disease.
- Nasal steroids are the most potent treatment in allergic and non-allergic rhinitis.
- In children topical sodium cromoglicate is given as first-line therapy.
- Systemic steroids are sometimes used to treat severe rhinitis not responding adequately to other medications.
- Decongestants are recommended for occasional use only.
- Immunotherapy is indicated only when allergen avoidance and pharmacotherapy have failed to suppress symptoms adequately.

ALLERGIC EYE DISEASES

Allergic eye disease can be extremely painful and irritating, and rarely it can lead to loss of sight. The condition primarily affects the conjunctiva where the mucosa is superficial and experiences contact with allergic and irritant agents frequently. Allergic eye disease associated with rhinitis (seasonal and perennial rhinoconjunctivitis) is common, responds well to treatment, and is not sight-threatening. Other forms of allergic conjunctivitis, such as atopic keratoconjunctivitis and vernal conjunctivitis are uncommon but more protracted. With these conditions, involvement of the cornea may lead to loss of vision. Contact allergy to contact lenses (giant papillary conjunctivitis) and to medications instilled in the eye, may also occur.

ALLERGIC CONJUNCTIVITIS

Seasonal and perennial allergic conjunctivitis are similar to disorders in the nose. The prevalence and natural history is similar to allergic rhinitis (Fig. 1), although involvement of the conjunctiva in perennial rhinitis is usually mild and may not be clinically obvious. The cause of seasonal disease is allergy to the pollens of trees, grasses and weeds. The duration of symptoms varies according to pollen sensitivity and geographical location. Perennial disease is due to allergy to dust mite, animals and moulds and symptoms are more persistent (Table 1).

Pathogenesis

Allergic conjuctivitis is a typical IgE-mediated disease. IgE produced locally in response to allergen exposure binds to mast cells, which are found in increased numbers in the mucosa and substantia propria of the conjunctiva in these patients. Further exposure leads to degranulation and the secretion of preformed and newly-synthesized mediators. Histamine is the most important mediator causing vasodilatation and increased permeability. Symptoms of allergic conjunctivitis can be mimicked by instillation of histamine drops. Other mediators contribute. For example, tryptase activates complement cascade, and prostaglandins and leukotrienes cause conjunctival oedema. Eosinophils are also recruited (not normally found in conjunctiva) and perpetuate inflammatory reaction.

Clinical features

Allergic conjunctivitis often develops in children or young adults who already have some evidence of atopy. There may also be a family history of atopy. Symptoms include itching (a particularly disturbing symptom), watering and, erythema and oedema of the conjunctival mucosa (Table 2). Swelling of the eyelids produces the appearance of 'allergic shiners'. Examination with the help of a torch may reveal dilated capillaries and mucosal oedema. Small papillae may be seen on tarsal conjunctiva. Slit lamp examination performed by an opthalmologist gives a more detailed assessment of the conjunctiva and cornea.

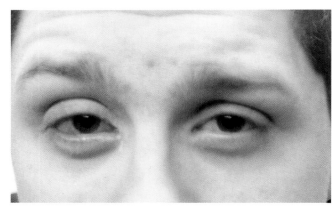

Fig. 2 **Vernal conjunctivitis in a highly atopic young man.**

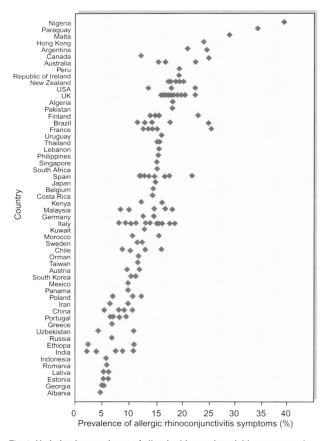

Fig. 1 **Variation in prevalence of allergic rhinoconjunctivitis symptoms in countries participating in ISAAC (International Study of Asthma and Allergies in Childhood) Study** (from: ISAAC Steering Committee 1998 Worldwide variation in prevalence of asthma, allergic rhinoconjunctivitis and atopic eczema. The Lancet 351: 1225–32).

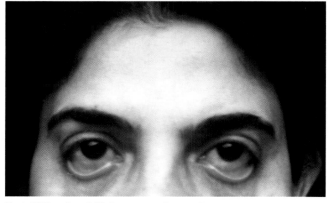

Fig. 3 **Mild conjunctivitis is common after wearing contact lenses.** This is an irritant reaction. In some patients it may progress to giant papilliary conjunctivitis.

Table 1 **Characteristics of different types of allergic conjunctivitis**

	Allergens	Immune reaction	Vision loss
Seasonal allergic conjunctivitis	Pollen	Type I	None
Perennial allergic conjunctivitis	Dust mite, mould, animals	Type I	None
Atopic keratoconjunctivitis	Uncertain	Types I + IV	Possible
Vernal keratoconjunctivitis	Uncertain	Types I + IV	Possible
Giant papillary conjunctivitis	Contact lens	Type IV	None

Table 2 **Cardinal features of allergic conjunctivitis**

- Allergic conjunctivitis is often associated with allergic rhinitis
- It is a typical IgE-mediated disease
- Pollens and dust mites are common causes
- Eye symptoms are more prominent in seasonal allergic rhinoconjunctivitis
- Symptoms include itching, burning and watery discharge
- The cornea is not involved and the disease is not sight-threatening
- Systemic antihistamine, topical antihistamine and topical cromoglicate are used for treatment

INVESTIGATIONS

Skin-prick tests

In seasonal rhinoconjunctivitis, the history often suggests the diagnosis and skin tests are not essential. In perennial disease, skin tests may be more helpful to identify and sometimes convince the patient of the allergic causes and the importance of allergen avoidance. Allergens include pollens of grasses, trees and weeds, dust mite, moulds and animal epithelia.

Cytology

Examination of a conjunctival scraping may occasionally be useful. The presence of eosinophils would confirm the diagnosis.

Conjunctival allergen challenge

This procedure is usually performed for research purposes. Allergen extract is instilled into the lower fornix of one eye and control solution into the other eye. Tear samples are collected from both eyes and carefully measured. There is usually an early response within half an hour where increased concentration of histamine and tryptase is observed. There is another peak in histamine concentration six hours later accompanied by elevation of eosinophilic cationic protein.

Treatment

It is crucial to give the patient a full explanation and education in methods of allergen avoidance and environmental control. The mainstay of treatment is topical mast cell stabilizing agents such as sodium cromoglicate, nedocromil sodium and lodoxamide. The major advantage of nedocromil is its twice-daily dose regimen, which improves compliance.

Oral non-sedating antihistamines are also effective, and have few side effects. Topical, new-generation antihistamine, such as levocabastine eye drops, are useful adjuvants and may be combined with vasoconstrictive agents to relieve hyperaemia. Topical steroids are only indicated in extreme situations, because of the sight threatening side-effects of glaucoma, corneal infection and cataract formation. Immunotherapy may be indicated in severe seasonal conjunctivitis.

VERNAL KERATOCONJUNCTIVITIS

Vernal keratoconjunctivitis is a self-limiting disease of atopic children and young adults (Fig. 2). In northern Europe, the disease is rare and usually seasonal (spring). In warmer climates the disease is relatively common and persists throughout the year. Activated T cells and eosinophils are crucial in its pathogenesis. A major basic protein secreted by activated eosinophils causes corneal ulceration. Symptoms include troublesome itching and burning of the eyes, photophobia and blurred vision. On examination giant papillae may be seen on the upper tarsal conjunctivae. Conjunctival hyperaemia, oedema and mucoid secretions are usually evident. Development of the corneal ulceration and scar formation leads to blindness in a significant proportion of patients. Topical mast cell stabilizers are used prophylactively with the addition of steroid and cyclosporin eye

drops for exacerbation. Surgery may be required for corneal plaques.

ATOPIC KERATOCONJUNCTIVITIS

Atopic keratoconjunctivitis is a chronic disease that affects adults with atopic eczema. Allergens, modified by antigen presenting cells, activate T-cells with the production of an array of lymphokines. Symptoms include itching, redness, discharge and photophobia. On examination hyperaemia and oedema of the conjunctivae is usually evident. The face and eyelids are usually affected with eczema.Chronic inflammation may lead to scarring, formation of papillae and keratopathy. Cataracts can develop as a consequence of the disease itself or treatment with topical steroids. Loss of vision is reported in up to one third of the patients. The treatment is difficult and unsatisfactory. It is essential to control the environment, removing allergens and other irritants. Associated facial and eyelid eczema should be treated along the standard lines. Topical mast cell stabilizer and steroids are frequently used.

GIANT PAPILLARY CONJUNCTIVITIS

The disease develops in patients using contact lenses, as the tarsal conjunctiva becomes sensitized to the allergens adhered to the outer surface of the lens. Itching and burning is common, and intolerance to the lens develops (Fig. 3). Later, the upper tarsal conjunctiva develops giant papillae as a result of continued exposure and inflammation. The histology is similar to vernal conjunctivitis, but corneal involvement does not occur. The disease is not sight-threatening. Treatment consists of discontinuing lens use, if possible, and topical sodium cromoglicate eye drops.

Allergic eye diseases

- Allergic eye disease associated with rhinitis (seasonal and perennial rhinoconjunctivitis) is common, and not sight-threatening.
- Vernal and atopic keratoconjunctivitis are uncommon but loss of sight is possible.
- Patients with allergic eye diseases often have a personal and/or family history of allergy.
- IgE, mast cells, T cells and eosinophils play a crucial role in the pathogenesis of allergic eye diseases.
- Symptoms include itching, watering,redness and burning sensation in the eyes.
- Examination of eyes reveals redness, oedema and papillae of the conjunctiva.
- Skin tests are usually positive.
- First-line therapy is environmental control, topical sodium cromoglicate and antihistamines.
- Steroid drops should only be prescribed by an opthalmologist.

ATOPIC DERMATITIS 1 – PATHOPHYSIOLOGY

Atopic dermatitis (AD) or atopic eczema is a chronic relapsing inflammatory skin disease (Fig. 1). It is frequently associated with asthma and allergic rhinitis as the third component of the atopic triad. It has a significant impact on affected children, their families, and the community at large. The factors contributing to family stress include sleep deprivation, loss of schooling and employment, time taken for the care of atopic dermatitis children and financial costs.

EPIDEMIOLOGY
Prevalence
AD is a common health problem for children and adolescents throughout the world. On average, it affects more than 10% of children at some point during their life, although most cases of AD in the community are mild. Recent data from the ISAAC study show a wide variation in prevalence in different countries. In children aged 6–7 years, the prevalence varied from less than 2% (Iran) to over 16% (Japan and Sweden). In adolescents (13–14 years) the prevalence ranged from less than 1% (Albania) to over 17% (Nigeria). Higher prevalences of AD symptoms were reported in Australia and Northern Europe, with lower prevalences in Eastern and Central Europe and Asia. Like other atopic diseases such as asthma and hayfever, the prevalence of AD has increased substantially over the last 30 years. Referral to secondary health care services is relatively infrequent as most cases are managed by general practitioners.

Natural history
AD starts early in life and nearly 60% of the patients develop the disease in infancy (Fig. 2). Vast majority of infants improve before the age of 5. However, many of these children develop respiratory allergic diseases such as asthma and allergic rhinitis. To some extent the prognosis depends on the severity, i.e. more severe disease starts early in life and tends to persist. There are also recent reports of recurrence of AD observed in adolescent patients who had apparently grown out of it during childhood. In adults, AD is usually seen as a continuum of disease from childhood and it is rare for it to appear for the first time during adult life.

AETIOLOGY
Development
The texture of the skin is abnormal with defective lipid barrier causing increased transepidermal water-loss. Whether this is due to abnormal metabolism of fatty acids is not clear. Genetic factors important for the development of AD include immunological abnormalities (atopy) and hypersensitivity of the skin. Environmental influences such as exposure to allergen and adjuvants, especially early in life, are critical in determining the disease expression. It is the complex interaction between genetic, immunologic and physiologic abnormalities with environmental influences that determine the clinical phenotype in each individual (Fig. 3). This view is strengthened by the wide variations in prevalence both within and between countries. Further exposure to allergen, infection and stress may induce exacerbation of the disease. The process is similar to that seen in other atopic diseases such as asthma and rhinitis, though the organ involved is different in each disease.

Role of allergens
The role of foods such as milk and egg in infancy, and aeroallergens such as house-dust mite in late childhood, is generally accepted. However, skin-prick test positivity, found in 80% of these children, does not always correlate with disease severity. Therefore, food challenges need to be carried out to detect the relevance of sensitization to these allergens. Approximately 50% of children with AD have clinical reactivity to food proteins. Young children and those with severe disease are more likely to be allergic to foods. Egg, milk, peanut, soy and wheat account for almost 75% of positive food challenges. AD can also be provoked by direct contact of the skin with food.

In older children and adults, food allergy is less important but sensitivity to aeroallergens, such as house-dust mites and moulds may be causative. On skin tests (prick and patch), sensitivity to mite antigens is found in 20–60% of patients in different studies. Allergen inhalation challenge in patients with asthma and AD can cause a flare-up of the skin lesions and avoidance of dust mites with bed covers has led to remission.

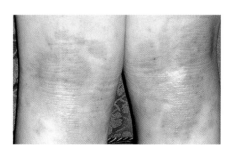

Fig. 1 **Flexural eczema in an atopic child, showing characteristic erythematous, excoriated lesions.**

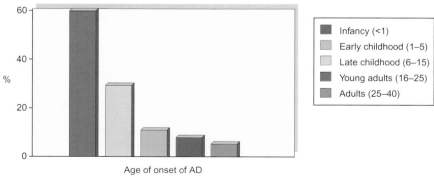

Fig. 2 **Atopic dermatitis starts early in life.** (Adapted from Wuchlich B 1996 Epidemiolgy and natural history of atopic dermatitis. Allergy Clin Immunol Int 8: 77–82.)

Role of infection

Patients with AD have increased tendency to develop viral, bacterial and fungal skin infections. *Staphylococcus aureus* and beta-haemolytic streptococci are the most common cutaneous pathogens. The immunological and inflammatory effects of *Staphylococcus aureus* include the release of exotoxins and exoenzymes and perhaps bacterial DNA-triggered mechanisms. Toxins from these organisms can act as superantigens to mediate an inflammatory skin lesion that consists predominantly of activated T cells and monocytes. Sudden aggravation of atopic dermatitis can be explained by this phenomenon.

PATHOPHYSIOLOGY

Pathogenesis

Atopic dermatitis skin tends to be dry and irritable with a low threshold for itching (dermal hyperreactivity). Immunological abnormalities include T cell dysregulation and elevated IgE levels. The decreased frequency of IFN-γ-producing CD4⁺ cells and increased IgE levels are central to the pathophysiology of AD (Th2-type reaction). Influx of activated T cells into the skin lesions is a hallmark of AD. These T cells secreting Th2-type cytokines (IL-4, IL-5, IL-3) cause the induction of local IgE responses and recruitment of inflammatory cells (lymphocytes and eosinophils) through increased expression of adhesion molecules (Fig. 4). Mediators from these inflammatory cells such as histamine, neuropeptides, and leukotrienes are responsible for oedema and pruritis. In chronic AD there is also evidence of increased expression of Th1-type cytokines such as IL-12, which promote infiltration of lymphocytes and macrophages.

Histological features

Even the uninvolved skin is abnormal, showing hyperkeratosis and T cell infiltrates. Acute lesions show marked intercellular oedema (spongiosis) of the epidermis and inflammatory cell infiltrate, predominantly of T lymphocytes, and occasionally monocytes. In the chronic lesions there is marked hyperkeratosis and inflammatory cell infiltrate consisting of Langerhans' cells, mast cells and eosinophils, in addition to lymphocytes. Chronic inflammation in AD is likely to involve a number of interdependent fac-

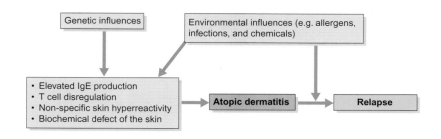

Fig. 3 **Pathogenesis of atopic dermatitis.** A combination of genetic and environmental influences determine the development and persistence of this inflammatory skin condition.

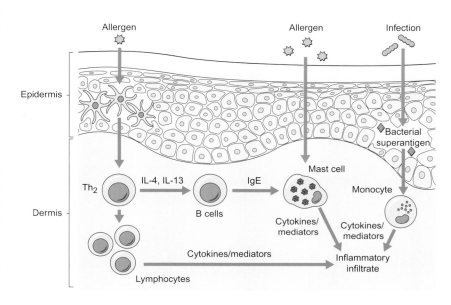

Fig. 4 **Immunologic mechanism involved in the pathogenesis of atopic dermatitis.** (Modified from Leung DYM 1995 Atopic dermatitis: the skin as a window into the pathogenesis of chronic allergic disease. J Allergy Clin Immunol 96: 302–19.)

tors, including repeated or persistent exposure to allergens and infection. The exotoxins secreted by *Staphylococcus aureus* act as both superantigens and allergens, thus contributing to persistent inflammation or exacerbation of AD.

Continuous adhesion-molecule expression may facilitate T cell extravasation in a non-antigen-specific manner, thus explaining the presence of increased T cell numbers in non-lesional skin of patients with AD.

Atopic dermatitis – Pathophysiology

- Atopic dermatitis is a chronic relapsing inflammatory skin condition.
- Dryness and intense itching are cardinal features.
- Frequently associated with other atopic diseases such as asthma and allergic rhinitis.
- Primarily a disease of early childhood.
- Affects 10–15% children at some stage during their life.
- Develops in infancy in 60% of children with the disease.
- There is increased transepidermal water-loss.
- Total serum IgE is increased in the majority of patients.
- There is influx of activated T cells (Th2 type) into the skin.
- A combination of physiological, immunological and environmental factors are important in the pathogenesis.

ATOPIC DERMATITIS 2 – CLINICAL FEATURES

The appearance of the atopic dermatitis (AD) skin varies according to the stage of lesion and presence of infection (Table 1). Distribution and pattern of the disease also varies according to age, with young children more likely to have acute lesions and older children and young adults having lesions in different stages. The disease runs a chronic or chronically relapsing course with intermittent exacerbation related to stress, exposure to allergens and irritants, and infection.

Intense pruritis is a hallmark of AD and the diagnosis should rarely be made if itching is not a prominent feature (Fig. 1). Itching and scratching is present during the day but is worse at night when sleep disruption is common. Patients with AD may have a reduced threshold for itching, which is then stimulated by mediators released from inflammatory cells. Other factors, which exacerbate itching, are reduced humidity, excessive sweating and exposure to allergens and irritants such as soap, detergents, acrylic and wool.

INVESTIGATIONS

Total serum IgE

A high total serum IgE confirms the presence of atopy in the patient but it is not particularly helpful in the diagnosis or management of AD. Skin-prick test (SPT) or measurement of specific IgE (RAST), indicating sensitization against specific allergens is more helpful.

SPT/RAST

Most children with atopic dermatitis are sensitized to food allergens (Fig. 2). SPT or RAST to a limited number of foods (milk, egg, peanut, soy, wheat and fish) is a useful screening test that can identify more than 90% of children with possible food allergy. The relevance of SPT positivity should be confirmed with food challenge or elimination/challenge diet, before a food avoidance diet is recommended. In older children and adults, allergy to house-dust mite, animal dander and moulds is important whereas food allergy is less frequent. These aeroallergens should therefore be included in the screening skin-test battery after the age of 2 years.

Table 1 **Morphological characteristics of atopic dermatitis**

- Acute lesions are papules and vesicles on an erythematous background with signs of erosions, bleeding and serous exudates
- Subacute lesions are erythematous and scaly papules on a dry background
- Chronic lesions are fibrotic papules on a lichenified (thickened) background
- Excoriation is often present due to scratching in all stages of AD
- Different stages of lesion may coexist in one individual
- Infection may alter the appearance with the presence of oozing or local abscesses
- Even uninvolved skin is often dry and scaly

Table 2 **Major and minor diagnostic criteria of atopic dermatitis (based on Hanifin and Rajka)**

Major features
- Pruritis and excoriation
- Typical appearance and distribution of skin lesions
  – facial and extensor involvement in infancy and early childhood
  – flexural involvement and lichenification by adolescence
- Chronic or frequently relapsing course (> 6 weeks)
- Personal or family history of atopic diseases

Minor features
- Dryness of skin (xerosis)
- Ichthyosis; keratosis pilaris; hyper linearity of palms
- Non-specific hand/foot dermatitis
- Scalp dermatitis e.g. cradle cap
- Allergic shiners
- Vernal conjunctivitis and keratoconus

Atopy patch test

It has been claimed that atopy patch test, i.e. application of allergen extract on the intact skin, is able to elicit eczematous skin reactions. Some investigators believe that atopy patch test with food and aeroallergen has a higher specificity and clinical relevance in AD, compared to SPT and RAST. However, this is as yet not part of the routine clinical testing in the evaluation of patients with AD.

Patch test

Patch test is done to detect delayed-type skin hypersensitivity reaction (contact dermatitis). It is claimed that contact sensitization occurs in nearly 40% of patients with AD. Positive reactions occur more frequently in adults than in children. The most frequent contact allergens are metals, fragrance, lanolin and emollients. The current practice is to perform patch tests only if there is a history suggestive of contact allergy. However, some investigators believe that patch testing should be done routinely to detect contact sensitivity, so that preventive measures can be taken at an early age.

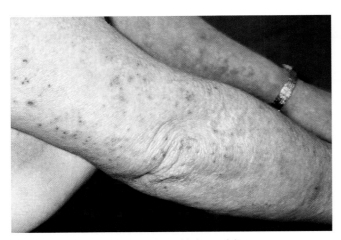

Fig. 1 **Chronic excoriating atopic dermatitis in an adult.**

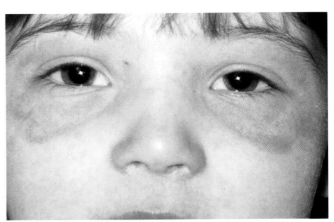

Fig. 2 **Peri-orbital dermatitis in an atopic child with allergy to house-dust mite, peanut and almonds.**

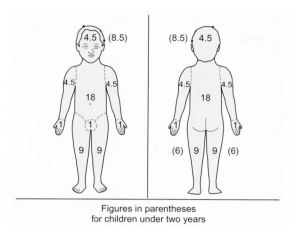

Fig. 3 'Rule-of-nine' to calculate the involvement of skin area as part of the SCORAD assessment.

Skin biopsy

Biopsy reveals infiltration of T-helper (Th) lymphocytes in all types of eczema (contact, drug-induced, etc.) and therefore it is not particularly helpful in making a diagnosis of AD. However, it can be helpful in excluding other morphologically similar skin diseases such as psoriasiform dermatitis and perivascular dermatitis.

DIAGNOSIS

Since there is no laboratory procedure to confirm a diagnosis of atopic dermatitis, different sets of clinical criteria have been developed for the purpose of making the diagnosis uniformly. The most commonly used are Hanifin and Rajka's, which have major and minor clinical criteria (Table 2). Three of four major criteria should be fulfilled to make the diagnosis of AD. Minor features are often present with atopic diathesis, but their presence is not essential for diagnosis. They are used only if the diagnosis cannot be established using the major criteria. Atopy can be detected in more than 90% of patients with personal or family history of atopic diseases, such as allergic rhinitis, asthma or AD, and confirmed by demonstrating the presence of IgE specific to common allergens on SPT or RAST.

CLINICAL ASSESSMENT OF DISEASE SEVERITY (THE SCORAD INDEX)

The SCORAD is a composite score developed to objectively assess the extent and severity of AD. This has the advantage of uniformity and consistency between observers and is reproducible. The three principal variables in this system include extent (A), intensity (B) and subjective symptoms (C). The rule-of-nine has been used to evaluate the extent of skin involvement (Fig. 3). Six items were selected for scoring of intensity, each graded from 0–3 (Table 3). Subjective symptoms were pruritis and sleep-loss, graded on a scale from 0–10.

Table 3 **Grading of intensity in SCORAD**

Items	Grade
Erythema Oedema/papulation Oozing/crust Excoriation Lichenification Dryness (uninvolved area)	Grade each item (Scale 0–3), using average representative area: 0 = absence 1 = mild 2 = moderate 3 = severe
Total intensity score	n

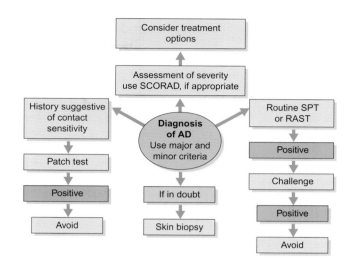

Fig. 4 **Management protocol** (if skin-prick test, patch test or challenge is negative, no further action is required).

Once the cumulative scores are available from each of the three variables, the SCORAD is derived by the following formula:

$$\text{SCORAD} = A/5 + 7B/2 + C$$

The SCORAD is used extensively in research studies but it may be clinically useful if objectivity is required in the assessment of severity, when a particular treatment option is being considered.

PROTOCOL FOR MANAGEMENT OF AD

Diagnosis is made clinically using the major and minor criteria. If the diagnosis is in doubt, skin biopsy may be helpful in excluding skin conditions with morphological similarities to AD. Skin-prick test should be done routinely to a battery of common allergens. The allergens are selected on the basis of age (food allergens in young children, with the addition of aeroallergens in older children and adults) and history (exacerbation on exposure to a particular allergen). Positive results to food allergens should be confirmed with food challenge before an exclusion diet is recommended. If the history suggests reactivity to contact sensitizers, patch test should be performed and, if positive, advice on avoidance to the chemical is given (Fig. 4). Treatment options are considered depending on the severity of the disease, assessed informally, or objectively using SCORAD.

Atopic dermatitis – Clinical features

- Appearance of AD skin varies according to the stage of the lesions and presence of infection.
- Acute lesions are erythematous papules and vesicles.
- Chronic lesions are fibrotic papules on a dry, thickened, excoriated skin.
- Dryness of the skin is characteristic.
- Face and scalp are often involved in infancy.
- Flexural eczema is more prominent in later childhood.
- Itching is a prominent feature.
- *Staphylococcus aureus* infection is a common complication.
- In young children, history and skin test may indicate the need for dietary manipulation.
- In difficult cases skin biopsy may help to exclude other diagnoses.

ATOPIC DERMATITIS 3 – TREATMENT

The management of atopic dermatitis (AD) includes topical and systemic treatments, as well as the avoidance of allergic and non-allergic trigger factors. The long-term effectiveness of management in AD depends on the understanding of the disease process by the patients, which improves compliance. Coping with the problem is easier if the patient or the parents have insight into the natural history of the disease, the role of trigger factors, and availability of treatment options. Standard first-line therapy consists of topical emollient and steroid, and antibiotics for infection.

AVOIDANCE

Irritants

AD skin is extremely sensitive and contact with detergents and other chemicals should be avoided. Oilatum should be used in the bath and use of soap should be restricted except for hygienic purposes or to clear infection. Warmth aggravates itching, so that indoor and water temperature should be kept relatively low, and warm, tight clothing should be avoided.

Food allergens

The role of elimination diet in AD is often questioned. Most studies support the view that a diet avoiding the causal food combined with suitable symptomatic treatment leads to remission of the skin manifestations. Most children below the age of 5 years with AD are sensitized to one or more foods on SPT or RAST. However, many of these positive tests are without clinical relevance. Common foods responsible for provoking symptoms are cow's milk, egg, wheat and nuts. If the history is suggestive of a reaction to one of these foods and SPT or RAST are positive, the food should be excluded. If there is doubt about the food responsible or the clinical relevance of a positive test, open or double-blind food challenges should be performed (Fig. 1).

Children with positive food challenges require elimination diets for at least 1–2 years, but a longer period of avoidance may be required. During follow-up, an open food challenge at 6–12 months intervals is justified, if intolerance is expected from the history. Accurate identification of children with a clinically relevant food allergy helps to prescribe specific diets on a scientific basis, avoiding dietary limitations which may be unnecessary or even harmful.

House-dust mite

Allergy to dust mites may be relevant in the pathogenesis of older children and young adults with AD. Studies have shown that house-dust mite avoidance is useful as part of the overall management of sensitized patients.

TOPICAL EMOLLIENT

The basis for topical treatment is the use of emollients, during and in between flare-ups, 2–3 times a day, in addition to their use after cleaning and bathing. Emollients hydrate the skin by reducing water-loss and itching. The choice of emollient is, to some extent, based on individual preferences. A change is also necessary when an emollient causes irritation, as sensitization may occur to a constituent of an emollient. Creams and lotions may be sufficient in the early stages but ointments are preferable for thick, excoriated skin. In severe cases, ointments are applied under occlusion (wet-wrap dressings) (Fig. 2) to minimize epidermal water-loss. However, the

Table 1 **Potencies of the topical corticosteroids preparations**

Potency	Examples
Mild	hydrocortisone 0.25–1 %
Moderately potent	clobetasone 0.05 %
	fluocortolone 0.25 %
Potent	betamethasone 0.1 %
	fluticasone 0.05 %
	mometasone 0.1 %
	triamcinolone 0.1 %
	diflucortolone 0.1 %
Highly potent	clobetasol 0.05 %
	halcinonide 0.1 %
	diflucortolone 0.3 %

Table 2 **Dermatological adverse effects of topical corticosteroids**

- Atrophy (thinning) of the skin
- Striae atrophicae and telangiectasia
- Contact dermatitis
- Perioral dermatitis
- Folliculitis, acne, rosacea
- Depigmentation
- Spread and worsening of untreated infection
- Rebound flare-up

Table 3 **Principals of topical corticosteroid therapy**

- Corticosteroids should not be used indiscriminately for itching
- Apply carefully on the affected area only
- Use for the minimum period necessary
- If possible, use mild steroids for infants and children, and on the face in adults
- Use relatively potent steroids initially (other than face) to achieve disease control
- Use of potent steroids should be followed by a weak steroid to avoid rebound
- If longer term use is anticipated, give a break of 2 days after 5 days' use
- Patient instruction in the appropriate use of topical steroids is essential

Fig. 1 **Approach to dietary management of young children with AD.**

Table 4 **Additional treatment strategies which may be used in specific situations**

Treatment	Indications	Comments
Antihistamine	Nocturnal itching	Not generally indicated in AD except a bedtime dose of sedative antihistamine which may reduce scratching at night
Tar	Mild to moderate AD	Anti-inflammatory properties; avoid use during exacerbation
Systemic steroids	Severe AD	Should be avoided because of adverse effects
Cyclosporin A	Severe AD	Effective but relapse may occur after cessation of therapy; potentially toxic
Azathioprine	Severe AD	Less toxic but probably less effective than ciclosporin A
Ultraviolet A (UVA) phototherapy	Severe AD, adults	May induce clinical remission; causes exacerbation in some patients due to increased temperature
Gamolenic acid	Moderate to severe AD	Increases skin hydration, beneficial only in a small subset of patients
Interferon-γ	Severe AD, adults	Clinical experience is limited
i.v. gamma-globulin	Steroid-dependent AD, adults	Being investigated

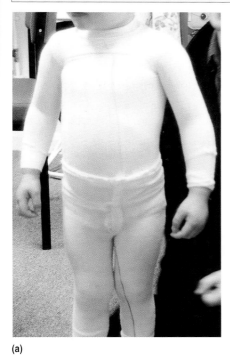

(a)

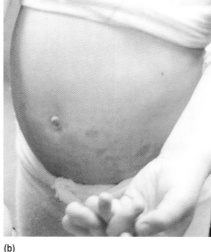

(b)

Fig. 2 **(a) and (b) Wet-wrap dressing is useful and effective in the treatment of moderate to severe generalized atopic dermatitis.**

skin underneath may become too itchy due to warmth. Topical cromolyn in a water-soluble emollient vehicle may have an anti-inflammatory effect.

TOPICAL STEROIDS

Topical steroids with their anti-inflammatory properties are the mainstay of AD treatment. They should be used, once or twice a day, on areas of disease activity, until remission is induced, which may take 1–3 weeks. They are available in various degrees of potency (Table 1). The efficacy of steroids and extent of absorption depends on the thickness of the skin. On the face, for example, it is advisable to use only mild potency steroids, such as hydrocortisone. On other areas mild to potent steroids may be used, depending on the severity.

The risk of local side-effects is directly related to the potency of the steroid and the length of the treatment (Table 2). These may be avoided to some extent if therapy principals are adhered to (Table 3). Significant systemic absorption may occur when moderate to higher potency steroid is applied to a large surface area for long periods.

ANTIBIOTICS

Staphylococcus aureus skin infection is common in AD and presents as oozing and pus formation. Anti-infective treatment depends on the extent of AD and severity of infection. Topical antibiotic (ointment or cream) is used for localized infection. Fusidic acid and tetracycline are suitable for the treatment of superficial infections of the skin caused by Gram-positive cocci. Thorough cleaning of the infected areas, with disinfectants such as 10% povidone–iodine, may be required. Disinfectants are mainly suitable for use on intact skin. Antimicrobial bath (e.g. with chlorhexidine 0.005%) is recommended for generalized infection, in addition to systemic antibiotics such as flucloxacillin or mupirocin, if the infection is severe. Anti-infective treatment is often combined with topical steroid therapy.

OTHER TREATMENT STRATEGIES

A number of other treatments are available, usually for severe AD not responding to standard treatment (Table 4). Treatments such as UVA phototherapy, ciclosporin and interferon-γ should only be given, and supervised, by specialists. Some patients and parents of children with AD seek complementary or alternative therapies. The use of unproven and unvalidated diagnostic and therapeutic procedures should be discouraged. Treatments based on irrational theories cause unnecessary long-term suffering to patients, and are harmful, because they withhold effective treatment modalities.

Atopic dermatitis – Treatment

- The principles of treatment of AD are:
  - avoidance of allergen and irritants
  - generous use of emollients for dryness
  - cautious use of topical steroids for exacerbation
  - antibiotics (topical and oral), for infection
- Avoid warm clothing and environment, as this worsens itching
- It is important to consider dietary factors in young children
- Cow's milk and egg are important allergens in early childhood
- Indiscriminate dietary elimination may be harmful
- Potency of topical steroids should relate to the area of the skin and severity of the disease
- Infection should be treated aggressively, as it damages skin and makes AD worse
- A number of treatment strategies are available for severe AD but these may have considerable adverse effects

CONTACT DERMATITIS

Eczema and dermatitis are often used synonymously to denote inflammation of the skin characterized by erythema, vesiculation and pruritus. Contact dermatitis (CD) is an eczema-like skin condition caused by direct contact with an external agent. Why some people develop CD after contact with the same agent, whereas others do not, is not clear. Genetic predisposition may be a factor. The clinical presentation depends on the nature of the offending agent and the reactivity of the subject. The lesions are usually confined to the site of contact.

CLASSIFICATION

Allergic contact dermatitis (ACD) is due to delayed hypersensitivity reaction (type IV). Irritant contact dermatitis (ICD) results from a chemical that damages the skin (Table 1). In photocontact dermatitis a chemical causes dermatitis only on interaction with sunlight (ultraviolet A).

EPIDEMIOLOGY

CD is a common condition; 5–10% of the population may be affected, although the vast majority of cases are mild. Repeated studies in the same population, several years apart, confirm a rise in prevalence. CD is most common in women of 20–40 years-of-age. Common agents causing CD include metals, rubber, cosmetics, cleaning agents, and topical medicaments.

PATHOGENESIS

Allergic contact dermatitis is a delayed hypersensitivity reaction involving CD4+ T lymphocytes (Th1 type). Langerhans' and dendritic cells present the antigen (often chemicals combined with proteins to form hapten) to lymphocytes (Fig. 1). This causes proliferation of T lymphocytes and sensitization of the skin to the

Table 1 **Characteristics of irritant contact dermatitis (ICD)**

- ICD is the most common form of contact dermatitis
- ICD can occur after a single exposure to a strong chemical or after repeated contact to milder agents, such as detergents
- Some substances act both as allergen and irritant
- ICD is often associated with other dermatological diseases such as atopic dermatitis and psoriasis
- The diagnosis is based on history and appearance of the skin
- Patch test is negative

Table 2 **Agents commonly responsible and their respective at-risk populations**

Groups	Allergen/irritants	At-risk population
Metals	Nickel, cobalt, chromium, mercury (thimerosal), aluminium	Those wearing earrings and other jewellery, industrial workers (leather, cement, dyeing and printing)
Topical medications	Antibiotics, anaesthetics, corticosteroids, formaldehyde and other preservatives such as lanolin in creams and ointments	Patients with skin diseases
Cosmetics and fragrances	Balsam of Peru, alcohols, lipids, stabilizers and preservatives in fragrances	Women more commonly than men
Detergents, soaps, preservatives	Chemicals such as formaldehyde	Cleaners, housewives, laboratory and health care workers
Plants	Poison ivy, Primula obconica and Compositae family, etc.	Gardeners, farmers, those using plant derivatives in cosmetics and topical medications
Rubber and its products	Thiuramins, latex gloves, shoes, tyres, balloons, undergarment elastic, rubber bands and condoms	Health care workers, industrial workers
Hair bleaches and dyes	Ammonium and potassium persulfates, paraphenylenediamine	Hairdressers
Synthetic glues and adhesives	Epoxy resins, colophony	Industrial workers

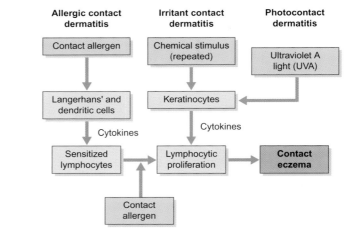

Fig. 1 **Pathogenesis of allergic, irritant and photocontact dermatitis.**

specific allergen. Subsequent exposure causes an eczematous reaction, which can be demonstrated by patch test.

Keratinocytes in the epidermis play an important role in irritant and photocontact dermatitis, as a variety of environmental stimuli, including chemical agents with or without ultraviolet A (UVA), can directly induce these cells to release inflammatory cytokines (IL-1, TNF-α) and chemokines (IL-8, IP-10). This results in the accumulation of T lymphocytes.

In acute CD, intercellular oedema leads to epidermal microvesiculation. The epidermis and superficial layers of the dermis are infiltrated heavily with lymphocytes. In chronic forms of the disease, histologic features are non-specific with thickening, hyperkeratosis and inflammatory cell infiltrate.

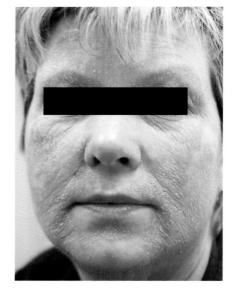

Fig. 2 **Contact eczema of the face in a hairdresser.**

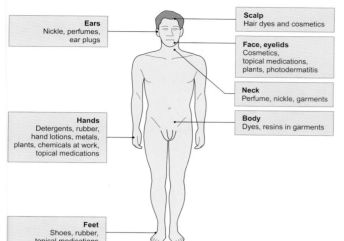

Fig. 3 **Areas of the skin affected by contact dermatitis and their common causes.** Face and hands are most commonly affected.

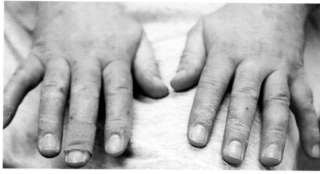

Fig. 4 **Contact eczema of hands with occupational exposure to epoxyresins confirmed on patch tests.**

CHEMICALS

The role of a substance in causing CD depends on its sensitizing capacity, frequency of use and the degree to which it penetrates the skin. Nickel is the commonest contact allergen, especially in women (Table 2). Ear-piercing is a strong risk factor for nickel allergy. Poison ivy/poison oak dermatitis is common in North America but not in Europe. The most frequent agents in Europe are nickel, potassium dichromate, cobalt, fragrance-mix, balsam of Peru, and thimerosal.

Occupation-related CD is common in certain professions such as hairdressers, cooks, bricklayers, mechanics and manufacturing and packaging workers. Rubber gloves are frequently worn in professions where contact with chemicals and/or allergens is common. Unfortunately, contact allergy to rubber and its products, including latex, has become common in recent years.

Fragrances, the *Compositae* family of plants, sunscreen and drugs such as phenothiazines are mainly responsible for photocontact dermatitis.

CLINICAL FEATURES

In the acute phase, the skin is erythematous and swollen with blistering and oozing in more severe cases (Fig.2). Later in the disease process, dryness, scaling and fissuring of the skin becomes prominent. The disease runs an intractable course over years, where chronic itching and scaling is interrupted by acute exacerbation. CD occurs usually on parts of the skin exposed to the outer environment. CD should always be suspected when eczematous lesions are present on hands, face and neck. Lesions affecting only the palms of the hands may be due to an endogenous form of eczema called pompholyx, where external allergen or irritants are not involved.

DIAGNOSIS

The distribution of the lesion often suggests the diagnosis and possible causes (Fig. 3). A detailed history including the patient's occupation and hobbies may reveal previously unsuspected contact allergens.

The patch test (see pages 28–29) is the key investigation in finding or confirming the cause of ACD. Any patients with chronic eczema, especially of hand and foot, or with a suggestive occupational history, should be patch tested (Fig. 4).

TREATMENT

The avoidance of contact allergens and chemicals and suppression of the reaction with corticosteroids form the basis of treatment (Table 3). Once the contact allergen is identified, specific advice on avoidance should be given. This may be difficult with certain allergens which are commonly encountered in household products, such as rubber. In occupation-related contact dermatitis, a change in occupation may be the only solution. However, improvement in working conditions and/or use of protective gear may be sufficient.

Table 3 **Principles of pharmacotherapy for contact dermatitis**

- In severe cases of acute dermatitis, a 2–3 week course of systemic steroids may be required
- Topical steroids should be used for mild acute dermatitis and for chronic disease
- Potent topical steroids are required for hands and feet
- Face and neck should be treated with mild-potency steroids
- Topical steroids may be used intermittently for subsequent exacerbation
- Regular long-term use of topical steroids should be avoided, because of potential toxic effects
- Creams and lotions are preferred in the initial stages
- Ointments are useful for chronic, dry, fissured skin
- Frequent use of emollient is recommended to prevent dryness and reduce itching
- Sensitization may occur to the topical medications
- Topical antihistamine, anaesthetics and antibiotics are not helpful
- If infection is suspected, oral antibiotics are preferred

Contact dermatitis

- Contact dermatitis may be allergic, irritant or due to UVA light.
- The condition is caused by direct contact with an external agent.
- Common sites include face, neck, hands and feet.
- The disease is mediated by CD4+ T lymphocytes.
- The most frequent agents in Europe are nickel, potassium dichromate, cobalt, fragrance-mix, balsam of Peru, and thimerosal.
- Hairdressers, cooks, bricklayers, mechanics and those in manufacturing and packaging industries are at a higher risk.
- During the acute phase, erythematous, itchy vesicles are formed.
- The skin is dry, scaly and fissured in the chronic phase.
- The disease runs a chronic course with intermittent exacerbations.
- Patch test is needed to discover or confirm the cause.
- Avoidance and topical corticosteroids form the basis of treatment.

FOOD ALLERGY 1 – INTRODUCTION

Adverse reactions to foods are extremely common. Only a small proportion of these are immunologically mediated and termed food hypersensitivity or allergy (Table 1). An accurate assessment of the prevalence of food allergy has been difficult because of the widely varying definitions. Self-reported questionnaire studies report a high prevalence with up to 20% of the adult population believing they are allergic to one or other food. This is seldom (< 2%) confirmed by a double-blind placebo-controlled food challenge. The prevalence also varies with the age and eating habits. Food allergy is relatively common in early childhood (5%), but rare in adults.

MECHANISM

Food proteins are broken down into small peptides and amino acids by digestive enzymes, which render them non-allergenic. However, small amounts of intact food protein may be absorbed through the normal gastrointestinal tract and elicit an immunological response. This occurs frequently in infants because of the increased permeability of the gastrointestinal mucosa and immaturity of the immune system. Secretory IgA lining the gastrointestinal mucosa inhibits abnormal immune responses but is deficient in early infancy. Therefore, food allergy is common in infancy and early childhood. IgG antibodies are formed normally but an exaggerated response may induce symptoms. Atopic individuals respond with the formation of IgE antibodies. These can be detected in the blood by in vitro tests or in the skin by skin tests. T cell responses, without the formation of antibodies, may cause delayed hypersensitivity reactions (Table 2).

COMMON FOOD ALLERGENS

Allergy to cow's milk and egg is common in infancy, although tolerance often develops to these foods before the age of 4 years. Some infants may become allergic to peanuts and tree nuts. Other food allergens in childhood include wheat, soy, fish and other seafood (Fig. 1). Nut and fish allergies tend to continue into adult life. Occasionally food allergy appears for the first time in adult life and may run a variable course. Other less common food allergens include cereals, fruits and vegetables.

Antigens from fish, peanut, and soy have been characterized. Cooked foods are usually less allergenic than raw foods as heat disintegrates some of the proteins. Cross-reactivity has been observed with some food antigens, and pollens and latex antigens.

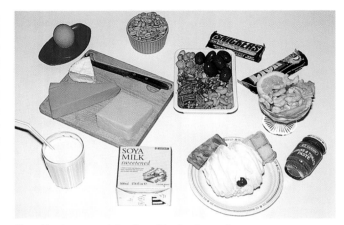

Fig. 1 **Foods commonly implicated in allergic reactions.**

MANIFESTATIONS OF FOOD ALLERGY

Allergic reactions to foods may affect many different organs and systems (Table 3). The gastrointestinal (GI) tract, including the oral mucosa and skin, is commonly involved. Airways are less commonly affected and the cardiovascular system may occasionally be affected in systemic anaphylactic reactions.

Anaphylactic reactions

Anaphylactic reactions are caused by IgE-mediated or immediate hypersensitivity reactions. These involve the classic pathway of mast cell and basophil degranulation with the release of mediators, particularly histamine. Theoretically, any food can cause anaphylaxis, but this is usually due to peanuts, tree nuts, milk, egg and fish. Peanut is the most common cause of food-induced anaphylaxis and death. A minute amount of the offending food hidden in a cooked meal may cause a serious reaction. In some cases, exercise following food consumption increases the risk of anaphylaxis.

An anaphylactic reaction usually occurs within minutes of exposure to the food, but may be delayed by up to 2 h. If the patient is very sensitive, a rash and itching may develop on mere contact with the skin or oral mucosa. Usual symptoms are acute urticarial rash, swelling and numbness of lips and tongue, followed by gastrointestinal symptoms of colic, vomiting and diarrhoea and respiratory symptoms of throat tightness, wheezing and difficulty in breathing. Hypotension, collapse and death may occur.

Oral allergy syndrome

Symptoms of numbness and pruritis of lips, tongue and oropharyngeal mucosa, swelling of the lips and perioral rash may be the initial manifestation of a systemic reaction to food. However, similar symptoms may be experienced on ingestion of certain fresh fruits in subjects sensitized to grass and tree pollens, when the progression to a systemic reaction may not occur.

Gastrointestinal symptoms

Gatrointestinal symptoms are common in food allergy and usually consist of nausea, vomiting, abdominal pain and diarrhoea.

Table 1 **Definitions**

Adverse food reactions	Any untoward reaction after ingestion of a food
Food allergy	Abnormal immunological response to food mediated by IgE (immediate hypersensitivity)
	Other immunologically mediated reactions
Food intolerance	Direct toxic or pharmacological effects
	Metabolic disorders
	Enzyme deficiency
	Other non-immunological reactions

Table 2 **Proposed immunological mechanism in food hypersensitivity reactions**

Component of immune system	Mechanisms	Effects
IgA	Secretory/protective	Reduce absorption of antigen and immunogenic responses
IgG (moderate response)		Normal
IgG (exaggerated response)	? type III reaction	? gastrointestinal symptoms/arthritis
IgE	Immediate hypersensitivity (type I) reaction	Anaphylaxis, acute urticaria, atopic eczema, wheezing, gastrointestinal symptoms
Ts (CD8+) lymphocytes	Immunosupressive	Promotes tolerance
Th (CD4+) lymphocytes	Delayed hypersensitivity (type IV) reaction	Cow's milk allergy, gluten-sensitive enteropathy

In children, malabsorption may cause failure to thrive. Other causes of diarrhoea and vomiting such as gluten and lactose intolerance, viral gastroenteritis, GI reflux and pyloric stenosis must be excluded.

Respiratory symptoms

Bronchospasm and stridor are common in acute allergic reaction. Chronic asthma and rhinoconjunctivitis may rarely be caused by food allergens.

Skin manifestations

Acute urticaria/angioedema – Development of an urticarial rash and erythematous swelling of the face and lips are a common feature of IgE-mediated allergy to food. This usually occurs within a few minutes to 2 h of ingestion and the cause and effect relationship is not difficult to establish.

Chronic recurrent urticaria – Chronic urticaria is a common disorder in both children and adults. It is rarely (1–2%) due to

Table 3 **Common foods implicated in food allergy**

Food groups	Food	Common reactions
Milk	Cow's, Goat's, soya	GI symptoms, eczema, anaphylaxis
Egg	Hen's	Urticaria/angioedema, eczema, anaphylaxis
Seafood	Fish, shrimp, prawn, lobster, crab	Urticaria/angioedema, GI symptoms, asthma, anaphylaxis
Legume	Peanut, soyabean	Urticaria/angioedema, asthma, anaphylaxis
Nuts	Hazelnut, brazil, walnut, pecan, almonds, cashew	Urticaria/angioedema, asthma, anaphylaxis
Fruits and vegetables	Apple, peach, pear, banana, orange, lemon, carrot, potato, kiwi, melon, celery, tomato	Oral allergy syndrome, urticaria/angiodema, rarely anaphylaxis
Cereals	Wheat, corn, rye, oat, barley	GI symptoms, urticaria

Table 4 **Atypical reactions to foods**

Occasional association
Irritable bowel syndrome
Inflammatory bowel disease
Migraine/headaches
Hyperactivity/behaviour problems in children

No proof of association
Enuresis
Otitis media
Arthritis
Fatigue/tension syndrome

IgE-mediated food hypersensitivity. Salicylates and food additives such as benzoates and azodyes have also been implicated in some cases of chronic recurrent urticaria but the mechanism is not clear.

Atopic eczema – Approximately one third of the young children with atopic eczema have a food-related IgE-mediated hypersensitivity, usually to cow's milk and egg. This is supported by high IgE and the presence of specific IgE, or positive skin tests to these food antigens and positive food challenges. Elimination of the food from the diet improves eczema. In other cases, delayed-type hypersensitivity may be involved when the SPT is negative and reaction to the food challenge may be delayed.

COW'S MILK ALLERGY AND INTOLERANCE

Approximately 4 % of infants react adversely to cow's milk. In less than half, evidence of IgE-mediated allergy is apparent, usually in those with an atopic family history. Symptoms are usually confined to the gastrointestinal tract and may include diarrhoea, vomiting, colic, rectal bleeding and failure to gain weight. Partial villous atrophy may occur. Occasionally, acute allergic reactions with systemic symptoms and anaphylaxis may occur. Most children tolerate cow's milk by the age of 2 years and it is uncommon to see cow's milk allergy or intolerance after the age of 4.

EGG ALLERGY

Allergic sensitization to egg protein occurs in 10% of children before the age of 2 years, often in those with a positive family history of atopy. However, clinical reactions occur in less than 3%. Symptoms vary from mild rash to anaphylaxis.

ATYPICAL REACTIONS TO FOODS

Food allergy is often blamed by patients for a number of diseases such as migraine and a wide variety of non-specific symptoms such as fatigue. Identification of food by tests that have no scientific basis enhance this perception. Food challenges are often negative and evidence of immunological mechanism is lacking in these cases. Patients should be reassured that foods are not responsible to save them from unnecessary dietary restrictions (Table 4). This is even more important in children whose normal growth and development may be affected.

Food allergy

- Immunologically mediated adverse reactions to food are termed food allergy.
- Food allergy is relatively common in early childhood but rare in adults.
- Major food allergens in childhood are milk, egg, peanut, soya, wheat and fish.
- Common food allergens in adults are peanut, tree nuts, fish and fruits.
- Allergic reactions to foods may affect the gastrointestinal tract, skin, respiratory and cardiovascular systems.
- Anaphylactic reactions to foods are usually due to peanut, tree nuts, egg, milk and fish.
- Acute urticaria/angioedema is a frequent manifestation of food allergy but chronic urticaria is rarely due to foods.

FOOD ALLERGY 2 – MANAGEMENT

PATIENT HISTORY

History is crucial in the diagnosis of food allergy. An assessment should be made of the validity of symptoms and the severity of the reaction. Important points to consider are outlined in Table 1.

A WORKING DEFINITION

Allergic reactions where typical skin, gastrointestinal, respiratory or systemic manifestations appear within 2 h of ingestion of the suspected food on more than two occasions strongly support the diagnosis of food allergy. This should, preferably, be confirmed with demonstration of sensitization to the suspected food(s) and/or food challenges (Fig. 1).

PHYSICAL EXAMINATION

Physical examination is usually not rewarding unless the patient presents during an acute allergic reaction, when acute urticaria/angioedema and signs of anaphylaxis may be found. In young children, atopic eczema may be a manifestation of food allergy, the distribution, severity and extent of which should be noted. In children, weight should be checked and any signs of malabsorption should be looked for.

DIAGNOSTIC TESTS
Skin-prick test (SPT)

SPT is a reproducible, quick and inexpensive test to confirm sensitization to one or more suspected foods. Extracts are available for most food allergens. However, they are less standardized than inhalant allergens and occasionally they need to be supplemented by prick-test of fresh foods. The choice of foods to be tested is based on the history and type of symptoms. For example, milk, egg and wheat should always be tested in an infant with atopic eczema and nuts should be included in the battery if a patient had an acute anaphylaxis.

A positive skin test denotes sensitization but not necessarily symptomatic allergy. Sensitization to food is commonly seen in patients who are able to tolerate the food without any adverse reaction. A history of clinical reaction to the food in addition to positive SPT is mandatory for the diagnosis of IgE-mediated food allergy. SPT is sometimes negative in the presence of a convincing history as other immunological mechanisms may operate.

Total IgE

Measurement of total IgE is not very helpful in identifying the causative food.

Specific IgE

Measurement of specific IgE in the serum by RAST (radioallergosorbent test) or enzyme-based immunoassays (ELISA) is useful in confirming sensitization. As for SPT, the relevance of this sensitization should be evaluated with history or food challenge.

Other immunological tests

Histamine levels in the blood or urine are occasionally used to confirm that an acute allergic reaction is indeed due to immediate hypersensitivity, as the blood histamine levels rise for a short period. In vitro tests such as basophil histamine release and mononuclear proliferation are primarily research tools and rarely useful in clinical situations (Table 2). Anti-gliadin antibodies may be useful in the diagnosis of gluten-sensitive enteropathy.

FOOD CHALLENGES

When the history suggests an acute or systemic reaction, food challenges should be performed under the supervision of personnel experienced in this procedure and where facilities for resuscitation are available. Challenges can be performed at home, under the guidance of a dietitian

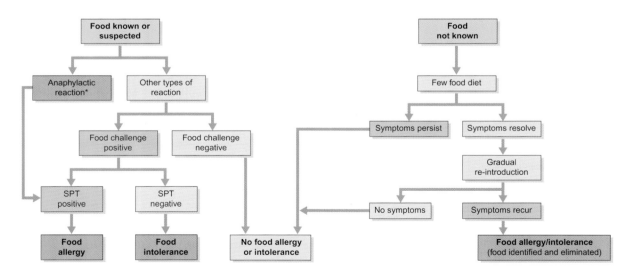

* If skin test is negative to the suspected food, a challenge should be performed

Fig. 1 **Algorithm for the diagnosis of food allergy.**

Table 1 **Points to consider in taking a patient's history**

Food	Although any food can cause allergy, cow's milk and egg (young children) and fish and nuts (all ages) are common allergens
Temporal relationship	Reactions occurring within 2 h of ingestion are more likely to be due to food allergy
Reproducibility	Two or more similar reactions after ingestion of the same food strongly suggest a causative relationship
Symptoms	Specific symptoms (acute urticarial rash, oropharyngeal itching and numbness, stridor, bronchospasm, abdominal pain, diarrhoea and vomiting) are more likely to be caused by food allergy than non-specific symptoms (headaches, tiredness, etc.)
Age of onset	Although food allergy can develop at any age, milk and egg allergy usually appear before the age of 2, and nut allergy during childhood
Other atopic diseases	Presence of other atopic diseases such as atopic eczema, asthma and allergic rhinitis occurs in the majority of patients
Family history of atopy	A history of atopy in the immediate family is a strong predictor for the development and persistence of food allergy

and allergist, when history suggests a delayed reaction without involving respiratory or cardiovascular systems.

Double-blind placebo-controlled food challenge (DBPCFC)

DBPCFC is the gold standard for the diagnosis of food allergy/intolerance. A small amount of suspected food is mixed in another food or drink to disguise its smell and taste. Food or drink portions are prepared with and without the suspected food and given to the patient in random order on two or more separate occasions. Both the patient and the physician assessing the reaction are unaware of the content of the food taken. Symptoms are recorded on visual analogue scale, or with predefined scores, and any signs are noted. Patients are usually monitored for 2 h and a diary is handed over to record any delayed symptoms.

Open challenge

An open challenge is sufficient to confirm food allergy where the reactions include objective signs such as the appearance of a rash or swelling, which can be confirmed by the physician. Although patient and observer bias may occur, open challenge is more convenient and less time-

consuming than the DBPCFC. Where the diagnosis is in doubt, DBPCFC is the only reliable alternative.

Elimination and challenge

Occasionally, several foods are suspected to cause adverse reactions, and DBPCFC may not be practical. In this case, elimination of these foods (under the supervision of a dietitian) for a trial period, while monitoring symptoms, is indicated. If there is significant improvement in symptom scores, then introduction of one food (or food group) at a predetermined interval, will help to identify the food responsible for the patient's symptoms. This procedure can also be used when a patient suspects food allergy but is unsure of the causative food (Fig. 1). A few food diet is given for a trial period. If successful, gradual introduction of the foods (or food groups) will identify the food responsible. Of course, if there is no improvement on a properly prescribed elimination diet, which had been adhered to, the patient should be reassured that food allergy is not responsible for the symptoms. The problem of patient and physician bias can not be overcome in these elimination/challenge diet procedures.

TREATMENT

Once food allergy is diagnosed and the food identified, treatment is primarily with elimination of the responsible food from the diet. For inadvertent exposure causing allergic reactions, adrenaline (epinephrine), antihistamines and corticosteroids are used. Self-injectable adrenaline (epinephrine) should be prescribed for patients that have a history of acute systemic allergic reaction.

Avoidance

A detailed explanation is essential for successful avoidance. Egg, milk, soy and nuts may be hidden in other foods and reading ingredient lists is essential. Alternative foods should be suggested and it is mandatory to make sure that the avoidance diet is nutritionally adequate. Soya milk or hypoallergenic formulae can be given for cow's milk allergy during infancy. The services of a qualified dietitian are extremely useful.

Pharmacotherapy with an antihistamine or oral sodium cromoglicate is not usually helpful to suppress the symptoms, if exposure to the offending food continues. Immunotherapy does not help and may indeed cause an acute allergic reaction.

Table 2 **Immunological tests in food allergy**

- Skin-prick test
- Total serum IgE
- Specific IgE (RAST or ELISA)
- Histamine levels in blood or urine
- Basophil histamine release
- Mononuclear proliferation assays

Food allergy – Management

- Cow's milk, egg, fish and nuts are common food allergens.
- Atopic eczema, asthma and/or allergic rhinitis often co-exist with food allergy.
- Family history of atopy is a strong predictor for the development of food allergy.
- SPT is a reproducible, quick and inexpensive method to confirm sensitization to the suspected foods.
- History supported by sensitization and/or positive challenge to the suspected food(s) confirms the diagnosis.
- Food challenges should be performed where facilities for resuscitation are available.
- DBPCFC is the gold standard for the diagnosis of food allergy/intolerance.

COW'S MILK ALLERGY

INTRODUCTION

Adverse reactions to cow's milk ingestion could be due to immunological,
metabolic, infective or other causes.
Cow's milk allergy (CMA) is defined as
an adverse reaction to cow's milk protein
with evidence of abnormal immune
response. The immune hypersensitivity
could be antibody-(IgE or IgG) or cell-
(lymphocyte) mediated. Adverse reaction
to cow's milk, due to non-immunological
causes, such as lactase deficiency, is
called cow's milk intolerance.

Cow's milk is often a major part of an
infant's diet. It is therefore not surprising
that CMA is the most common food
allergy in the first year of life. CMA is
reported in 5–15% infants but it can be
confirmed by challenge procedures in
only a third of these children. The prevalence of CMA during infancy is probably
2–3% in the general population but
nearly 10% in atopic infants. Most of
these children outgrow their reactivity
before the age of 5 years. Risk factors for
the development of CMA include family
history of atopy and early introduction of
cow's milk.

MECHANISM

Any food protein may be allergenic if it
can be absorbed intact or as substantial
fragments through the gut mucosa and
then evoke an immune (allergic) response.
Cow's milk has more than 20 constituent
proteins, but those which are commonly
responsible for allergic reactions are β-
lactoglobulin, caseins, bovine serum albumin, γ-globulin and α-lactalbumin. The
intrinsic properties of the protein and the
processing (especially thermal processing) may have an effect on the allergic
potential.

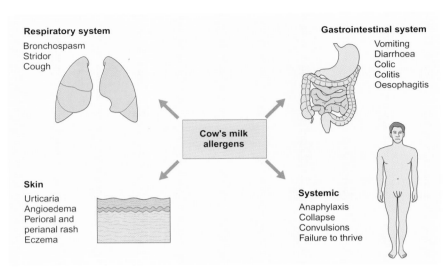

Fig. 1 **Common manifestations of cow's milk allergy.**

In some patients gut mucosal immunity may be abnormal with defective
secretory IgA function. This enhances
absorption of intact cow's milk proteins.
The development of a local immune reaction causing increased intestinal permeability allows further absorption of
antigen. These antigens then evoke anti-
body- or cell-mediated hypersensitivity
reactions resulting in clinical manifestations of CMA.

CLINICAL FEATURES

CMA can affect many organ systems
(Fig. 1). Several distinct syndromes are
recognized (Table 1). Other food allergies are also common in these children
(Fig. 2).

DIAGNOSIS

Diagnosis is made primarily on clinical
grounds (Fig. 3). The gold standard
for the diagnosis of cow's milk allergy is

double blind-placebo-controlled challenge. In some cases, an open challenge
may be adequate if the history is highly
suggestive. However, this is not always
required and may not be advisable if
there is a history of systemic reaction or
anaphylaxis. Skin tests and/or RAST are
of value in differentiating IgE-mediated
allergy from other causes. Other tests
may be required to exclude cow's milk
allergy and to establish other causes of
gastrointestinal symptoms or failure to
thrive, such as stool-test, endoscopy,
sweat-test, etc.

TREATMENT

The treatment of CMA is its elimination
from the infant's diet. This restores normal
gut permeability with reduction in absorption of other food allergens. Removal of
antigenic stimuli also causes reversal of
immune dysfunction with fall in cow's
milk IgG and IgE levels. Soya milk,
protein hydrolysate or amino acid-based

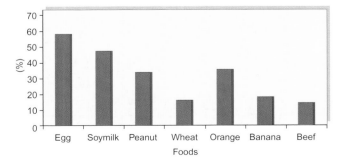

Fig. 2 **Sensitization to common foods in children with cow's milk allergy.**
From Bishop JM, Hill DJ, Hoskings CS 1990 J Pediatrics.

Table 1 **Syndromes associated with cow's milk allergy**

Syndromes	Features
Immediate type	IgE-mediated symptoms of urticaria, angioedema, bronchospasm, stridor and anaphylaxis may occur immediately after ingestion of small amounts
Gastrointestinal	Delayed hypersensitivity – vomiting, diarrhoea and colic occur hours to days later, usually after ingestion of larger amounts of cow's milk
Eczema	A combination of IgE- and cell-mediated hypersensitivity; chronic eczema improves after exclusion of cow's milk
Colitis	Probably lymphocyte-mediated with evidence of eosinophilia, diarrhoea and rectal bleeding are prominent features

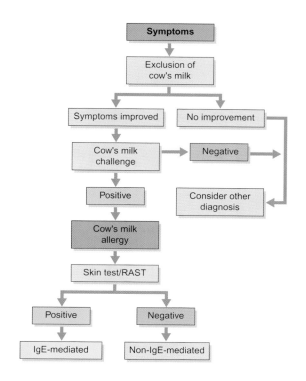

Fig. 3 **Algorithm for the diagnosis of cow's milk allergy.**

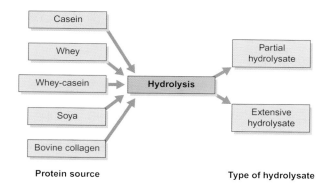

Fig. 4 **Protein sources for the production of partial and extensive hydrolysate.**

allergic patients to assess their allergenic potential, in addition to standard nutritional evaluation and laboratory and animal testing for antigenicity.

HFs are generally well tolerated although there are several reports of allergic reactions including anaphylaxis. eHF is safer but less palatable than pHF. The latter is not generally recommended for the treatment of CMA. Children with CMA should be skin tested with eHF before this is prescribed. A negative reaction indicates eHF is safe to use. Children with positive skin-test result to the eHF should be further evaluated by an open challenge in a hospital setting where facilities for resuscitation are available. Alternatively, they could be given amino acid-based formulae.

PREVENTION OF CMA

Avoidance of cow's milk in early infancy has been shown to reduce the development of CMA in at-risk infants. Exclusive breast-feeding should be encouraged in all infants. Since intact cow's milk protein can pass into the breast milk, the lactating mother should avoid excessive intake of milk products herself. If breast-feeding is not feasible, or as supplement, soya milk, hydrolysate or amino acid-based formulae may be used. There are, however, problems of designing suitable hydrolysates that are low in antigenicity and good in taste.

formulae may be used as alternatives to cow's milk. The choice of substitute milk depends on the allergenicity, nutritional composition, palatability and cost.

Soya milk may safely be used in many children with CMA. However, 5–10 % children with CMA are also allergic to soya protein and some children with CMA become allergic to soya milk after its introduction.

Hypoallergenic formulae

Allergic reactions require large protein molecules (antigens) to stimulate the production of antibodies. To reduce allergenicity, the source protein can be broken down into small peptide molecules and amino acids by enzyme hydrolysis. This process has been used successfully in the production of hydrolysed formulae (HF). The peptides of HF should be as short as possible. In extensively hydrolysed formulae (eHF), 95% of peptides have a molecular weight below 1500 Dalton and < 0.5% of the remaining peptide is above 6000 Dalton. Partially hydrolysed formulae (pHF) have 2–18% peptides above 6000 Dalton. These larger peptides may elicit allergic reaction. pHF have a higher capacity to bind to human serum IgE antibodies of cow's milk-allergic children, to induce positive skin tests and provocation tests. These infant formulae are based on animal or vegetable protein (casein, whey, soya and bovine collagen) and are used extensively in children with cow's milk allergy or intolerance (Fig. 4). Amino acid-based formulae do not have peptide and are therefore safe to use in children with CMA.

Some HFs are not optimal in nutritional content. The process to reduce allergenicity may modify amino acid content or reduce its bioavailability. Changes in the absorption of calcium, zinc and copper have been found. All infant formulae promoted as 'hypoallergenic' should also be tested in milk-

> **Cow's milk allergy**
> - CMA is common in the first years of life.
> - Both IgE-mediated and cell-mediated mechanisms are involved.
> - Skin and gastrointestinal and respiratory systems may be involved, and anaphylaxis may occur.
> - Diagnosis may require cow's milk challenge.
> - Treatment requires elimination of cow's milk from the infant's diet.
> - Hypoallergenic (extensively hydrolysed or amino acid-based) formulae are recommended as substitute milk.
> - In high-risk infants prevention of CMA is with longer periods of exclusive breast-feeding and use of hypoallergenic formulae as supplement.

ALLERGY TO PEANUT AND TREE NUTS

INTRODUCTION

Allergy to nuts is a common and well-known problem. Peanut (PN) and tree nut (TN) allergies are potentially life-threatening, rarely outgrown, and appear to be increasing in prevalence. Nut allergy is characterized by more severe symptoms than other food allergies and by high rates of symptoms on minimal contact. PN is the most common cause of severe or fatal food-associated anaphylaxis.

PN (*Arachis hypogaea*) is a legume and not a 'true' nut. The clinical features of PN allergy are more closely related to those of TN allergy than other legumes such as peas. Indeed 30% of patients allergic to PN are also allergic to one or more TN. Common TNs include brazil nut, hazelnut, walnut, cashew nut, almond, pecan and pine nut (Fig. 1).

PREVALENCE

Sensitization to PN occurs early in life. In a study of unselected 4-year-old children, 1% were sensitized to PN and 0.2% to one or more TNs. A history of clinical reaction to PN was obtained in only half of those who were sensitized. Allergy to nuts represents around 25% of food allergies in older children and adults. In about half of them the first reaction occurs before the age of 2, and in 90% before the age of 15. PN affects more than half of all nut-allergic individuals.

An increase in morbidity and mortality from PN allergy has been reported in the last two decades. The increase in prevalence may reflect a general increase of atopy but increased consumption of PN allergens, especially in the form of peanut butter, may be responsible.

NATURAL HISTORY

PN allergy appears early in life, often following cow's milk and egg allergy. By the age of 3 years PN becomes an important allergen as children grow out of milk and egg allergies (Fig. 2). Recent data suggest that PN allergy is presenting earlier in life, possibly reflecting increased consumption of PN by pregnant and nursing mothers. Allergy to TN appears somewhat later, but still commonly in the first 10 years of life. It is uncommon for nut-sensitive patients to lose their clinical reactivity, even after several years' abstinence.

CLINICAL FEATURES

The allergic reactions may vary in severity from mild urticaria to severe anaphylactic episodes and death (Table 1). Allergic reactions to nut frequently occur on first known exposure and may be life-threatening. Accidental ingestion is common and frequently occurs outside of the home. About one-third of PN-sensitive patients have severe reactions to PN which occur within a few minutes of ingestion. The major feature accounting for life threatening reactions is laryngeal oedema. Severe symptoms are more common in adults and those with asthma.

Exposure to a small amount of PN or TN may induce a severe systemic reaction (Fig. 3). The majority of patients react

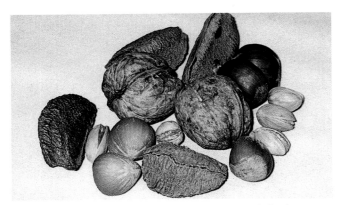

Fig. 1 **Nuts are becoming an increasingly common cause of allergic reactions to food.**

to less than 1 g which may be present hidden in other foods. In some individuals, even contact with PN on unbroken skin can cause an immediate local reaction. Exercise-induced anaphylactic reactions occur in some patients only when certain foods, commonly nuts, have been eaten before exercise.

Patients allergic to grass or tree pollen, particularly birch pollen, may develop symptoms of numbness and swelling of the lips and tongue and throat tightness following ingestion of TN (the oral allergy syndrome). Although laryngeal oedema rarely occurs, these patients do not get systemic anaphylaxis. The reaction is thought to be a result of cross-reactivity of antigens between pollens and nuts.

INVESTIGATIVE METHODS

Skin-prick test (SPT)

Using a commercial standardized extract, SPT is a cheap, reproducible and safe way of detecting sensitization. SPT has a good negative predictive value, i.e. a negative reaction largely excludes IgE-mediated allergy. A wheal diameter of > 5 mm is

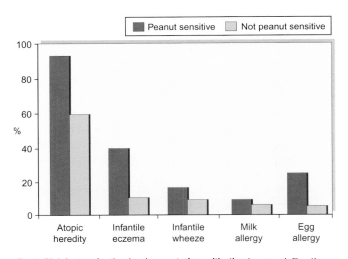

Fig. 2 **Risk factors for the development of sensitization to peanut.** Family history of atopy is the strongest risk factor. Eczema and wheeze during early infancy and allergy to milk and egg are other indicators. (Data from: Tariq S, Stevens M, Mathews S, Ridout S, Twiselton R, Hide DW 1996 Cohort Study of peanut and tree nut sensitisation by age 4 years. Br Med J 313, p514–517.)

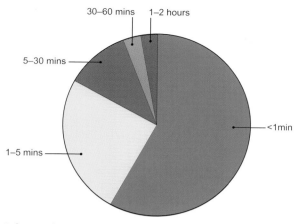

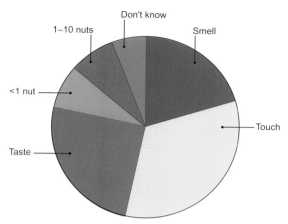

Fig. 3 **Survey of Brazil nut allergy. (a) Timing of reaction; (b) Amount of Brazil nut producing reaction.**

Table 1 **Clinical features of nut allergy**

Local (skin, oral mucous membrane)	Localized erythema and swelling of skin, numbness and swelling of lips and oral mucous membrane
Skin	Generalized urticaria, angioedema and atopic dermatitis
Gastrointestinal	Vomiting, diarrhoea and abdominal pain
Respiratory	Wheezing, throat tightness, coughing and dyspnea
Cardiovascular	Tachycardia, hypotension and collapse

a good indication of clinical reactivity but reactions of less than 5 mm are not helpful. The size of wheal on SPT predicts reactivity but not severity of reaction. Some of the extracts are not standardized and in these situations native or freshly prepared extracts from the nut might give a better result.

Specific IgE test

As an alternative to SPT, specific IgE antibodies can be measured by radioallergosorbent test (RAST) or similar methods. The cross-reactivity of nut antigens can be investigated with RAST inhibition test.

Oral challenge test

In spite of the development of numerous in vivo and in vitro diagnostic techniques for food allergy, the oral challenge test is still the 'gold standard'. Labial food challenge is a modification of oral challenge, which is simple, rapid to perform and is associated with a low risk of systemic reaction. A positive reaction is indicated by labial oedema with perioral urticaria. Systemic reactions are rare. Labial food challenge should be the first stage of an oral challenge in nut allergy. A positive result indicates the presence of nut allergy, but a negative result should be further investigated by open or blind oral challenge.

DIAGNOSIS

A convincing history of an acute reaction (at least one organ system involved within 60 min of ingestion) to PN or TN in the presence of sensitization to that nut (positive SPT or RAST), is diagnostic and oral challenge is not required. If the history is ambiguous and/or evidence of sensitization is lacking (negative or small reaction on SPT or absence of or low level of specific IgE on RAST), then oral challenge test is needed to confirm the diagnosis. An open challenge is sufficient in most cases but

double-blind placebo-controlled challenges may occasionally be required. Children who have had a positive SPT to peanut and have not knowingly eaten it should have an open challenge. A number of these children can eat peanut safely.

TREATMENT

Although the ideal treatment is avoidance, this is not always possible because of hidden exposures. Hidden sources of nuts include cookies, candy, pastry, a variety of chocolates and sweets and Asian and vegetarian foods. The nut-allergic patient should be instructed to carefully read labels of foods. Education on avoidance and treatment measures is imperative.

Nut-sensitive individuals must carry and be able to self-administer adrenaline (epinephrine) at the first sign of a systemic reaction, while awaiting medical help. Antihistamines may be used for mild reactions and oral allergy syndrome. A 'medic-alert' bracelet may be helpful. Emergency care providers should be aware of cricothyrotomy as a life-saving procedure where intubation and ventilation are not possible. Immunotherapy has not been successful as the rate of systemic reactions is unacceptable.

In the emergency department, treatment of an acute reaction should include repeated doses of adrenaline (epinephrine), antihistamines and corticosteroids, as well as availability of oxygen, mechanical ventilation, vasopressors, and intravenous fluids.

Allergy to peanut and tree nuts

- PN and TN allergies are potentially life-threatening, and rarely outgrown.
- Sensitization to PN occurs early in life.
- Nut allergy appears to be increasing in prevalence.
- Cross-reactivity is common among nuts.
- Exposure to a small amount of PN or TN may induce a severe systemic reaction.
- In the absence of a convincing history, oral challenge test is the gold standard of diagnosis, performed under expert supervision.
- PN and TN products are common foods in the diet and avoidance may prove difficult.
- Nut-sensitive individuals must carry and be able to self-administer adrenaline (epinephrine.)

ACUTE ALLERGIC REACTIONS AND ANAPHYLAXIS

Allergic reactions vary widely in severity from mild pruritis and urticaria to circulatory failure and death. An acute allergic reaction with one or more life-threatening features, such as respiratory difficulty or hypotension, is termed anaphylaxis. Reactions with troublesome but not immediately life-threatening reactions, such as generalized urticaria/ angioedema and bronchospasm of mild to moderate severity, may be called severe allergic reactions.

Anaphylaxis and anaphylactic deaths are becoming more common, especially in children and young adults. A recent report suggested a yearly incidence of 1–3 per 10 000 population. Nearly 500 people die from anaphylaxis every year in the USA.

CAUSES AND MECHANISM

Common causes of anaphylaxis include foods (e.g. nuts and shellfish), drugs (e.g. antibiotics and NSAIDs), insect venom and latex. Foods are the commonest cause of anaphylaxis and there have been several reports of deaths due to anaphylactic reactions to peanuts and tree nuts. Both IgE-mediated and non-IgE-mediated immunological mechanisms have been described (Fig. 1). The commonest is an IgE-mediated anaphylactic reaction. Exposure to the protein leads to degranulation, releasing mediators such as histamine (Table 1). These mediators increase the formation of nitric oxide (NO) which produces smooth muscle relaxation and increases vascular permeability, leading to hypotension and intravascular volume depletion.

Non-IgE-mediated reactions are sometimes called anaphylactoid reactions. Activation of the complement cascade may result in the formation of anaphylatoxins (e.g. C3a and C5a) which can release mediators from mast cells and basophils. Certain substances, such as radiocontrast media, can directly stimulate the release of mediators from mast cells and basophils.

Idiopathic anaphylaxis

In approximately 20–40% of cases, the cause remains obscure despite extensive investigations. Some of these patients have recurrent episodes. The mechanism

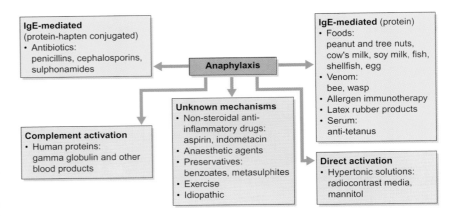

Fig. 1 **Mechanisms and causes of anaphylactic reactions.**

Table 1 **Mediators of anaphylaxis released from mast cells and basophils**

- Histamine
- Prostaglandin D_2
- Leukotriene C_4
- Platelet activating factor
- Tryptase
- Chymase
- Heparin

Table 2 **Factors which increase the risk of a severe anaphylactic episode**

- Previous anaphylaxis
- Bronchial asthma
- Personal history of atopy
- Family history of atopy
- Non-compliance with avoidance diet (away from home, denial of the problem)
- Exercise following meal
- Glucocorticoid therapy
- Beta-blocker therapy
- ACE inhibitor therapy

is unknown but it is suggested that either there is an intrinsic defect in mast cells with release of mediators, or a circulating histamine-releasing factor is present.

CLINICAL FEATURES

The type and severity of symptoms depends on the patient's sensitivity and the route, quantity and rate of administration of the antigen. Those who are highly sensitive may react even to the smell and/or touch of the food. A number of factors increase the risk of severe reactions or make the treatment more difficult (Table 2).

Anaphylaxis can affect virtually any organ in the body, but the skin and respiratory, gastrointestinal and cardiovascular systems are most commonly affected (Fig. 2). The onset of action may be rapid. There may be generalized pruritis, urticaria, swelling of the lips and tongue, feeling unwell and a sense of doom. Swelling of the larynx and glottis may lead to stridor. An asthma-like condition may develop with severe bronchospasm resulting in hypoxia and hypercapnia. Hypotension and cardiovascular collapse is usually due to vasodilatation and enhanced vascular permeability but

arrhythmias may also occur. Dizziness and loss of consciousness occur as a result of cerebral hypoperfusion.

The diagnosis of anaphylaxis is clinical. Previous history of anaphylaxis and the circumstances and exposure to possible triggers immediately before the reaction help to establish the diagnosis. Other causes of collapse or loss of consciousness should be excluded, such as vasovagal syncope, seizures, myocardial infarction and arrhythmias and acute respiratory difficulty such as foreign-body aspiration or pulmonary embolism. Absence of any cutaneous manifestations (erythema, urticaria and angioedema) argues against the diagnosis, as these are present in over 90% of patients. Elevated blood levels of mast-cell tryptase may help if the diagnosis is in doubt. Serum tryptase peaks at 1 h and remains high up to 5 h after the onset of anaphylaxis.

MANAGEMENT

An assessment should be made of the severity, and reaction classified as mild to moderate, severe or anaphylactic.

Treatment of anaphylaxis

Adrenaline (epinephrine) given subcutaneously or intramuscularly is the first-line

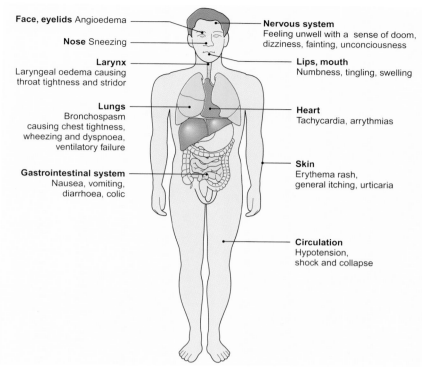

Face, eyelids Angioedema

Nose Sneezing

Larynx
Laryngeal oedema causing throat tightness and stridor

Lungs
Bronchospasm causing chest tightness, wheezing and dyspnoea, ventilatory failure

Gastrointestinal system
Nausea, vomiting, diarrhoea, colic

Nervous system
Feeling unwell with a sense of doom, dizziness, fainting, unconciousness

Lips, mouth
Numbness, tingling, swelling

Heart
Tachycardia, arrythmias

Skin
Erythema rash, general itching, urticaria

Circulation
Hypotension, shock and collapse

Fig. 2 **Anaphylaxis affects most systems and organs in the body.**

therapy. It is the most useful drug to counter the dangerous effects of large amounts of histamine and other mediators released into the bloodstream. Absorption is better through the intramuscular route. The usual dose is 0.3–0.5 ml of 1:1000 solution. The dose can be repeated after 15–30 min if response is not adequate. Early treatment is crucial and may often need to be given outside the hospital setting. However, treatment with adrenaline (epinephrine) should not be relied upon as the complete treatment and medical help should always be sought.

Other therapies include antihistamine such as chlorphenamine (chlorpheniramine) 10 mg i.v., followed by intravenous steroids such as hydrocortisone 100 mg. An assessment should be made of the circulatory status and intravenous fluids are administered (Fig. 3). Treatment of bronchospasm (nebulized bronchodilators) and arrhythmia (antiarrhythmics) may be required. Oxygen may be required for patients with respiratory symptoms and mechanical ventilation instituted for refractory respiratory failure. Standard cardiopulmonary resuscitation should be instituted in case of cardiac or respiratory arrest.

Long-term management

The patient should be referred to an allergy specialist to establish the cause of anaphylaxis and for appropriate advice on management. A detailed history is taken and skin-prick test performed to confirm the IgE-mediated allergy.

It is important that patients are prepared for accidental exposure. Treatment with adrenaline (epinephrine) at the onset of a reaction is effective and patients should be given a syringe loaded with adrenaline (epinephrine), for self-injection, or for use by friends and relatives. This is available in two strengths: for adults, 0.3 ml of 1:1000 solution and for children, 0.3 ml of 1:2000 solution. The dose can be repeated after 15 min if the response is inadequate. Patients and their caregivers should be instructed in the use of these syringes. Children should lead a normal life, and not be stigmatized by their problem. It is also important to stress that the availability of adrenaline (epinephrine) is not a substitute for avoidance.

Treatment of severe allergic reactions

Systemic reactions without life threatening features, such as generalized urticaria and angioedema and bronchospasm may be treated with antihistamine and hydrocortisone while the patient is observed in a medical facility.

Treatment of mild or localized reactions

Reactions confined to skin or oral mucosa such as localized urticaria or swelling and numbness of the lips can be treated with oral antihistamine, and those at risk of recurrent episodes should keep a supply of non-sedating antihistamine.

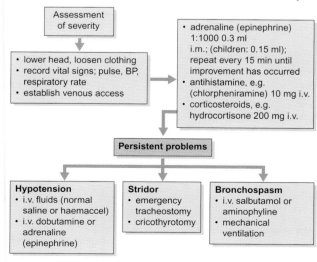

Assessment of severity

- lower head, loosen clothing
- record vital signs; pulse, BP, respiratory rate
- establish venous access

- adrenaline (epinephrine) 1:1000 0.3 ml i.m.; (children: 0.15 ml); repeat every 15 min until improvement has occurred
- antihistamine, e.g. (chlorpheniramine) 10 mg i.v.
- corticosteroids, e.g. hydrocortisone 200 mg i.v.

Persistent problems

Hypotension
- i.v. fluids (normal saline or haemaccel)
- i.v. dobutamine or adrenaline (epinephrine)

Stridor
- emergency tracheostomy
- cricothyrotomy

Bronchospasm
- i.v. salbutamol or aminophyline
- mechanical ventilation

Fig. 3 **Management of anaphylaxis.**

Acute allergic reactions and anaphylaxis

- Acute allergic reactions vary considerably in severity from mild rash to circulatory collapse.
- Severity of reaction depends on patient's sensitivity and the quantity and route of administration of the antigen.
- Foods such as nuts are the commonest cause of anaphylactic reactions.
- Any system or organ may be involved.
- Hypotension, laryngeal oedema and severe bronchospasm are life-threatening features.
- Adrenaline (epinephrine) is the most important drug for anaphylaxis.
- Antihistamine and hydrocortisone are other useful treatments.
- Patients at risk of anaphylaxis should carry self injectable adrenaline (epinephrine).

ACUTE URTICARIA AND ANGIOEDEMA

Urticaria is characterized by the appearance of well-demarcated, erythematous, palpable, itchy lesions with a pale centre (Fig. 1). These lesions are variable in size and shape and may be localized or generalized. They can involve any area of the skin and last for a few hours. Angioedema is the swelling of the subcutaneous or submucosal tissues (Fig. 2). It usually occurs on the face, but occasionally involves the extremities. Swelling of the tongue or larynx may cause respiratory difficulty. Urticaria and angioedema affect approximately 20% of the population at least once in their lifetime.

In acute urticaria and angioedema, the lesions appear quickly (over minutes) and resolve within hours, leaving no trace. One or more episodes may occur but if they continue beyond 6 weeks, it is arbitrarily classified as chronic urticaria. Acute urticaria/angioedema is more common in children and young adults and is often due to IgE-mediated allergy.

PATHOPHYSIOLOGY

The underlying pathophysiology of urticaria is mast-cell activation and degranulation through immunological and non-immunological mechanisms, with the release of histamine and other mediators (Fig. 3). Histamine has a direct effect on H_1-receptors on the blood vessels, causing vascular dilatation and increased vascular permeability with subcutaneous and submucous oedema formation (wheal). It also stimulates cutaneous sensory nerves, causing itching, and the axon reflex generates the flare response.

The histological features are primarily due to the dilatation and engorgement of cutaneous blood vessels and lymphatics with little cellular (eosinophil) infiltrate. This causes extravasation of the fluid with widening of the dermal papillae, flattening of the rete pegs and swelling of the collagen fibres.

DIAGNOSTIC APPROACH

Urticaria and angioedema are frustrating problems for physicians and their patients, as the cause may not be obvious. A thorough history and physical

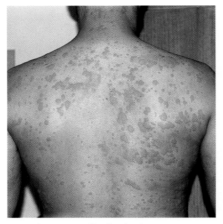

Fig. 1 **Acute generalised urticaria – cause unknown.**

examination may provide clues to the cause. Events immediately before the appearance of urticaria, such as ingestion of a food or drug, an insect-bite or contact with a chemical or irritant, should be carefully explored. No single investigation can determine the cause of acute urticaria and angioedema. However, in the presence of a suggestive history, the demonstration of specific IgE antibodies by skin-prick test or RAST may be helpful. Other tests, such as challenge procedures, patch test and intradermal tests may also be indicated (Fig. 4). Despite careful history and appropriate investigations, the cause remains obscure in nearly 50% of patients.

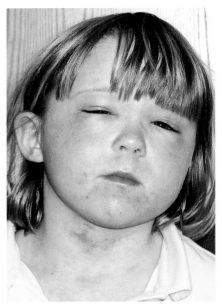

Fig. 2 **Acute allergic reaction with angiodema in a child who reacted to contact with a horse.**

CAUSES

In children, acute viral infections are known to be associated with acute urticaria (Table 1). These episodes improve with the resolution of infection and do not necessarily recur with future viral infections. Acute urticaria and angioedema are also common manifestations during anaphylactic or anaphylactoid reactions. The causes in these situations are similar to those for anaphylaxis and include foods, drugs, latex,

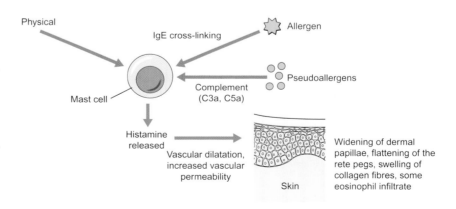

Fig. 3 **Mechanism of autoimmune urticaria/antioedema.** Anti-FcεRI antibody stimulates mast cell receptor directly, while anti-IgE antibody through IgE is bound to mast cell receptors. This results in degranulation with the release of histamine and other mediators.

insect-bite, etc. In some cases, no cause can be found (idiopathic anaphylaxis).

Food allergy is an important cause of acute urticaria and angioedema. The mechanism is usually IgE-mediated type I hypersensitivity reaction. History alone may be diagnostic if a cause and effect relationship can be established, with reactions occurring soon after the ingestion of the food on more than one occasion. Common foods implicated in acute urticaria and angioedema are milk, egg, fish, nuts and fruits. If in doubt, an oral food challenge or standard elimination procedure for suspected allergy to food or food additives may be helpful. This should only be done under appropriate medical supervision. A positive skin-prick test to a food such as egg or peanut supports the diagnosis only in the presence of a suggestive history, whereas a negative skin test makes IgE-mediated allergy highly unlikely.

Drugs are another important cause of acute urticaria and angioedema (Table 2). Antibiotics and cyclo-oxygenase inhibitors, such as aspirin and other non-steroid anti-inflammatory drugs (NSAIDs), are common offenders. However, a number of drugs including diuretics, antihypertensives, tranquilizers and muscle relaxants may produce the reaction. Drug-induced urticaria is usually IgE-mediated, but some drugs may act directly on mast cells. These include morphine, codeine and radiocontrast media. Urticaria and angioedema due to aspirin and NSAIDs may result from an imbalance between prostaglandins and leukotrienes. Angioedema due to angiotensin-converting enzyme inhibitors is probably mediated by bradykinin which accumulates as a

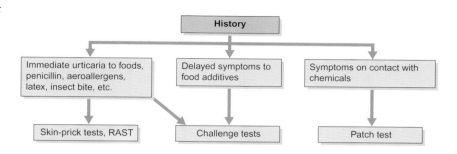

Fig. 4 **Approach to diagnosis in a patient with acute urticaria or angioedema.**

Table 1 **Causes of acute urticaria / angioedema**

Cause	Examples
Foods	Milk, egg, nuts, seafood, fruits such as strawberry, spices
Drugs	Antibiotics, aspirin, NSAIDs, ACE inhibitors
Viral infections	
Insect stings	Bee, wasp
Allergen immunotherapy	Pollen or dust mite allergen extract
Others	Latex, blood products, radiocontrast media
Idiopathic	

result of decreased degradation. Rarely, egg-containing vaccines may cause acute reactions in egg-allergic patients.

Allergy to inhaled allergen does not usually cause urticaria. However, some patients who are highly sensitive to an aeroallergen, e.g. grass pollen or cat dander, may develop urticaria on direct contact. Allergy to latex can cause urticaria, both on contact with skin, or following inhalation of latex allergen.

TREATMENT

The cause of acute urticaria should be identified and avoided whenever possible. The acute episodes are usually self-limiting. Effects of histamine in the skin can be blocked by H_1 histamine receptor antagonists. The second generation of non-sedating or mildly sedating antihistamines has proved useful in the management of these cases. For prolonged or persistent urticaria or angioedema, a short course of oral steroid can be used in addition to antihistamines. The extended use of systemic corticosteroids should be avoided because of significant adverse effects. If there are life-threatening features such as laryngeal oedema or anaphylaxis, adrenaline (epinephrine) should be given. However, adrenaline (epinephrine) should be used with extreme care in elderly subjects due to the possibility of concomitant ischaemic heart disease.

Table 2 **Drugs commonly implicated in urticaria and angioedema**

Type of drug	Examples
Antibiotics	Penicillin, cephalosporins, sulphonamide, tetracyclines
Cyclo-oxygenase inhibitors	Aspirin, NSAIDs (e.g. ibuprofen)
Anti-hypertensives	ACE inhibitors, β-blockers, diuretics
Opiates	Morphine, codeine
Non-prescription medicines	Vitamins, cold remedies
Chemotherapeutic agents	Doxorubicin, bleomycin
Psychotropics	Sedatives, tranquilizers
Immunotherapy allergen extracts	Pollen, house-dust mite, insect venom
Vaccines	DPT

Acute urticaria and angiodema

- Urticaria is characterized by palpable, itchy lesions of variable size and shape.
- Mast cell degranulation, with the release of histamine and other mediators, is the primary event in urticaria and angioedema.
- Acute urticaria and angioedema is commonly due to IgE-mediated allergy.
- A detailed history may provide clues to the underlying cause.
- Food and drugs are common causes.
- Treatment should be with non-sedating antihistamines with or without a short course of oral steroids.
- Lingual or laryngeal swelling may cause respiratory difficulty and require treatment with adrenaline (epinephrine).

CHRONIC URTICARIA AND ANGIOEDEMA 1 – AETIOLOGY AND PATHOPHYSIOLOGY

Chronic recurrent urticaria is defined as frequent episodes of urticarial rash (nettle rash or hives) which continues for more than 6 weeks. The rash itself is indistinguishable from the lesions seen in acute urticaria (erythematous, itchy wheals) but individual lesions may persist for longer than 12 h. Angioedema is the swelling of the subcutaneous or submucosal tissues primarily affecting face, lips and tongue. Angioedema occurs with chronic urticaria in nearly half of patients, although occasionally it may occur alone. Angioedema associated with chronic urticaria is rarely life-threatening. Chronic urticaria and angioedema is more common in adults than in children. Contrary to popular belief, most patients with chronic urticaria are not allergic to a foreign substance. The disease is usually self-limiting and follows a remitting and relapsing course for a variable period from months to years. Infections, drugs, stress or menstrual cycle may trigger a relapse.

PATHOPHYSIOLOGY

The skin mast cells play a central role in chronic urticaria and angioedema, with the release of histamine and other mediators. Histamine is the most important mediator in all forms of urticaria. However, other mast cell mediators such as leukotrienes may be involved. Histamine causes itching and increased vascular permeability, which produces localized wheals. Other inflammatory cells, including lymphocytes, eosinophils and neutrophils are also involved. Neutrophils accumulate early in the evolution of a wheal, but eosinophil activation may be more persistent.

It is likely that there is an autoimmune basis for up to 30% of patients with idiopathic urticaria. In these patients, autoantibodies, of the IgG type, against the high-affinity IgE receptor (FcεRI) or occasionally to IgE, or both, are found. This functional autoantibody causes activation of mast cells and basophils via FcεRI, directly or through IgE, inducing the development of wheals (Fig. 1). Autoantibody-positive and -negative patients are clinically indistinguishable except that the presence of autoantibodies indicates a more severe disease.

CAUSES

Chronic urticaria and angioedema can result from multiple causes, although in most patients (60%) the cause remains obscure (idiopathic urticaria) (Fig. 2). Many of the causes are the same as those of acute urticaria. Indeed, if acute urticarial episodes continue for longer than 6 weeks, by definition, it becomes chronic urticaria. A number of factors have been identified including intolerance to food, adverse reactions to drugs, autoimmune disease, physical factors, contact with chemicals and some infections such as *Helicobacter pylori* (Table 1).

Table 1 Causes of chronic urticaria and angioedema

- Idiopathic
- Physical
- Cholinergic
- Autoimmune
- Urticaria vasculitis (associated with other autoimmune diseaes, e.g. SLE)
- Foods and food additives
- Drugs (NSAIDs, ACE inhibitors)
- Contact with chemicals
- Infections (viral, parasitic, *Helicobacter pylori*)
- Malignancy (e.g. lymphoma)
- Aeroallergens
- Hereditary angioedema (C1 esterase deficiency)

Table 2 Types of physical urticaria

- Dermographism
- Delayed pressure urticaria
- Cholinergic urticaria
- Heat urticaria
- Solar urticaria
- Cold urticaria
- Aquagenic urticaria

Physical factors

Patients with urticaria caused by physical agents account for roughly one-fifth of all cases. There are several different types of physical urticaria (Table 2). In dermographism, stroking the skin firmly produces a wheal, but in delayed pressure urticaria, the wheal appears on sites of prolonged pressure, such as the buttocks. Cholinergic urticaria takes the form of a widespread rash following exercise, emotion or heat, with excessive stimulation of cholinergic nerves. Exposure to water (aquagenic urticaria), sun (solar urticaria) and cold (cold urticaria) are other examples (Fig. 3).

More than one agent may precipitate urticaria in a given individual. Urticarial response can be easily reproduced in the sensitive patient and generally lasts less than 1 h. Systemic features such as flushing, dizziness, headaches, and even hypotension may occur during severe episodes. Identification of the causative physical agent is necessary for effective avoidance.

Foods

Food additives may be the cause of chronic urticaria in 10–20% of patients. In children, preservatives such as benzoates and colouring agents (e.g. azodyes) play a more important role than in adult patients, where naturally occurring

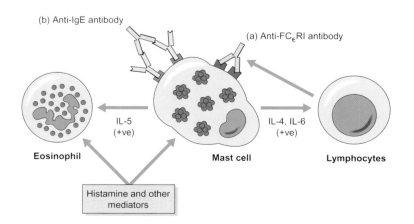

Fig. 1 **Mechanism of the development of autoimmune urticaria and angioedema.**

pseudoallergens in fruits and vegetables (e.g. salicylate) are mainly responsible. IgE-mediated food allergy (e.g. to fish and nuts) rarely causes chronic urticaria. It may occur in an occasional patient with multiple food hypersensitivity when inadvertent exposures occur frequently despite attempts at avoidance.

Drugs

In some patients, drugs (such as aspirin, quinine, opiates and chlortetracycline) degranulate mast cells directly.

Contact chemicals

The wheal occurs at the site of contact, such as the face for cosmetics and hands for detergents. A number of chemicals are implicated, including plants, cosmetics, household goods and industrial chemicals. On patch tests, the presence of contact urticaria increases the likelihood of a delayed reaction to the same allergen.

Vasculitis

The rash is similar to chronic idiopathic urticaria, though the individual lesions may last longer and leave residual scarring. Urticaria vasculitis should be suspected when systemic features (arthralgia, fever, nephritis, etc.) are present and response to antihistamine is poor. Acute-phase proteins are raised and antibodies to nucleus or its components may be present. If there is suspicion, the lesion should be biopsied to reveal evidence of vasculitis. These patients need full investigation for autoimmune diseases, such as lupus erythematosus, and require treatment with colchicin or oral steroids.

C1 esterase inhibitor deficiency

This diagnosis should be suspected when angioedema occurs without urticaria. The disorder is characterized by a deficiency in C1 esterase inhibitor (C1 INH). The deficiency can be caused by impaired synthesis due to a genetic defect, or acquired due to increased degradation from autoantibodies to C1 INH. People deficient in C1-INH present with recurrent angioedema without urticaria. Although rare, hereditary angioedema is a potentially life-threatening disorder. Bradykinin is believed to be the main mediator of symptoms. Activation of coagulation leads to the generation of thrombin whose vasoactive effect can thus influence oedema formation.

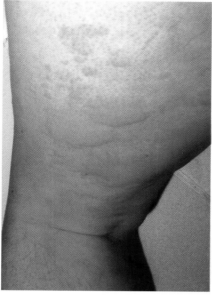

Fig 2 **Chronic idiopathic urticaria in an adult.**

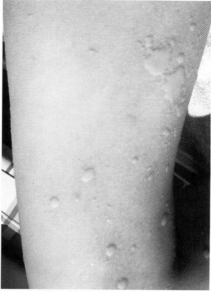

Fig 3 **Cold urticaria in a young woman.**

Manifestations include gastrointestinal, subcutaneous, and respiratory oedema. Factors that trigger episodes vary. Symptoms typically last 48–72 h, but they can last from hours to days.

Idiopathic anaphylaxis

Idiopathic anaphylaxis is a disease where no identifiable antigen initiates an anaphylactoid reaction. Idiopathic anaphylaxis can present at any age. Patients usually present with urticaria, angioedema, or generalized flushing. Respiratory difficulty due to wheezing or angioedema may occur and this can be life-threatening.

Mastocytosis

Mastocytosis is a rare chronic disorder characterized by an excessive number of apparently normal mast cells in the skin, and occasionally in other organs. Clinical presentation varies from a pruritic rash to unexplained collapse and sudden death. Patients with mastocytosis often have a long history of chronic and acute symptoms that were unrecognized. The disease shows slow progression, and malignant transformation is rare.

Characteristic skin lesions, urticaria pigmentosa, are brownish-red macules, distinct from chronic urticarial rash, that appear on the trunk and spread symmetrically. Other skin manifestations include generalized pruritus, wheal formation and recurrent flushing episodes. Skin lesions may or may not accompany systemic mastocytosis. Systemic disease may involve the gastrointestinal tract, the bone marrow (anaemia, thrombocytopenia) or other organs. When the disease is suspected, skin biopsy should confirm the diagnosis.

Chronic urticaria and angioedema – Aetiology and pathophysiology

- Chronic urticaria is defined as frequent episodes of itchy wheals which continue for longer than 6 weeks.
- Angioedema associated with chronic urticaria is rarely life-threatening.
- In approximately 80% of patients, the cause remains unknown (idiopathic urticaria). Half of these may be due to physical factors (physical urticaria) or autoantibodies (autoimmune urticaria).
- Common causes include food additives, drugs and chemicals.
- Rare causes include vasculitis, C1 esterase inhibitor deficiency and masteocytosis.
- Chronic urticaria is rarely due to IgE-mediated allergy.
- Histamine is the primary mediator but others such as bradykinin and prostaglandins may be involved.

CHRONIC URTICARIA AND ANGIOEDEMA 2 – MANAGEMENT

Patients with chronic idiopathic urticaria suffer moderate to severe impairment of quality-of-life, as assessed by standardized questionnaires. It should be realized by the physician and, emphasized to the patient, that a cause is not found in the great majority of cases. This does not mean that a cause should not be looked for, as detection and removal of the cause can be extremely rewarding. However, an extensive battery of investigations is unlikely to yield useful information. As in many disciplines in medicine, a careful history is the most important first step that determines the need and type of investigation required. Physical examination may confirm the diagnosis if the rash is present at the time of consultation. It may also give clues to any underlying disease such as lymphoma, thyroid disease or connective tissue disorders.

DIAGNOSTIC APPROACH

If the history clearly indicates physical urticaria such as dermographism, cold or heat urticaria, further investigations are unrewarding (Fig. 1). A simple challenge test should establish these diagnoses; stroking or scratching the skin (dermographism) or placing an ice cube on the skin (cold urticaria) results in wheal formation. If the history indicates food additives as a possible cause, an oral provocation test, preferably double-blind (DBPCFC) should be arranged. If facilities for food challenge do not exist, a diet free of additives and salicylates may be tried for a period of 4–6 weeks. If significant improvement occurs on avoidance, and symptoms recur on reintroduction, the diet should be prescribed for an extended period (6–12 months). If a drug is suspected, discontinuation of the drug should lead to amelioration of the symptoms. When the history is suggestive of contact urticaria, a patch test with the substance is recommended to confirm the diagnosis. In contrast to acute urticaria, food allergy rarely causes chronic urticaria, except in an occasional patient with multiple hypersensitivity to foods, which they cannot avoid completely. In these patients, and in those with a history of contact allergy to

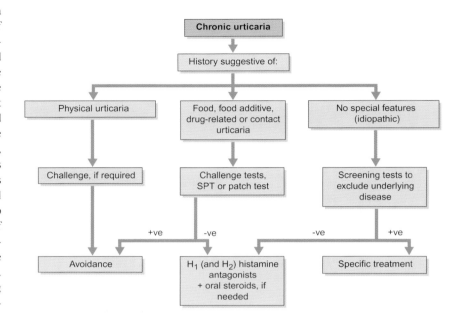

Fig 1. **Flow-chart for the management of chronic recurrent urticaria.**

animal saliva or dander, skin-prick test or RAST for specific IgE may yield useful information, avoiding the need for provocation tests.

If no triggers are identified on history, a complete physical examination and a few screening blood tests (to exclude underlying disease) should be performed (Fig. 2). This may reveal the possibility of malignancy or connective-tissue disease. Further investigations are directed towards establishing the underlying cause if an abnormality is detected on examination or screening blood tests. Skin biopsy should be considered if there is evidence of an underlying cause, or the response to standard treatment is poor, to look at the types of inflammation present (lymphocyte or neutrophil predominance) or evidence of vasculitis or mastocytosis.

TREATMENT
Non-specific
Patients are often in considerable distress with pruritus and uncomfortable lesions. Itching is worse in warm conditions. A cooler temperature at night helps. Emollients, such as aqueous cream, may

reduce itching. Patients should be reassured that there is no permanent damage to the skin or other organs and the condition usually resolves spontaneously (Table 1).

Avoidance
If a cause (including a physical factor) has been identified, advice on avoidance should be given with a verbal, and preferably written, explanation. For patients with intolerance to food additives (benzoate, azodyes) and salicylates, a handout listing common foods containing these chemicals, prepared and monthly updated by a dietitian, is extremely helpful. Once identified, drugs and contact allergens are relatively easy to avoid.

Suppression
In the majority of patients, no causative factor can be identified, despite a thorough history and appropriate investigations (idiopathic, including autoimmune urticaria). In these patients, the mainstay of treatment is to suppress the disease with regular oral antihistamines (H$_1$ antagonists) while awaiting spontaneous resolution, which happens in the majority

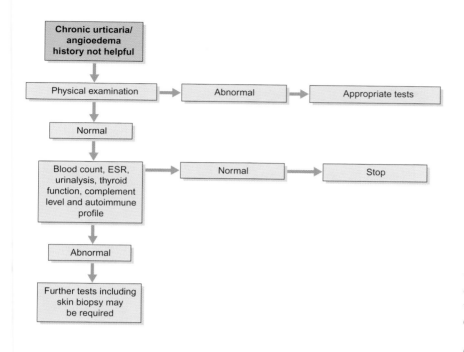

Fig. 2 **Algorithm for investigating patients with chronic urticaria without any specific triggers in history.**

Table 1 **Management points**

- The fact that a patient has used a food or drug before, without adverse effects, does not exclude it as a cause of urticaria, as sensitization may occur after repeated use
- Infections, stress and drugs, such as aspirin, are common triggers and should be avoided
- Physical urticaria may coexist with chronic idiopathic urticaria
- Avoid tight fitting clothes, belts, shoes, etc.
- Chronic urticaria of more than 6 months duration is less likely to resolve spontaneously
- Avoid antihistamine in pregnancy, as safety records are lacking but if essential, use chlorphenamine (chlorpheniramine) as the drug with the best safety record
- An underlying disease should be looked for if the response to antihistamine is poor
- Biopsy of the lesion may help in deciding appropriate treatment in difficult cases

of patients within 2–3 years. Antihistamines are also useful in those where the causative factor cannot be avoided completely (e.g. physical urticaria). In these patients, antihistamines can be used regularly or as needed, depending on the frequency of episodes.

The second generation, non-sedative antihistamines are preferred for their reduced side-effects. There is not much to choose between them, though patients vary in their response and sometimes a change is required to suit an individual. Loratadine or cetirizine, both 10 mg once a day, are used commonly. If the response is inadequate, an H_2-antagonist (e.g. ranitidine 150 mg twice a day) may be added. Some patients respond better to the addition of ketotifen with its antihistaminic and anti-inflammatory properties. If nocturnal itching remains a significant problem, a sedative antihistamine, such as chlophenamine (chlorpheniramine) 4 mg or the antidepressant doxepin, given at night, has been shown to be useful. Oral steroids should generally be avoided, however they may be given at a short course, such as prednisolone 30 mg daily for a maximum of 3 weeks, to treat a severe relapse. Very rarely, long-term steroid treatment is required for resistant disease. The dose should be kept to a minimum, and steroid-sparing agents, such as ciclosporin, may be considered.

In difficult cases, not responding to standard treatment, a biopsy may be helpful. If there is evidence of vasculitis, steroid or other specific treatment may be required. In a minority of patients where biopsy shows neutrophil as opposed to lymphocyte predominance, drugs such as colchicine or dapsone may be helpful. Severely affected patients with autoimmune urticaria can be treated with plasmapheresis, intravenous immunoglobulin or ciclosporin. Both the diagnosis and treatment in these cases require special expertise.

C1 esterase inhibitor deficiency

Treatment includes prophylactic therapy with attenuated androgens such as stanozolol. These can stimulate the production of C1 INH. Side-effects include hirsutism, weight gain and coagulation defects. Acute episodes can be medical emergencies, and airway management should be a priority. The treatment of choice in an acute episode is administration of plasma concentrate of C1 INH, although patients with an acquired defect frequently need very high doses.

Mastocytosis

Drug therapy is initiated to reduce the severity of the attacks and to block the action of inflammatory mediators. The mainstay of therapy is histamine H_1 and H_2 blockers and the avoidance of triggering factors.

Chronic urticaria and angioedema – Management

- Patients are often in considerable distress and their quality of life is affected.
- The diagnostic approach depends on history and stepwise management.
- The cause should be established with challenge tests, when required.
- A large battery of routine or screening investigation does not yield useful information.
- Avoid cause (if identified) and triggers.
- Oral antihistamine (H_1 antagonists) remains the mainstay of treatment.
- Add H_2 antagonists, if needed.
- Use oral steroids only as a short course, if possible.
- Ciclosporin, i.v. immunoglobulin and plasmapheresis may rarely be required.
- Be optimistic, majority of chronic idiopathic urticaria resolve spontaneously.

INSECT ALLERGY

Allergy to stinging insects such as the honeybee, wasp, hornet, yellow jacket and fire-ant may cause severe allergic reactions including anaphylaxis. Bee allergy is mostly seen in beekeepers and their families, whereas wasp allergy is commoner among the general population. Allergy to bee and wasp occurs in most parts of the world.

PREVALENCE

Insect stings account for nearly a quarter of cases of severe systemic anaphylaxis referred to in an allergy clinic. In the USA at least 40 deaths are reported every year due to insect allergy, in addition to others which may have gone unrecognized. A positive skin test or specific IgE to insect venom may be present in 15% of an unselected population, but most such individuals have had no systemic reactions to stings. The clinical significance of this sensitivity is uncertain, although the risk of a systemic reaction may be higher in these subjects. Allergy to insect sting takes a variable course and often improves with time (Table 1).

Bee and wasp venoms are antigenically different and there is little cross-reactivity. Sensitization to bee allergen usually requires several stings, whereas sensitization to wasp can occur after a few or a single sting. The reasons why severe allergic reactions to bee and wasp stings develop in only a small number of exposed individuals are not completely understood, but differences in T cell responses to venom antigens are likely to be important. Bee venom-specific IgG correlates directly with the degree of exposure to bee venom.

CLINICAL FEATURES

Localized reaction, consisting of erythema and wheal formation is not uncommon in non-allergic subjects after insect sting. Those with allergy to an insect respond more aggressively with either a large local or systemic reaction. A large local reaction usually develops over the next few hours. This consists of widespread erythema, spreading from the site of sting, and oedema of the subcutaneous tissue of varying size. A whole limb may be swollen and in extreme cases blister formation and infection may occur. If the site of sting is the lips, tongue or inside of the mouth, life-threatening laryngeal oedema may occur.

Systemic reaction usually starts within 10 min of a sting. During a systemic reaction, organs and systems distant from the site of sting may be involved. The severity varies, but it may include generalized pruritis, urticaria and angioedema, dyspnoea due to laryngeal oedema or bronchospasm, hypotension and collapse.

RISK FACTORS

Beekeepers are at risk of repeated stings and often become sensitized, with a higher risk of reaction on subsequent stings. Allergic beekeepers show higher levels of bee venom-specific

Table 1 **Characteristics of allergy to insect sting**

- Presence of a skin test reaction or specific IgE to insect venom does not necessarily indicate a clinical reaction on future sting
- Severity of the reaction depends on the patient's sensitivity, amount of venom injected and the site of sting
- Severity of reaction does not correlate well with the size of skin-test reaction or the level of specific IgE. However, no allergic reaction can occur if skin test is negative and specific IgE is not detected
- The likelihood of a reaction on subsequent sting generally decreases with each passing year, however, in a particular patient it is difficult to predict the outcome
- There is little cross-reactivity between bee and wasp-venom allergy

serum IgG, lower skin sensitivity, and lower levels of bee venom-specific serum IgE, than other bee venom-allergic patients. It is not possible to accurately predict the type of reaction on subsequent stings but some risk factors have been identified (Table 2).

DIAGNOSIS

Diagnosis is based primarily on the history. Large local reactions should be distinguished from systemic allergic reactions. Positive venom skin tests, or the detection of venom-specific IgE antibodies confirm the diagnosis and are helpful in identification of the responsible insect. Skin tests are more reliable than the measurement of specific IgE. Skin-prick tests are routinely done, but if the test is negative, some authorities recommend intracutaneous test with up to 1.0 mg/ml concentration of venom, before skin test is regarded as negative. In many cases, the patient is unable to identify the offending insect accurately, and therefore skin tests should be performed for the venom of wasp, honeybee and hornet. Challenge testing (deliberate insect sting or injection of pure venom) is not required for the diagnosis.

MANAGEMENT OF ACUTE REACTIONS

A large local reaction may be treated with oral or parenteral antihistamine depending on the severity (Table 3). The treatment needs to be continued for several days, and occasionally a short course of oral steroid may be needed. The treatment of a systemic allergic reaction is similar to that of other causes (e.g. drugs or nuts) of acute allergic reaction. Life-threatening features (laryngeal oedema, severe bronchospasm or hypotension) require intramuscular adrenaline (epinephrine).

FURTHER MANAGEMENT

Precautions can be taken to reduce the risk of future stings. Appropriate clothing and footwear should be worn when working outside or walking in the countryside, and plants and areas which attract these insects should be avoided. All patients should be given antihistamines. Those with a generalized reaction should also be given self-injectable adrenaline in a

Table 2 **Risk factors for a severe or systemic reaction**

- History of previous systemic reaction
- Beekeepers; the risk is higher for new beekeepers and those who develop nasal or respiratory symptoms while working at hives
- A history of atopy
- The pre-season presence of high concentrations (> 1.0 kU/L) of venom-specific IgE
- Short time of onset of reaction after stinging (< 30 min)
- High number of prior stings (> 3)
- Age (> 18 years)

pre-loaded syringe. Education and training in self-administration is crucial. A large local or mild generalized reaction can be treated with oral antihistamine immediately after the sting. If the response is not adequate, or systemic features appear, adrenaline (epinephrine) should be given and medical advice sought.

IMMUNOTHERAPY

The indication for immunotherapy depends on clinical symptoms, in vivo and in vitro testing and risk of re-sting. Patients with a history of moderate to severe systemic allergic reaction should be offered venom-specific immunotherapy (Fig. 1). In these patients the risk of a systemic reaction on subsequent sting is reduced from 60% to <5% following successful immunotherapy. The presence of venom specific IgE must be demonstrated with a positive skin test before commencing immunotherapy. Various regimens are recommended. Conventionally, gradually increasing doses of venom extracts are given at weekly intervals, beginning with 0.1 mg, to reach the maintenance dose of 100 mg (equivalent to two stings). This dose is then injected at monthly intervals for approximately 3 years. There is a 10% risk of reaction during immunotherapy and this treatment should only be given at specialized centres with experience, and where facilities for resuscitation are at hand. Several shorter regimens, reaching the maintenance dose in hours, days or weeks (rush immunotherapy) have been shown to be effective, although the risk of reaction is higher.

Venom immunotherapy is equally effective in beekeepers who tolerate it better than other bee-allergic patients. The majority of allergic beekeepers can continue bee keeping successfully under the protection of venom immunotherapy.

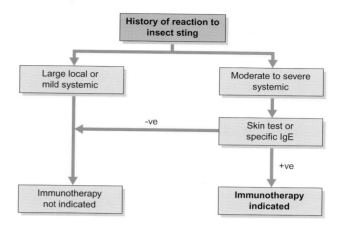

Fig. 1 **Indications for venom-specific immunotherapy.**

Discontinuation of venom immunotherapy appears to be safe if venom-specific antibodies can no longer be detected. For the remaining patients, a treatment period of 3–5 years may suffice. The residual risk of a systemic reaction is 5–10%. Risk factors may include history of a systemic reaction during venom immunotherapy, persistent strongly positive skin test sensitivity, and the severity of the pre-treatment reaction. After discontinuation of immunotherapy, a clinical sting challenge can be considered to estimate the likelihood of reaction on future stings. However, this is rarely needed in clinical practice.

Table 3 **Immediate management of reaction to insect sting**

Type of reaction	Features	Treatment
Large local	Itching, erythema and oedema of the area of sting	Oral antihistamine ± oral steroids for 3–7 days
Mild systemic	Generalized urticaria/angioedema	Oral or parenteral antihistamine
Moderate systemic	Urticaria, angioedema, bronchospasm	Parenteral antihistamine and hydrocortisone, inhaled bronchodilator
Severe systemic	Laryngeal oedema, severe bronchospasm, hypotension, loss of consciousness	Intramuscular adrenaline (epinephrine), parenteral antihistamine and hydrocortisone, IV fluids, intubation and ventilation if required

Insect allergy

- Insects responsible for allergic reactions include bees, wasps, yellow jackets, hornets and fire-ants.
- Most insect stings produce local reactions including erythema, swelling, itching and pain.
- Those allergic to a particular insect's venom may react with large local or mild to severe systemic reactions (urticaria, angioedema, bronchospasm, laryngeal oedema and hypotension).
- Children are at lower risk of systemic reaction than adults.
- At least 40 deaths due to insect allergy are reported each year in the USA.
- Individuals with a history of systemic reaction are at increased risk.
- Skin test to venom extracts is useful in evaluating allergy to stinging insects.
- All patients with a history of reaction should be given antihistamine for 'as required' use.
- Those with a history of systemic reaction should be given self-injectable adrenaline (epinephrine) and immunotherapy should be considered.
- Venom-specific immunotherapy is an effective form of treatment for individuals at risk of insect-sting anaphylaxis.

DRUG ALLERGY 1 – GENERAL PRINCIPLES

INTRODUCTION

An adverse reaction to drugs is any unwanted effect of medication (Table1). Patients often consider drug allergy to be synonymous with adverse reaction. Drug allergy is an adverse reaction resulting from an immunological response to the drug or its metabolites, and accounts for approximately 10% of all reactions. These reactions result in predictable patterns of organ-specific or systemic manifestations that usually recur on subsequent exposure to the same drug.

Allergic reactions can be life-threatening and are avoidable in most cases. Risk factors for allergic drug reactions include age, type of drug, degree of exposure, and route of administration. Around 10–15% of patients report drug allergies, but self-reporting is much higher than confirmed reactions, which occur in 1–3% of hospitalized patients.

MECHANISMS

Drugs are usually low-molecular-weight substances unable to stimulate the immune system per se. To be recognized by the immune system, the drug or its metabolites have to combine with a protein molecule to form a drug–protein complex (drug combined in this fashion is called hapten). Initial exposure leads to sensitization, with the production of specific IgE antibodies or T memory cells. Subsequent exposure may cause a clinical reaction (Fig. 1).

Allergy to a drug may be due to any of the four types of immune reaction (Table 2). Many drugs can cause direct release

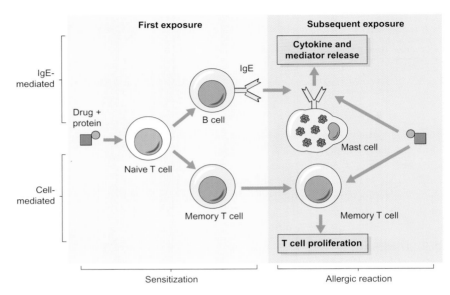

First exposure   **Subsequent exposure**

Fig. 1 **Mechanism of drug allergy.** Drug combines with large protein molecules (hapten) to stimulate either IgE response (immediate hypersensitivity), or T lymphocyte response (delayed hypersensitivity).

of histamine and other mediators from mast cells. In many instances however, the exact mechanism remains obscure. Sometimes, the clinical manifestations are those of allergy, though evidence for involvement of the immune system is lacking (pseudoallergy or allergy-like reaction).

DIAGNOSIS

The problems in identifying and managing drug allergy are myriad, primarily because of the number of possible agents involved, the lack of objective diagnostic methods, and the varied signs and symptoms that may occur. Diagnosis of an adverse reaction and identification of its cause require an

index of suspicion, knowledge of common reactions to drugs, and appropriate investigations, including skin test and challenge with the suspected drug.

History

A systematic approach should be adopted in the evaluation of patients with drug allergy. A detailed history should be obtained and a physical examination should be performed. The physician must determine if the reaction demonstrates features common to immunologic reaction (Table 3). A maculopapular or urticarial rash is more likely to be due to an allergic reaction to drugs than, for

Table 1 **Types of adverse reactions to drugs**

Toxic	Excessive pharmacological effect (over-dose)
Side-effects	Undesirable pharmacological effects
Intolerance	Lowered threshold to pharmacological effects
Idiosyncrasies	Metabolic and enzyme deficiency
Drug allergy	Immunologically mediated adverse reactions to drugs
Allergy-like reactions (pseudo allergic)	Symptoms of adverse reaction suggestive of allergy, such as rash or angioedema, with uncertain pathogenesis

Table 2 **Immunopathological classification of drug allergic reactions**

Type of immune reaction	Example	Clinical features
Immediate hypersensitivity	β-lactam antibiotics, insulin	Anaphylaxis, urticaria, angioedema
Cytotoxic antibodies	Methyldopa	Haemolytic anaemia, thrombocytopenia
Immune complex	Antilymphocytic globulin	Serum sickness, vasculitis
Delayed hypersensitivity	Steroid creams and ointments	Contact dermatitis
Pseudoallergic	Radiocontrast media, aspirin	Rash, anaphylaxis, bronchospasm

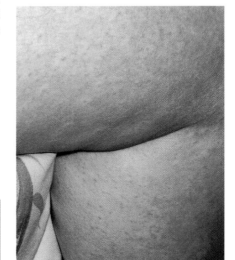

Fig. 2 **Cutaneous manifestation of drug allergy, a typical maculopapular rash.**

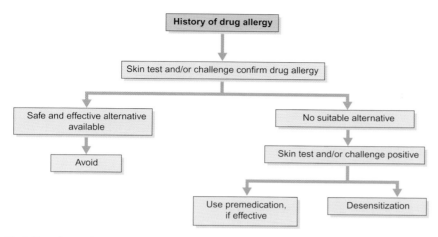

Fig. 3 **Flow diagram for the management of drug allergy.**

Table 3 **Clinical manifestations of drug allergic reactions**

Organ/system	Manifestations
Systemic	Anaphylactic (laryngeal oedema, hypotension, shock), fever, vasculitis, lymphadenopathy, serum sickness
Skin	Urticaria, angioedema, maculopapular rash, pruritis, dermatitis (contact, photosensitivity, exfoliative), erythema multiforme and Stevens–Johnson syndrome, fixed drug eruptions, toxic epidermal necrolysis
Lung	Bronchospasm, alveolitis, fibrosis
Hepatic	Hepatocellular damage, cholestasis
Renal	Interstitial and glomerulonephritis, nephrotic syndrome
Blood	Thrombocytopenia, haemolytic anaemia and neutropenia

example, nausea or headache (Fig. 2). The temporal relationship of exposure to drug and the development of symptoms should also be established. Other important information includes medication usage, previous drug exposure, current illnesses and family and personal history of drug allergy. Atopics are not at increased risk of having drug allergy. However, the reaction may be more severe or anaphylactic in these patients.

Skin tests

Skin tests are used widely in the evaluation of drug allergy. However, apart from the penicillin group of antibiotics, appropriate reagents containing most antigenic determinants are not available. Therefore, the test often takes the form of an intradermal provocation test with the suspected drug. For safety, a skin-prick test should always be performed first. If negative, gradually increasing doses of the drug may be given intradermally at specified intervals and the response carefully monitored. Patch test may be useful in some patients with cutaneous reactions.

In vitro tests

Measurement of specific IgE with radioallergosorbent test (RAST) may be helpful in some cases of drug allergy such as penicillin and insulin. However, both false-positive and false-negative reactions may occur and these are less reliable than skin tests. Measurement of specific IgG and IgM antibodies may be helpful in some drug-induced thrombocytopenia, agranulocytosis and haemolytic anaemia. Assays of basophil histamine release on exposure to specific drug antigen correlate with skin test, but these are cumbersome to perform. The measurement of mediators such as histamine and tryptase in blood, or their metabolites in urine, is occasionally needed to elucidate the nature of the allergic reaction (high levels indicate mast cell/basophil degranulation).

Challenges

Both oral and parenteral challenges are performed depending on the type of drug and the intended use. Initially, a small dose is given with 5–10-fold increases. The interval between doses depends on the rate of absorption and the type of allergic reaction. Protocols have been devised for common drugs requiring challenge, such as β-lactam antibiotics.

MANAGEMENT

In the absence of quick and reliable tests, consideration should be given to use a safe and effective alternative if there is a history of allergy to a particular drug (Fig. 3). If there is no suitable alternative, the allergy should be confirmed with skin test and/or challenge. If allergy to the drug is confirmed, the benefit and risk of using the drug either with pre-medication (e.g. radiocontrast media) or after desensitization (e.g. penicillin) should be carefully evaluated.

Desensitization protocols have been devised for many drugs including penicillin, sulphonamides, insulin and aspirin. Initially, the drug is diluted to 1:10 000 or 1:100 000 and given orally or parenterally. The dose is gradually increased twofold and given every 15–30 min. The full dose can usually be achieved in 6–8 h. Challenge and desensitization are sometimes combined in one procedure, so that if a reaction is observed in the challenge protocol, the increment is slowed to the desensitization level, while carefully watching for any reaction.

Drug allergy – General principles

- Drug allergy is an adverse reaction resulting from an immunological response to a drug or its metabolites.
- Approximately 10% of drug reactions are immunologically mediated.
- Patients often consider drug allergy to be synonymous with adverse reaction.
- Allergy to a drug may be due to any of the four types of immune reaction.
- The exact mechanism of allergic reaction to many drugs remains unknown.
- If there is a history of allergic reaction to a drug, a safe and effective alternative should be considered.
- Allergy skin tests (prick and intradermal) are key to the evaluation of patients with suspected allergic reactions to drugs.
- Oral or parenteral challenge is the only way to confirm or exclude many drug allergies.
- Pre-medication may reduce the risk of reaction in allergy to radiocontrast media.
- Desensitization is possible with many drugs such as the penicillin group of antibiotics, sulphonamides and insulin.

DRUG ALLERGY 2 – COMMON DRUGS

β-LACTAM ANTIBIOTICS

The penicillin group of antibiotics, particularly amoxicillin, is used extensively in clinical practice. It is therefore not surprising that hypersensitivity reactions to β-lactam antibiotics (penicillins and cephalosporins), are the most common allergic reaction to drugs. These antibiotics have a common β-lactam ring, the side-chain structure being specific to each antibiotic. The vast majority of reactions (> 90%) are due to antibodies against the β-lactam ring and hence the cross-reactivity. Rarely, allergy to one but not the other β-lactam antibiotic occurs due to antibodies to side-chains and other unique chemical-ring structures.

The prevalence of allergy to β-lactam antibiotics is reported variously to be 1–8%. Most reactions are mild but severe reactions may occur. Anaphylaxis to this group of antibiotics causes 400–800 deaths annually in the USA. Allergy to β-lactam antibiotics is most commonly an IgE-mediated drug reaction. Other immunological mechanisms have also been described.

Penicillin group

Only 10–20% of patients with a history of allergy to penicillin are proven on tests. Although patients with a history of penicillin allergy are at a higher risk, most severe reactions occur in individuals with no such previous history. Sensitization may have occurred on a previous therapeutic course.

Penicillin is metabolized into penicilloyl (major determinant, 95%) and some minor determinants such as penicilloate and penilloate. Skin tests should be done to major and minor determinants as well as commercially available penicillin G. Skin tests are safe and reliable and preferable to in vitro detection of specific IgE. The probability of reaction during subsequent therapy, following a negative skin test, is less than 5%, and these reactions are usually minor.

Cross-reactivity

Patients with allergy to penicillin are usually sensitized to the β-lactam ring and therefore may react to other β-lactam antibiotics such as other penicillins, cephalosporins, carbapen and monobactam. However, the incidence of reaction varies with each antibiotic. For example, the risk of reaction in a patient with proven allergy to penicillin may only be 10% with cephalosporins.

Diagnosis and management

If there is history of a reaction to β-lactam antibiotics, another group of antibiotic with equivalent efficacy should be used. If

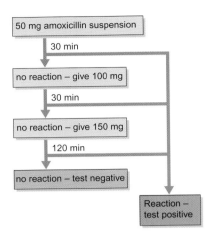

Fig. 2 **Protocol for oral challenge with β-lactam antibiotic – amoxicillin suspension is usually used for ease of administration.** Dose in children is reduced (50% of adult dose in children aged 5 years or over). Dose increment should be more gradual in patients with a history of anaphylaxis.

this is not possible, skin tests should be done to confirm or exclude the presence of allergy (Fig. 1). It should be remembered that patients tend to lose their sensitivity after successful avoidance and those who had a reaction several years ago may not remain allergic. If the previous reaction was doubtful or minor (dermal) in nature and skin tests are negative, it is generally considered safe to use the β-lactam antibiotics. If the reaction was definite with systemic features, oral challenge is required

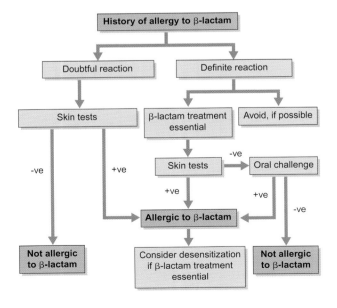

Fig. 1 **Management protocol for allergy to penicillin group of antibiotics.**

Table 1 **Protocol for parenteral penicillin desensitization**

Injection*	Benzylpencillin conc. (U/ml)	Volume (ml)	Route#
1	100	0.1	ID
2		0.2	SC
3		0.4	SC
4		0.8	SC
5	1000	0.1	ID
6		0.3	SC
7		0.6	SC
8	10 000	0.1	ID
9		0.2	SC
10		0.4	SC
11		0.8	SC
12	100 000	0.1	ID
13		0.3	SC
14		0.6	SC
15	1 000 000	0.1	ID
16		0.2	SC
17		0.2	IM
18		0.4	IM
19	1 000 000 U/h	Continuous IV infusion	

*Dose-interval between injections should not be less than 20 min
#ID intradermal; SC subcutanoeus; IM intramuscular; IV intravenous
(adopted from Weiss ME, Adkinson Jr. NF: Immediate hypersensitivity reaction to penicillin and related antibiotics. Clinical Allergy 18: 515, 1988)

Table 2 Allergy-like reactions to aspirin and nonsteroidal anti-inflammatory drugs (NSAIDs)

Reaction	Manifestations	Cross-reactivity*	Possible treatment strategies
Respiratory	Asthma, rhinitis, sinusitis and nasal polyps	Usual	Anti-leukotriene antagonists, desensitization
Skin	Urticaria and angioedema	Usual	Desensitization up to 75 mg asprin
Eyelids	Periorbital oedema	Common	Avoid
Anaphylactoid	Laryngeal oedema, bronchospasm, hypotension	Uncommon	Strictly avoid

*Between aspirin and different NSAIDs

Table 3 Suggested pre-medication before the use of radiocontrast media in high-risk patients

Drugs	Time before procedure
Prednisolone 50 mg orally OR	13 h, 7 h and 1 h
Hydrocortisone 200 mg i.v.	
Diphenhydramine 50 mg i.v.	1 h

Table 4 Some other drugs causing allergic or allergy-like reactions

Drugs	Mechanism	Reaction	Suggested treatment
Streptokinase	IgE-mediated	Anaphylactic reaction	Use tissue plasminogen activator
Insulin	IgE-mediated	Local, anaphylactic	Desensitization
Angiotensin-converting enzyme inhibitors	Pseudoallergy	Cough, angioedema	Avoid
Muscle relaxants such as d-tubocurarine	Both IgE-mediated and non-IgE-mediated	Anaphylactic reaction	Avoid
Corticosteroids	Immediate and delayed hypersensitivity	Rash, anaphylaxis	Use a different corticosteroid

despite negative skin tests (Fig. 2). Drug challenge should only be performed where staff are trained in dealing with any adverse reactions. Challenge should be avoided if the previous reaction was severe anaphylaxis or erythema multiforme.

If the allergy is confirmed, and it is essential to use this group of antibiotics, desensitization may be carried out. Desensitization involves administration of gradually increasing doses of the specific antibiotic (intravenously or orally) until a therapeutic dose is tolerated (Table 1).

A reaction to β-lactam antibiotics should be treated on standard lines, depending on the clinical features and severity. The drug should be discontinued and another group of antibiotics should be substituted. Desensitization remains an option if β-lactam use is essential.

SULPHONAMIDES

Sulphonamides may cause maculopapular or urticarial rash, erythema multiforme, Stevens–Johnson syndrome and toxic epidermal necrolysis. The exact mechanism is not known. There is no test available (apart from challenge) and sulpha drugs should be avoided in patients with a clear history of reaction. In patients with human immunodeficiency virus (HIV) related disease, the drug is valuable in the prophylaxis and treatment of *Pneumocystis carinii* infection. Unfortunately, the risk of reaction is related to the degree of T cell deficiency

and therefore increases many-fold in these patients. Desensitization has been performed successfully in many patients, with gradually increasing doses over several days. However, severe reactions have been induced during desensitization.

NON-STEROIDAL ANTI-INFLAMMATORY DRUGS (NSAIDs)

Allergy-like reactions are common with aspirin and NSAIDs. Cross-reactivity may occur with some types of reactions (Table 2). Aspirin and NSAIDs should be avoided in patients with a history of reaction to aspirin. If aspirin or NSAIDs are essential in a patient with a history of allergy, desensitization may be indicated.

RADIOCONTRAST MEDIA

Intravenous administration of radiocontrast media may produce allergy-like

reactions in 5–10% of an unselected population, and in 30% of those with a previous history of reaction. Most of these reactions are minor, but life-threatening reactions may occur. Others at risk include asthmatics and those on β-blockers. The newer, low-osmoler or non-ionic contrast media is less likely to produce a reaction and should be used in those who are at high risk. Pre-treatment with prednisolone and antihistamine further reduces the likelihood of a reaction in the high-risk group (Table 3).

LOCAL ANAESTHETIC AGENTS

Allergy-like reactions to local anaesthetic agents are reported relatively commonly but are rarely proven. Most reactions are probably toxic (dose-related) pharmacological effects, or due to anxiety. In a patient with presumed allergy to local anaesthetic, skin-prick testing followed by challenge (increasing subcutaneous doses of the suspected agent) is a safe and useful procedure.

OTHER DRUGS

A brief description of some other drugs causing allergic reactions is given in Table 4.

Drug allergy – Common drugs

- Most IgE-mediated allergic reactions to β-lactam antibiotics are directed against the β-lactam ring.
- Skin tests to major and minor determinants are valuable in the diagnosis of penicillin allergy.
- Challenge is the definitive test to confirm or refute allergy to antibiotics.
- Desensitization is possible for both β-lactam and sulpha group of antibiotics.
- Aspirin and NSAIDs may cause allergy-like reactions such as rash, angioedema and asthma and rhinitis.
- Allergy to anaesthetic agents is rarely proven on subcutaneous challenge.
- In patients with a history of reaction to radiocontrast media, pre-medication and use of non-ionic media is recommended.
- A significant number of deaths following reaction to β-lactam antibiotics and radiocontrast media are reported annually.

LATEX ALLERGY

INTRODUCTION

The increased incidence of latex allergy, a potentially life-threatening condition, has been of mounting concern over recent years. Latex allergy has become an important occupational health problem, particularly among healthcare workers. This may be due in part to increased awareness, but the use of latex gloves and other latex products has increased several-fold during the last two decades due to concerns about AIDS and hepatitis.

Rubber products are used in various occupations and household work (Fig. 1). Rubber gloves protect hands from noxious agents and prevent cross-contamination. Most rubber gloves are made of latex from the rubber tree (*Hevea brasiliensis*). Other chemical substances (such as thiurams) are added to the latex in the manufacturing process to act as accelerators, antioxidants and stabilizers.

HISTORICAL PERSPECTIVE

Delayed hypersensitivity to rubber chemicals such as thiuram causing contact eczema has been known for sometime. In 1986, Frosch and co-workers reported that contact urticaria to rubber gloves is due to IgE-mediated allergy. Later in that year, Axelsson and colleagues reported five patients who developed systemic anaphylactic reactions to natural rubber latex (NRL). All were sensitized to NRL on skin-prick tests or radioallergosorbent test (RAST).

PREVALENCE

The prevalence of latex allergy in the general population is approximately 1%. However, in some high-risk populations the prevalence is much higher (Table 1). It is an increasingly important problem in healthcare workers, a group which uses gloves frequently. The prevalence of sensitization ranged, in most studies, from 5–12% and symptoms on exposure to latex were reported in 6–7%.

Children with spina bifida are exposed to latex rubber products frequently with repeated surgical procedures and use of urinary catheters. Approximately half of them are sensitized to latex on skin tests and 25% manifest allergic reaction on exposure.

Predisposing factors to the development of latex allergy include a history of atopy or allergy and frequent exposure to latex products (Table 2).

LATEX ALLERGEN

Identified allergens in natural rubber latex include latex proteins from the rubber tree that remain in manufactured products, as well as smaller molecules that remain from the latex purification and manufacturing process. There are more than 150 polypeptides in natural rubber latex, and 35 or more can act as allergens and are recognized by IgE antibodies in the sera of latex-sensitive subjects. Complete or partial amino-acid sequence data have now been obtained for 20 or more allergens, and have facilitated cloning of genes and development of allergen-specific antibodies.

In latex-sensitive adults, hevein (Hev b6), rubber elongation factor (Hev b1) and Hev b5 are reported as major allergens, while in children with spina bifida, latex particle proteins are important allergens. Latex proteins absorbed to powder in latex surgical and examination gloves may be aerosolized and inhaled. Powder-absorbed latex proteins are thought to be important in causing sensitization in susceptible individuals, as well as triggering symptoms in previously-sensitized patients.

CLINICAL FEATURES

A history of itching, swelling and redness (urticaria) after contact with rubber products such as rubber gloves, balloons and barrier contraceptives, may indicate the possibility of an allergic reaction to latex (Fig. 2). Many patients present with contact eczema of the hands. Clinical effects of latex allergy include local dermal reactions, urticaria, angioedema, rhinoconjunctivitis, bronchial asthma, eczema and potentially life-threatening anaphylactic reactions.

Operating rooms often have a large number of latex-containing products. Respiratory symptoms of latex allergy in healthcare workers have been reported in rooms with a detectable allergen load in the air. Anaphylactic reactions are most

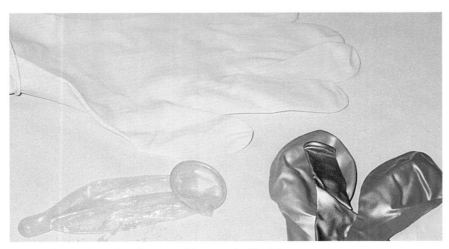

Fig. 1 **(a) Commonly used products containing natural rubber latex.**

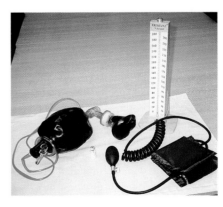

(b) Latex-containing products are regularly used in hospital.

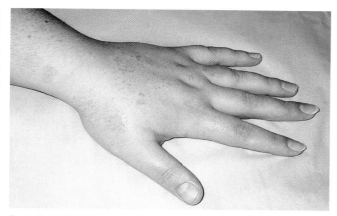

Fig. 2 **Hand urticaria.**

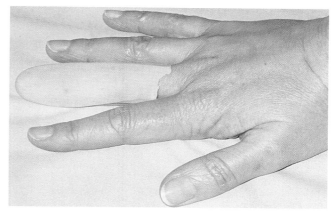

Fig. 3 **Latex glove-finger challenge.**

Table 1 **Prevalence of latex allergy within the medical professions**

Professions	Prevalence
Surgical nurses	28.3%
Surgeons	9.2%
Regular floor nurses	5.8%
Technicians	5.2%
Physicians	4.6%
Laboratory researchers	4.5%
All	6.8%

(*Data from Lai CC, Yan DC, Yu J, Chou CC, Chiang BL, Hsieh KH. Latex allergy in hospital employees. J Formos Med Assoc 1997 Apr 96(4):266–271)

Table 2 **Risk factors for latex allergy**

- Presence of atopic diseases such as hayfever, asthma and dermatitis
- Allergy to foods such as banana, avocado and kiwi fruits
- Healthcare profession
- Patients who had repeated surgical procedures esp. bladder catheterization
- Patients with a history of anaphylaxis of unknown origin
- Female gender

common in the perioperative period, where latex protein may be absorbed directly into the bloodstream of the patient during a surgical procedure. Latex allergy has resulted in progressive asthma and disability of healthcare professionals, with accompanying loss of income caused by their inability to work in their chosen profession.

In latex allergic patients, food allergy may occur from cross-reactivity with antigens in some fruits and vegetables including kiwi, pear, orange, almond, pineapple, apple, tomato and banana.

DIAGNOSTIC METHODS

The diagnostic efficiency of skin test with natural latex extracts is significantly higher than that of latex-specific serum IgE determination. Skin-prick test to latex can be safely performed with natural latex extract, latex extracts obtained from gloves and commercially available extracts. The sensitivity and specificity of the natural latex and commercially available extracts is high (85–90%) but natural latex is not standardized. The sensitivity of latex-specific serum IgE determinations with RAST or immuno-CAP system is 75–80% with variable specificity.

False-negative tests can occur with immunological tests, and in the presence of a suggestive history but a negative skin test, a challenge test is recommended. In the absence of challenge test, a history of at least two episodes of dermal or respiratory symptoms on exposure to latex products is sufficient to make a diagnosis irrespective of the skin-test result.

Challenge tests should always be performed where facilities for resuscitation are available. These tests are not standardized and several different protocols have been suggested. A use-test may be sufficient where there is a history of dermal reaction on direct contact, for example, wearing a glove finger and examining its effect on the skin (Fig. 3). In those with respiratory symptoms, repeated spirometry after shaking the powdered gloves resulting in a drop in FEV_1 of at least 20% would be regarded as a positive challenge.

TREATMENT AND PREVENTION

Treatment consists primarily of avoidance of latex products. Those with latex allergy and children with spina bifida should be provided with a latex-free environment. Wider measures to address latex allergy should include measures to decrease exposure to latex in naïve subjects, to prevent sensitization. These measures may include finding acceptable substitutes for latex in many products. Latex-free gloves and other products are expensive. Eliminating powdered latex gloves from the workplace reduces latex allergen load in the air below the detection limit. This allows personnel sensitized or allergic to latex to be asymptomatic in their work place and reduces the risk of sensitization in others.

Latex allergy is not generally considered to be a major health problem. Education is needed to reduce avoidable morbidity. Other measures include development of latex-free equipment and products and clear labelling of products that contain latex. Methods to reduce antigenicity of latex in the manufacturing process are being investigated.

Latex allergy

- The prevalence of latex allergy has increased in the past decade.
- Allergy to latex could be life-threatening.
- High-risk groups are healthcare workers and those with multiple surgical procedures.
- Powdered latex gloves are important in causing sensitization and symptoms.
- Clinical effects include urticaria, angioedema, eczema, rhinitis, asthma and anaphylaxis.
- Skin test with latex allergen extract is the preferred immunological test.
- If in doubt, the diagnosis can be confirmed by latex allergen challenge.

INDEX

C000098139

Using the *Teach Yourself in 24 Hours* Series

Welcome to the *Teach Yourself in 24 Hours* series! You're probably thinking, "What, they want me to stay up all night and learn this stuff?" Well, no, not exactly. This series introduces a new way to teach you about exciting new products: 24 one-hour lessons, designed to keep your interest and keep you learning. Because the learning process is broken into small units, you will not be overwhelmed by the complexity of some of the new technologies that are emerging in today's market. Each hourly lesson has a number of special items, some old, some new, to help you along.

Minutes

The first 10 minutes of each hour lists the topics and skills that you will learn about by the time you finish the hour. You will know exactly what the hour will bring—with no surprises.

Minutes

Twenty minutes into the lesson, you will have been introduced to many of the newest features of the software application. In the constantly evolving computer arena, knowing everything a program can do will aid you enormously now and in the future.

Minutes

Before 30 minutes have passed, you will have learned at least one useful task. Many of these tasks take advantage of the newest features of the application. These tasks use a hands-on approach, telling you exactly which menus and commands you need to use to accomplish the goal. This approach is found in each lesson of the *24 Hours* series.

Minutes

You will see after 40 minutes that many of the tools you have come to expect from the *Teach Yourself* series are found in the *24 Hours* series as well. Notes and tips offer special tricks of the trade to make your work faster and more productive. Cautions help you avoid those nasty time-consuming errors.

Minutes

By the time you're 50 minutes in, you'll probably run across terms you haven't seen before. Never before has technology thrown so many new words and acronyms into the language, and the Term Review element found in this series will carefully explain each and every one of them.

Minutes

At the end of the hour, you may still have questions that need to be answered. You know the kind—questions on skills or tasks that come up every day for you but that weren't directly addressed during the lesson. That's where the Q&A section can help. By answering the most frequently asked questions about the topics discussed in the hour, Q&A not only answers your specific question, it provides a succinct review of all that you have learned in the hour.

Teach Yourself
MICROSOFT
EXCEL® 97

in 24 Hours

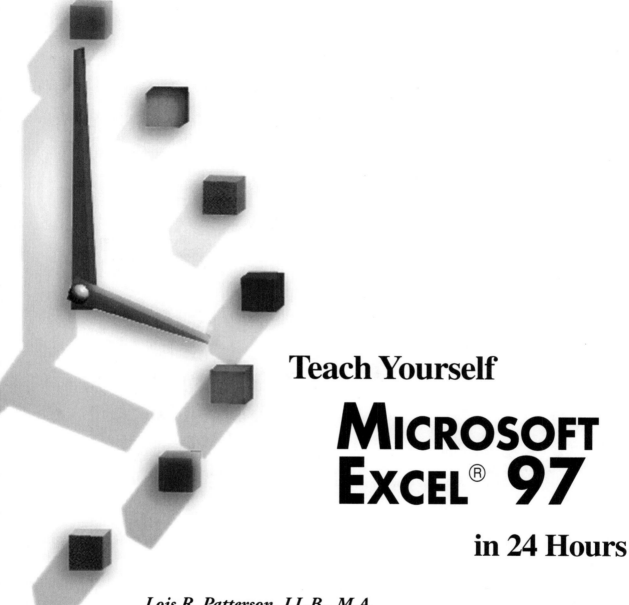

Teach Yourself

MICROSOFT
EXCEL® 97

in 24 Hours

Lois R. Patterson, LL.B., M.A.

SAMS
PUBLISHING

201 W. 103rd Street
Indianapolis, Indiana 46290

Publisher and President   Richard K. Swadley
Publishing Manager   Dean Miller
Director of Editorial Services   Cindy Morrow
Director of Marketing   Kelli S. Spencer
Assistant Marketing Managers   Kristina Perry, Rachel Wolfe

Acquisitions Editor
Cari Skaggs

Development Editor
Brian-Kent Proffitt

Production Editor
Alice Martina Smith

Indexer
Kevin Fulcher

Technical Reviewer
Angela Murdock

Editorial Coordinator
Katie Wise

Technical Edit Coordinator
Lynette Quinn

Resource Coordinator
Deborah Frisby

Editorial Assistants
Carol Ackerman
Andi Richter
Rhonda Tinch-Mize

Cover Designer
Tim Amhrein

Book Designer
Gary Adair

Copy Writer
David Reichwein

Production Team Supervisors
Brad Chinn
Charlotte Clapp

Production
Jeanne Clark
Sonja Hart
Gene Redding
Deirdre Smith

Overview

Contents

Acknowledgments

My editors once again deserve most of the credit. **Cari Skaggs** as acquisitions editor gave me the opportunity to write this book, and I very much wish to thank her for that. **Brian Proffitt** as development editor, **Alice Martina Smith** as copy editor, and **Angie Murdock** as technical editor all worked very hard to offer suggestions and improvements. I am responsible for all errors remaining, of course.

Hazel Pendray has helped so much with her special friendship and care for my children. My husband, **Paul**, and children, **Anne** and **Andrew**, have continually demonstrated their patience and loving encouragement—I hope to make it up to them.

About the Author

Lois Patterson is a freelance writer, Web designer, and researcher living in Vancouver, British Columbia, Canada. She has completed a degree in law and a master's degree in English with an emphasis on medical writing, and she has studied English and math as an undergraduate. She wrote Volume 1, *HTML*, of the *Web Publishing and Programming Resource Library* (published by Sams.net Publishing). When not working, she surfs the World Wide Web and spends time with her family. You can send e-mail to her at lpatter@greatstar.com.

Tell Us What You Think!

As a reader, you are the most important critic and commentator of our books. We value your opinion and want to know what we're doing right, what we could do better, what areas you'd like to see us publish in, and any other words of wisdom you're willing to pass our way. You can help us make strong books that meet your needs and give you the computer guidance you require.

Do you have access to CompuServe or the World Wide Web? Then check out our CompuServe forum by typing GO SAMS at any prompt. If you prefer the World Wide Web, check out our site at http://www.mcp.com.

JUST A MINUTE

> If you have a technical question about this book, call our technical support line at 317-581-3833.

As the publishing manager of the group that created this book, I welcome your comments. You can fax, e-mail, or write me directly to let me know what you did or didn't like about this book—as well as what we can do to make our books stronger. Here's the information:

Fax: 317-581-4669

E-mail: opsys_mgr@sams.samspublishing.com

Mail: Dean Miller
          Sams Publishing
          201 W. 103rd Street
          Indianapolis, IN 46290

Introduction

Microsoft Excel is the world's most commonly used spreadsheet program. Excel 97 has many powerful new features and has been designed to integrate with the rest of the Office 97 suite.

Part of the fun of using Excel is that you can always think of new applications for it. You can use it for your annual company report, your household budget, your meal planner—you can even create games and graphics with it. Excel is a fun program to use, and this book captures that aspect of it.

Who Should Read this Book

This book has been designed to be helpful for both beginning users and those with previous Excel experience. This text is helpful as a guide, as well as a tutorial. The reader of this book is assumed to be intelligent, but no familiarity with Excel or other Office programs is expected.

To use this book and Excel 97, you need a suitable computer, Windows 95, and Excel 97. Otherwise, all you need is a desire to learn Excel quickly and easily.

Does Each Chapter Really Take an Hour?

You can learn the concepts presented in each chapter in one hour. If you want to experiment with what you learn in each chapter, it may take longer than an hour to finish a chapter. However, all the concepts presented in this book are straightforward. If you are familiar with Windows applications, you can progress more quickly through the chapters.

How to Use this Book

This book is designed to teach you topics in one-hour sessions. All the books in the Sams *Teach Yourself* series enable the reader to start working and become productive with the product as quickly as possible. This book can do that for you!

Each hour, or chapter, starts with an overview of the topic that informs you what to expect in the lesson. The overviews help you determine the nature of the lesson and whether the lesson is relevant to your needs.

Each lesson also has a main section that discusses the lesson topic in a clear, concise manner by breaking down the topic into logical component parts and explaining each component clearly.

Embedded into each lesson are Time Saver, Caution, and Just a Minute boxes that provide additional information.

TIME SAVER

Time Savers inform you of tricks or elements that are easily missed by most computer users. You can skip them, but the Time Saver frequently shows you an easier way to do a task.

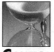

CAUTION

A Caution deserves at least as much attention as a Time Saver because Cautions point out problematic elements of the application. Ignoring the information contained in a Caution box can have adverse effects on the stability of your computer. Caution boxes are the most important informational sidebars in the book.

JUST A MINUTE

The Just a Minute boxes are designed to clarify the concept being discussed. These boxes elaborate on the subject; if you are comfortable with your understanding of the subject, you can bypass these boxes without danger.

Workshop Sections

The Workshop section at the end of each lesson defines terms introduced in the lesson and also provides Questions and Answers and Exercises that reinforce concepts learned in the lesson and help you apply them in new situations. Although you can skip this section, we advise you to go through the exercises to see how you can apply the concepts to other common tasks.

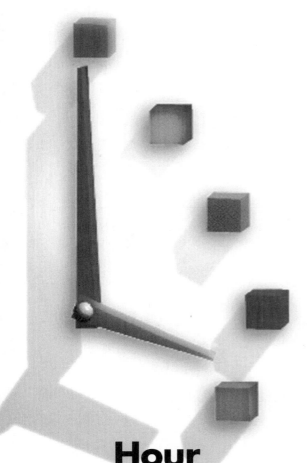

PART

I

Excel: The Preliminaries

Hour

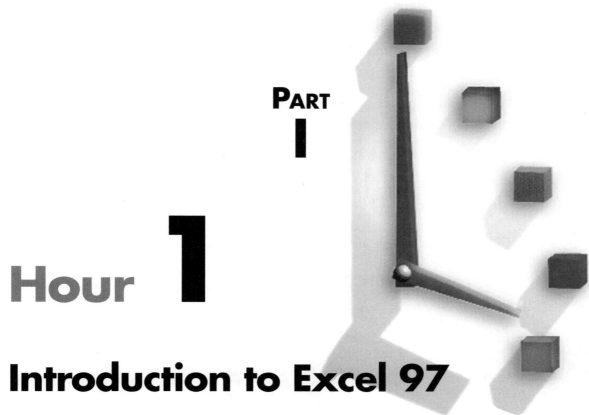

Hour 1

Introduction to Excel 97

What's so great about Microsoft Excel? Currently, it is the world's most popular spreadsheet program. Microsoft Excel's interface is intuitive and easy to use, although all its numerous features and functions can be intimidating. However, you can easily master the basics of Excel, and once you've done that, it's relatively straightforward to learn the more complex aspects of the program.

The History of Spreadsheets

Before there were typewriters, writers used pen, ink, and paper (or whatever writing implements were handy) to create their masterpieces. Accountants used the same tools to prepare their balance sheets. The Mesopotamians wrote their accounts on cuneiform tablets. Charts and graphs, if used, were created painstakingly with paintbrushes or special pens.

Spreadsheet programs do for figures, statistics, data charts, and forms what word processors do for writing. A *spreadsheet* is like an automated ledger. There is no need to add and subtract columns of numbers by hand, or even with a calculator. Excel can do it for you. You can see Excel as interactive scratch paper that never gets crumpled or messy.

The first spreadsheet, VisiCalc, was introduced in 1978 for the Apple II. VisiCalc was considered one of the first "killer apps," meaning that the need to use VisiCalc was a compelling reason to purchase a computer. Lotus 1-2-3 was introduced in 1983 and held the largest market share for a considerable period of time. In 1987, Quattro Pro and Excel were released; both used graphical user interfaces (GUIs). Microsoft Excel has taken over the spreadsheet market for a variety of reasons and is often considered the most fully featured and easy to use of all the spreadsheet programs available. If you have data in other formats, it is easy to convert to and from Microsoft Excel format.

Referring to Excel as a *spreadsheet program* gives too limited a notion of what Excel can do. Excel can be used for numerous purposes, as you can see from a few of the templates offered freely on the Web. Baarns Publishing has created the spreadsheet shown in Figure 1.1 that you can use to calculate how much and what kind of candy to purchase for Halloween. This spreadsheet also includes a variety of Halloween recipes. Baarns Publishing also produces another spreadsheet: a clever hangman game, shown in Figure 1.2.

Figure 1.1.

A Halloween candy calculator created by Baarns Publishing.

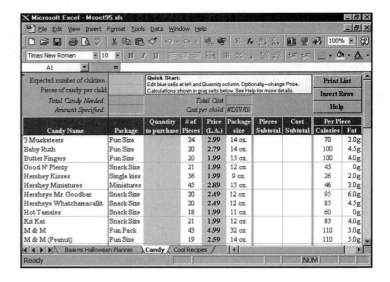

You can use Excel to create invoices or to analyze scientific data. Excel spreadsheets are used for invoice templates, holiday planners, recipe collections, home mortgage calculations, profit-and-loss statements, tax preparation, music tutorials, software tutorials, and more. Figure 1.3 shows a business planner template, created by Microsoft, which can be customized to your own particular needs. You can create similar applications—or very different ones. The uses of Excel are limited only by your imagination and the time you have available.

Figure 1.2.

A hangman game created by Baarns Publishing.

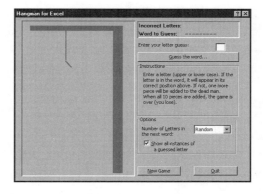

Figure 1.3.

A business planner created by Microsoft.

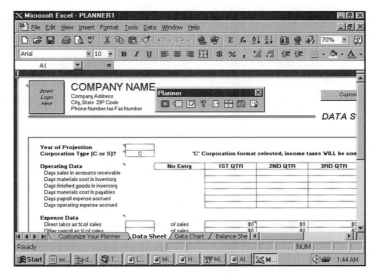

When you are working out a problem with paper and pencil or keeping records by hand, you can erase, add, multiply, or do anything you want with your figures. However, it's hard to keep your work attractive while constantly changing data, and it's hard to bring back your old data if you are constantly crossing it out or erasing it. Excel combines the ease of working by hand with the data permanence inherent to computer programs. Transferring the ease of working with a pencil, paper, and calculator to a computer program is a daunting task, but Microsoft Excel has done a superb job. Excel's capabilities allow you to speedily duplicate the work that would previously have required heaps of paper, lots of time, and a dedicated staff of graphic artists, mathematicians, and accountants. That's not to say you have to use Excel for complex situations—it works well for both simple and complicated uses.

You can use Excel for just about any situation in which you want to create a report, use formulas, keep records, or do calculations. Excel can be used for statistical analysis, mathematical analysis, forecasting, regression analysis, and more.

The capabilities of Microsoft Word and Excel overlap to some degree. You can create attractive templates, charts, and so forth with both programs, and you can create functional data tables in Word. However, Word lacks the analytical capabilities of Excel, and Excel lacks the publishing capabilities of Word. It is quite possible to use the two programs together, embedding or linking between Word documents and Excel documents. You can also use Excel to create forms and charts that do not require any sort of calculation.

As Microsoft says, you can "turn your numbers into answers" with Excel. As with any other software program, Excel cannot do all your thinking for you. You have to know what you want to achieve. However, Excel's capabilities show up best in much larger spreadsheets than it is possible to show in this book. Imagine calculating payroll data for a given week, if the 16,000 or so employees in your company are paid hourly and have irregular schedules. Excel makes this process easy. You can automate data entry and other routine tasks so that new entries can readily be added and deleted.

What can't you do with Microsoft Excel? Well, there's no doubt that database programs such as Microsoft Access are more suited to certain types of data storage and data retrieval. However, you can use database programs and Excel together, as discussed in Hour 19, "Using Excel with Databases." Microsoft PowerPoint is particularly well suited for creating presentations, and you can copy Excel charts or data into these presentations.

Excel makes it easy to move data to and from different parts of the spreadsheet. You can run any number of analyses on the data without having to write the data out in a different form. You can create a complex formula and apply it instantly to any or all of your data. You can draw relationships between different kinds of data, and these relationships can change when you enter new data.

The term *spreadsheet* is a generic term used in accounting to refer to the presentation of data in columns and rows. In Excel, the term *worksheet* refers to a traditional spreadsheet—but you can also create Excel worksheets that bear no similarity to traditional spreadsheets at all. An Excel worksheet can consist of games, plain text, graphics, or other types of information.

Planning Strategies for Excel Worksheets

When you think of using Excel, consider the following questions:

- ☐ What do you want to achieve?
- ☐ Who will see your information?
- ☐ What do you want to do with the information?

Looking at examples is a good way to see what you can do with Microsoft Excel. It truly is a multifeatured program, and its uses cannot be easily categorized. You can see some examples of what Excel can do at the Microsoft Web site at http://www.microsoft.com/excel/ and the Baarns Web site at http://www.baarns.com/. Some software and publishing companies offer Excel templates for sale for a variety of purposes.

When creating Excel worksheets, don't try to cram too much information into a single spreadsheet; use white space judiciously.

If your spreadsheet is huge by necessity, use graphics and other features to delineate different areas and make the document easy to navigate. Formatting worksheets is discussed in Hour 6, "Formatting and Protecting Worksheets"; adding graphics and other multimedia is discussed in Hour 8, "Adding Graphics and Multimedia to Your Excel Documents."

Excel enforces organization to some extent, but make sure that you have a good idea of what data should be included and excluded, and how you want the final product to look. Remember that Excel also allows you to hide parts of a spreadsheet from view.

Of course, one of the virtues of Excel is that it is so easy to change the appearance of your spreadsheets and so easy to alter the data contained within them. You can transpose rows with columns and vice versa. You can add and delete graphics. Excel can chart the same data in dozens of different ways. You can play around with Excel as much as you want to get different effects—and doing so can be very useful when you are initially learning the program and when you are learning new features.

Microsoft has added many new features to Excel 97 and has made the program even simpler to use than earlier versions. With Excel 97, it's easier to edit your work, the graphical capabilities are improved, you can save your settings more easily, formulas are easier to develop, and the integration between Excel and other Office 97 applications is tighter.

The overriding principle to keep in mind when learning Excel is that it doesn't hurt to experiment—at least if you've backed up your work. It isn't possible to show all Excel's capabilities in this book, and there are many undocumented features. In Excel 97, the online help is more useful than ever, and you will probably find that you can have many questions answered on the spot.

Summary

Microsoft Excel can't do all your number-crunching for you any more than Microsoft Word can do your writing for you. Excel can, however, make your work as a number-cruncher easier; the program is ideally suited for preparing and presenting data in an orderly and meaningful fashion. Learning how to use Excel facilitates the process of data organization, presentation, and analysis immensely.

Workshop

Term Review

backup   A duplicate copy of your working file. You save the backup in another location so that you can recover your work if something happens to your working copy (such as a hard drive failure or malicious destruction of data). You should keep backup copies of all your important files.

spreadsheet   In accounting parlance, a *spreadsheet* refers to the presentation of data in columns and rows.

template   A preformatted file you can reuse as many times as necessary to create documents. Templates save time because much or all of the formatting and text you otherwise have to create from scratch are already present.

worksheet   In Excel, a *worksheet* is often an electronic form of a spreadsheet, but the term *worksheet* can also refer to many other possible types of presentations. You can create worksheets that contain games, graphics, text, or other types of data.

Q&A

Q What is Microsoft Excel 97 and what can it do?

A Microsoft Excel 97 is the world's most popular spreadsheet program. It can be used to organize and manipulate numbers and other data. It can be used for a variety of purposes, from holiday planning to mortgage calculation to analysis of scientific experiments.

Q Is Excel hard to use?

A No. Although you may have a slightly higher initial learning curve than with a word processing program, Excel is basically like interactive scratch paper or an automated ledger.

Q What should you keep in mind when creating spreadsheets?

A You should develop your organizational plan before you start, particularly with a large project. However, it's easy to modify your worksheets and make formatting changes as you go.

Q How does Microsoft Excel 97 differ from previous versions of Excel?

A Excel 97 is coordinated better with other Microsoft programs and with the Internet. It is easier to edit changes, there are improved graphical capabilities, and there are many new features in this version.

Q What's the most important thing to remember when learning Excel?

A Don't be afraid to experiment. If your data is important, however, make sure that you have backups—preferably in more than one location.

Hour **2**

Installing Excel 97

The first thing you have to do with your sparkling new software package of Microsoft Office or Microsoft Excel is to install it. You may have one of the several Microsoft Office 97 packages (Standard, Professional, or Small Business), or you may have only Microsoft Excel 97. You may have an upgrade package. (An *upgrade package* is one that requires you to have one of a number of different programs already installed on your machine. There are a couple dozen programs that make you eligible for the upgrade, including office suites, word processors, spreadsheets, presentation graphics programs, and databases. The eligible programs are listed on the side of the upgrade package.)

Here are the listed requirements for Microsoft Excel:

- ☐ A computer with a 486 or higher processor
- ☐ Microsoft Windows 95 or Microsoft Windows NT Workstation 3.51 Service Pack or later
- ☐ 8M of RAM for use with Windows 95 and 16M of RAM for use with Windows NT Workstation
- ☐ 36M of hard disk space for a typical installation (space requirements range from 22M to 64M, depending on the options chosen); Office 97 requires between 73M and 191M of disk space

As always, the more RAM you have, the better your system will run. Twenty-four megabytes of RAM is considered by many to be the comfortable minimum. In addition, having a generous amount of hard disk space available makes Excel run better, particularly if you are short on RAM.

Beginning the Installation from a CD-ROM

Let's start at the very beginning, a very good place to start.

Turn on your computer. Start Windows 95, if your system does not do that automatically. Turn off your virus-detection utility if you are using one, and close any programs you may be running, including those that start automatically.

If you are already in Windows 95, close all the programs that you are running, including virus-detection utilities.

Insert the CD-ROM that came with the software package you purchased in your computer's CD-ROM drive and close the drive drawer.

Windows 95 includes a feature called AutoRun, which causes Windows to recognize CD-ROM discs you insert in your disc drive automatically. AutoRun also begins execution of the program on the CD-ROM. Unless you have turned off this feature, AutoRun is enabled. If you have AutoRun enabled, you automatically get the first screen of the installation program shown in Figure 2.1 (you see a similar screen if you are installing only Excel 97).

Figure 2.1.

*The first installation
screen.*

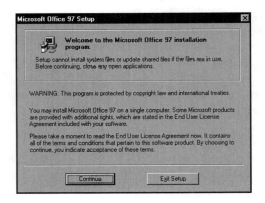

If you don't have AutoRun enabled, click the Start button on the Windows 95 toolbar. Select Settings | Control Panel and double-click the Add/Remove Programs icon. You see the Add/Remove Programs Properties dialog box. Select the Install/Uninstall tab if it is not already selected, and click the Install button. You see the Install Program from Floppy Disk or CD-ROM dialog box. You are then asked to insert the CD-ROM. Do so and click Next. The installation wizard then looks for the correct program to install. Click Finish when the correct program is located. You then see the screen shown in Figure 2.1.

2

Although it may seem like a nuisance, it is a good idea to actually read the End User License Agreement, just as the installation program tells you to do. Click the Continue button to see it. The License Agreement gives you details about the legal consequences of creating copies, using the software on other computers, and so forth. Click OK when you are finished reading the License Agreement.

JUST A MINUTE

If you purchase Microsoft Office or Microsoft Excel and do not have a CD-ROM drive, you can still use the program. There is a coupon inside the package that you can send away to Microsoft to receive the 3.5-inch disks.

Once you have the disks, insert Disk 1 in floppy drive A. Click the Start button on the Windows 95 taskbar, select Run, and enter `a:\setup`. You can then continue the installation process described in the following sections. You will be prompted to switch disks frequently, but otherwise the procedure is the same as the one described here.

Choosing Your Installation

After you read the License Agreement, you are prompted for your name and organization. The default entries are the name and organization entered when Windows 95 was installed. Make any necessary changes to this information and click OK. You are then asked to confirm your name and organization. Click OK. The installation program then asks you to enter the 11-digit CD-Key number found on the back of your CD-ROM package. Type this information and click OK. The installation program displays your product-ID number. Write this number down and save it in case you need it (although it is also accessible from within the program, once the program is installed).

For Upgrade Version Users

If you are not using an upgrade version of Office 97 or Excel 97, you can skip to the next section. As mentioned earlier in this hour, *upgrade packages* of Office 97 or Excel 97 require you to have one of a couple dozen or so programs already installed on your hard drive. Microsoft has provided the upgrade package to encourage users of previous Microsoft products to upgrade to Excel 97 and to encourage users of products from competing companies to switch allegiances. Some of the programs that make you eligible for an upgrade include Corel WordPerfect Suite 7, Microsoft Word 6, and Lotus 1-2-3, among numerous others.

If the installation program cannot find the old program or programs, you are asked to enter the path of the old program. For example, if you installed the old program in your `D:\Somefile` directory, enter that path when prompted to do so. The installation program can usually find the old program, but may have difficulty if you have chosen a directory other than the default, or if you have installed the program on another hard drive. Click OK when done.

Choosing an Installation Directory

After you have recorded your product-ID number, the installation program prompts you for the installation directory, as shown in Figure 2.2.

Figure 2.2.

Choosing the installation directory.

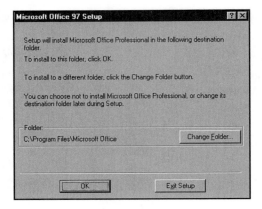

You may want to change the default directory for several reasons. Perhaps you don't have enough disk space to install the program on drive C and prefer to use another drive. Or perhaps you simply prefer to keep all your programs on a different drive. Most of the time, however, you will want to keep the default directory:

```
C:\Program Files\Microsoft Office
```

If you want to keep your old copies of Microsoft Office or Excel on your system, choose a different directory path for the installation of Office 97 or Excel 97. You can choose whatever path name you want. Here are two suggestions, depending on whether you are installing Office 97 or Excel 97:

```
C:\Program Files\Office 97
C:\Program Files\Excel 97
```

If you have a hard drive D or another hard drive on which you want to install the program, just substitute D for C and continue with the installation.

JUST A MINUTE

From a functional point of view, there's little reason to keep old versions of programs. The new version can do everything the old version can—and it can save files in the old format as well. Nevertheless, many users like the comfort and familiarity of using their old versions of programs, particularly for older files.

2

Choosing Installation Options

Once you have entered your identification information and chosen your directory path, you see a dialog box of options (see Figure 2.3). If you are installing only Microsoft Excel or if you are installing Microsoft Office 97 from floppy disks, you will not see the Run from CD-ROM option in the dialog box on your screen.

Figure 2.3.

The installation options.

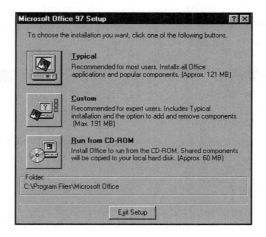

Here are the installation options from which you can choose if you are installing Office 97:

☐ **Typical.** The standard, no-brainer installation is Typical. This installation option contains the components that Microsoft considers to be used by typical users. Remember that you can always add and remove components as needed. If you want to do a Typical installation of Microsoft Office, including Microsoft Access, you require 121M of free disk space on your hard drive.

☐ **Custom.** If you choose the Custom installation, you can install any or all of the programs that come with Office 97, such as Excel, Word, PowerPoint, and Access. You will see the Microsoft Office 97 - Custom dialog box shown in Figure 2.4. Select (check) the components you want to install and deselect (uncheck) the components you do not want to install. For example, if you don't want to install PowerPoint, clear its checkbox.

If you have enough disk space and you want to be sure that you install everything you might need, click Select All and then click Continue. If you choose more options than you have disk space for, you see a dialog box informing you of that fact. Keep in mind that you probably will not want to use every last megabyte of disk space for your Excel program; having free disk space makes the program run better and faster.

☐ **Run from CD-ROM.** The Run from CD-ROM option takes up the least space on your hard drive. However, the programs run more slowly this way.

Once you have chosen the programs you want to install, you can decide which components of each program you want to install. Excel (as well as each of the other Office programs) has a number of optional components. Each component takes additional disk space, of course.

To choose which components of Microsoft Excel you want to install, highlight Microsoft Excel and choose Change Options. You see a dialog box like the one in Figure 2.5. The various components you can install are listed in Table 2.1.

Figure 2.4.

The Custom Installation dialog box.

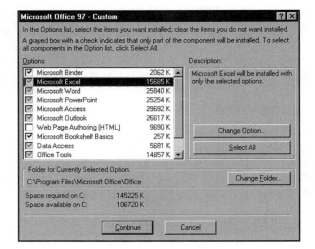

Figure 2.5.

The components of the Excel 97 program.

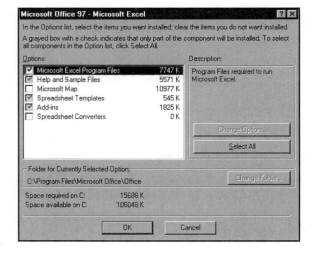

2

Table 2.1. Excel 97 components.

Option	Description
Microsoft Excel Program Files	This component is essential if you want to run Excel.
Help and Sample Files	Install this component if you want to access online help and view the sample files included with Excel.
Microsoft Map	This component is needed if you want to use the map-creation program that displays geographical data in a handy format.
Spreadsheet Templates	This component includes templates for invoices and customer information forms.
Add-ins	Excel includes a number of add-ins you can choose to install. These add-ins add different capabilities, such as statistical analysis functions, additional database and World Wide Web features, file converters, and more.

JUST A MINUTE

If you are installing Excel 97 and choose the Custom installation, you get a slightly different dialog box than the one in Figure 2.5. Most of the options available with a plain Excel 97 installation are listed in Table 2.1. Here are some other options that may be available to you:

☐ **Data Access.** A component that improves your ability to integrate Excel with databases.

☐ **Office Tools.** A component that includes several helpful authoring and correction tools.

☐ **Converters and Filters.** A component that converts files to and from Excel 97 format and other formats.

Select the box for each of the components you want to install. Alternatively, click Select All to install all the components.

Several of the components, such as the Add-ins component, are each made up of several components. For example, to install one or more of the add-in programs, select Add-ins and click Change Options to display a list of the options. Select the add-in programs you want to install and click Continue to return to the Microsoft Excel dialog box.

When you have made your choices in the Microsoft Excel dialog box (refer to Figure 2.5), click Continue to return to the Custom dialog box (refer to Figure 2.4). When you have made all the choices you want to make in the Custom dialog box, click Continue.

Whether you have chosen Typical, Custom, or Run from CD-ROM, follow the remaining prompts presented by the installation program. The rest of the program installation proceeds automatically. If you have old versions of Microsoft Office or Microsoft Excel, the installation program asks whether or not you want to keep the old program components.

When you are nearly finished, you see the dialog box in Figure 2.6, telling you to either click Restart Windows to complete the installation, to click Online Registration to register the product, or to click Exit Setup to go back to Windows. The installation is not complete until you restart Windows.

Figure 2.6.

Complete the installation process by restarting Windows.

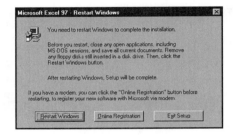

If you click Online Registration, the Registration Wizard appears (see Figure 2.7).

Figure 2.7.

The Registration Wizard dialog box.

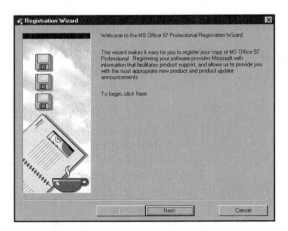

Many users never register their software. If you do, however, you may get special offers and benefits not available otherwise. If you have a modem, you can use the Registration Wizard after you finish installing Office or Excel. The online registration process helps you complete the process easily without the hassle of remembering to fill out and mail the registration postcard.

2

If you don't choose to complete the online registration after you initially install the software, you can always run Setup again later and register online, as described in the next section.

Using the Microsoft Office or Excel Maintenance Program

After you have installed Microsoft Office or Excel, you may want to add or remove components, reinstall the program if the files are damaged, or remove the program completely. To do any of these, run the install program just as you did when installing the software initially; this time, however, the installation program recognizes that the software is already installed and displays a dialog box of maintenance options, as shown in Figure 2.8.

TIME SAVER

To start the installation program, insert the CD-ROM into the appropriate drive. If you have AutoRun enabled, you automatically see the screen in Figure 2.8. If you don't have AutoRun enabled, click the Start button on the Windows 95 toolbar, select Settings | Control Panel, and choose Add/Remove Programs; click Install on the Install/Uninstall tab; the screen shown in Figure 2.8 appears. If you are using 3.5-inch disks, insert Disk 1 in floppy drive A; click the Start button on the Windows 95 taskbar; select Run, and enter `a:\setup` to begin the installation program and display the dialog box shown in Figure 2.8.

Figure 2.8.

The Microsoft Office maintenance program.

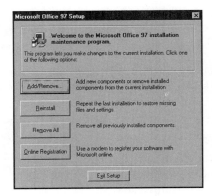

Installing Additional Components Later

As you work with Microsoft Excel, you may find that you need a component you did not install when you installed the rest of the program. This can happen if you selected a subset of Excel's features when you initially installed the program. To add a component at some later time, start the maintenance program as described in the preceding section. From the dialog box of options, click Add/Remove to see the dialog box shown in Figure 2.9.

Figure 2.9.

Adding components.

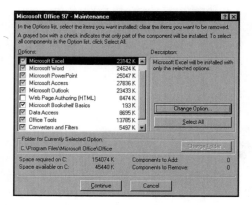

If you want to install all the components, click Select All and then click Continue. Even if you have installed some of the components previously, Excel recognizes that this is the case and installs only the ones you do not have.

If you want to install or remove particular components, highlight Microsoft Excel and click Change Option to see the dialog box shown in Figure 2.10. Highlight the components you want to add or remove. If you want to install everything, click Select All and then click OK.

If you want to add only parts of a component (as you can do with the Add-ins component), highlight the component name and click Change Option to see the different parts of that component. Choose the parts you want and click Continue. You return to the screen shown in Figure 2.9. Continue selecting components in this way until you have marked all the components you want to install. Click OK when done.

If you want to delete a component, display the appropriate dialog box as explained in the preceding instructions and clear its checkbox. If you want to delete part of a component, highlight the component name and click Change Option to see a list of the different parts of that component. Clear the checkboxes for the elements you want to delete and click Continue. Continue selecting components in this way until you have cleared the checkboxes for all the components you want to delete. Click OK when done.

2

Figure 2.10.

*Choose the options you
want to add or delete.*

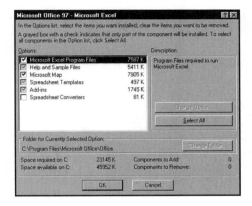

Uninstalling Microsoft Office or Excel

If you want to uninstall the entire Office 97 or Excel 97 package, start the maintenance
program to see the screen shown in Figure 2.8. Click Remove All; follow the prompts to delete
the entire application.

JUST A MINUTE

You can also uninstall Microsoft Office or Excel by choosing Control Panel
from the Start menu. Click Add/Remove Programs and choose the appropriate entry, depending on your system.

TIME SAVER

If you have downloaded templates from the Microsoft site and installed
them, you can use the maintenance program to remove them from your
system if you want. Start the maintenance program; from the dialog box
of options, select Add/Remove. The template names are listed
in the dialog box that appears; select the ones you want to remove and
click OK.

Repairing Damaged and Missing Files

It sometimes happens that you accidentally delete important Microsoft Office system files;
it may also happen that your hard drive is damaged, invalidating or rendering useless some
of your files. You can experience moments of panic when you realize your files are missing
or damaged if your four-year-old has been clicking away in Windows Explorer or for any of
a myriad of other reasons.

You can repair or replace the damaged or missing *application* files using the maintenance program. Notice that the following procedure does not work if you are missing *data* files; for these emergencies, you will have to resort to your data backups. You learn how to make backups of your data in Hour 3, "Introduction to the Excel Environment."

To repair or replace the damaged application files, insert the Office 97 CD-ROM in the appropriate drive. If AutoRun is enabled, you see the opening screen for the maintenance program. If AutoRun is not enabled, type **d:\setup** (substitute the appropriate drive letter for your CD-ROM drive). If you are using 3.5-inch disks, insert Disk 1 in the appropriate drive and type **a:\setup** or **b:\setup** from the Start | Run menu.

From the maintenance program's main list of options, select the Reinstall option. This option reinstalls your programs and repairs your missing and damaged files. Just follow the prompts and respond to the dialog boxes as you did with the initial installation. Of course, the data files you have created on your machine will not be restored from the CD-ROM if they are missing, but you do have backups elsewhere, don't you?

Upgrade Users: Keep All Versions of Your Software

If you have purchased an upgrade version of Microsoft Office or Excel 97, remember to keep the disks from the *original* application. You may need these to recover from a hard disk crash or system failure; the upgrade version of the program cannot be installed unless it recognizes components from an earlier version of the application.

In addition, you cannot sell the original application without selling the upgrade with it; doing so violates the terms of your End User License Agreement. Be sure to read the agreement if you have any uncertainties about whether you should purchase additional licenses for Microsoft Excel if you install the program on multiple computers or have multiple users on a single computer.

Technical Support

The instructions in this chapter should work for most systems in most situations. However, given the variety of computer systems and configurations, there are always exceptions. You can access the Microsoft Knowledge Base on the Web at http://www.microsoft.com/kb/ to search for help with different programs, including Excel. Microsoft has set up a database you can use to enter a search query and then read detailed articles pertaining to the problem you queried about. You can also enter as a search query any error message you may have seen. Although you do not get custom-tailored help from this source, you can find answers for the vast majority of problems you will encounter.

Summary

The main thing you have to consider when installing Microsoft Office or Microsoft Excel is how much disk space you have available. Of course, you may not have any use for many of the options, so you can make choices about which components you want to install. Microsoft has made the installation process easy. If you just follow the prompts, your program installs successfully in almost all cases. You can customize the installation if you want, and you can always add or remove components later.

Workshop

Term Review

upgrade   A software program that relies on the presence of a previous version of the software, or the presence of a competitor's version, in order to install the program. Upgrades are usually cheaper than the full software program.

Q&A

Q What is the "typical installation" of Microsoft Office or Microsoft Excel?

A This installation includes the features most commonly used by Microsoft Office or Microsoft Excel users—at least in Microsoft's judgment of the matter. If you choose this installation option (or any of the others, for that matter), remember that you can always add or remove components later.

Q What is the Run from CD-ROM installation option?

A This installation option does not put entire programs on the hard drive. Instead, it installs enough of the programs on your drive so that you can run them when you insert the CD-ROM in the appropriate drive.

Q What is the Custom installation option?

A With this option, you can pick and choose which components of Microsoft Office or Microsoft Excel you want to install on your drive. You can also choose to install everything with this option.

Hour 3

Introduction to the Excel Environment

If you've used other Microsoft Office products such as Microsoft Word, you will find much about Excel to be very familiar. Most Windows 95 programs share a number of similarities in their toolbars and menus. This chapter is a basic introduction to operating Excel and creating a workbook.

Starting Excel

Excel documents are called *workbooks*. To create a new Excel workbook, first start Excel: Click the Start button in Windows 95, move your mouse over the Microsoft Excel icon, and click it. If you haven't changed your default settings in Excel, Excel opens with a new document, as shown in Figure 3.1.

Figure 3.1.
A typical Excel screen.

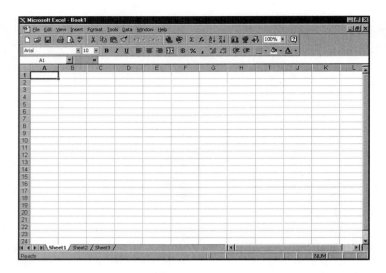

JUST A MINUTE

> Excel documents are called *workbooks*; each workbook is a separate file. The terms *Excel document*, *Excel workbook*, and *Excel file* are used interchangeably throughout this text.

Here are two other approaches to starting Excel from Windows 95:

- ☐ Click the Start button on the Windows 95 toolbar, select Run, and type **excel** in the Run dialog box.
- ☐ Click the Start button and select New Office Document. Double-click the Blank Workbook option in the New Office Document dialog box that appears, or select one of the other tabs, such as Spreadsheet, to open the type of document you want.

Using Excel's Toolbars

Now that you've opened the program, let's look at the parts of a typical Excel screen, shown in Figure 3.2. Many of these components are common to other Windows 95 applications as well.

At the top of the document is the Windows 95 *title bar*. The title includes the program name and the filename of the current workbook. In this example, the document has not been saved under any filename, but Excel has given it the name Book1 (because it is the first workbook opened in this particular session).

At the bottom of the screen is the *status bar*. Depending on whether the currently highlighted cell has any data in it, the status bar reads either Ready or Edit.

3

Figure 3.2.

*Parts of an
Excel screen.*

Name box   Title bar   Main menu bar   Standard toolbar   Formatting toolbar

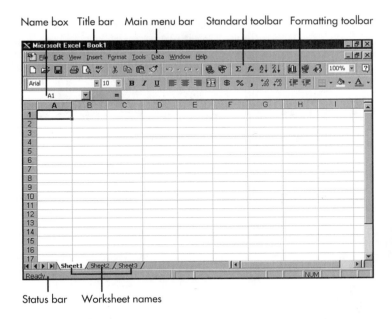

Status bar   Worksheet names

The menu bar at the top of the screen that begins with File and ends with Help is called the *main menu bar*, or often simply the *main menu*. Each of the entries on the main menu has a corresponding pull-down menu. Try clicking each entry on the main menu bar to see its pull-down menu. Many of the entries on the pull-down menus have their own *submenu*, or *cascading menu*. For example, select the Insert menu and then select Picture to see the cascading menu shown in Figure 3.3.

Figure 3.3.

*The Insert | Picture
cascading menu.*

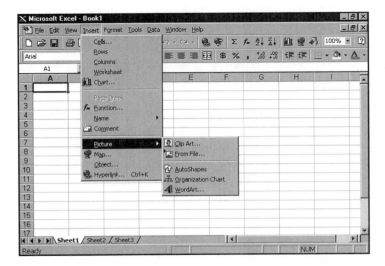

The toolbar underneath the main menu, with its pictorial icons, is called the *Standard toolbar*. The toolbar underneath the Standard toolbar controls fonts and the formatting of text. It is called the *Formatting toolbar*.

Table 3.1 lists the different toolbars available in Excel along with their functions.

Table 3.1. Some commonly used Excel toolbars.

Toolbar	Description
Worksheet menu bar	The standard main menu toolbar located across the top of the worksheet by default, with the entries File, Edit, and so on.
Chart menu bar	The same as the worksheet menu bar except that the Chart option replaces the Data option.
Formatting	The toolbar with the font control icons, cell formatting icons, and pattern tools.
Standard	This toolbar includes the icons for New, Open, Save, Print, and numerous other commonly used tools. By default, it is located under the worksheet menu bar.
Drawing	This toolbar contains various drawing tools and is located, by default, at the bottom of the worksheet.

Other toolbars—some of which are discussed elsewhere in this book—are PivotTable, Chart, Reviewing, Forms, Stop Recording, External Data, Auditing, Full Screen, Circular Reference, Visual Basic, Web, Control Toolbox, Exit Design Mode, Word Art, Picture, Shadow Settings, and 3D Settings.

Display and Placement of Toolbars

Like most Windows 95 applications, Microsoft Excel allows a great deal of latitude in how you display or place your toolbars. Toolbars take up screen space; you can hide them if you prefer to have extra space for your worksheets. Just click the right mouse button over the toolbars to see the menu shown in Figure 3.4. Click the checkmark in front of the toolbar you want to remove from view. Alternatively, you can select View | Toolbars from the main menu and click the checkmark in front of the toolbar you want to remove from view. You can add toolbars to or delete toolbars from your screen at any time by checking or unchecking the ones you want to add or delete from either of these menus.

3

Figure 3.4.

The Toolbar menu that appears when you right-click a toolbar.

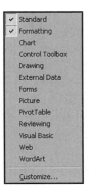

Many users like to have the Drawing toolbar handy, particularly if they use graphics in their worksheets, as described in greater detail in Hour 8, "Adding Graphics and Multimedia to Your Excel Documents." The other toolbars can be handy to bring up when you are doing certain tasks. For example, the Control Toolbox toolbar is helpful when you are creating controls, the Chart toolbar is helpful when you are creating charts, and so forth.

Repositioning Toolbars and Making Them Float

The main menu bar, the Standard toolbar, and the Formatting toolbar all appear at the top of a worksheet by default and extend across the width of the Excel window. Other toolbars that you use for manipulating various features of Excel, including such toolbars as Chart and PivotTable, "float" by default in the worksheet space itself and do not take up the full space of the Excel window.

You can change the defaults, however. You can place toolbars along the side of the Excel window, or you can reposition them anywhere you like in the worksheet. You can convert fixed toolbars to floating toolbars, and floating toolbars to fixed toolbars. The form of the toolbar display does not affect how it works.

To change the location and form of a toolbar, position the mouse pointer on the edge (or any inactive part) of the toolbar, click, and drag the toolbar to its new location. If you drop the toolbar in the worksheet, it will "float," as shown in Figure 3.5. If you take a floating toolbar, drag it to the top of the screen, and drop it there, it becomes fixed.

JUST A MINUTE

Drag and drop means that you position the mouse cursor over an object, press the left mouse button, and hold it while you move (drag) the mouse pointer to the object's new location. When you release the mouse button, you "drop" the object in the new position.

Figure 3.5.

*A floating main
menu bar.*

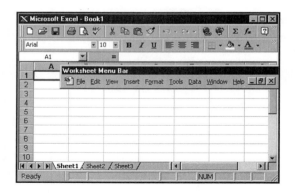

You can alter the positions of toolbars by dragging and dropping them below or above other toolbars. You cannot position toolbars one on top of the other; however, floating toolbars can overlap.

Accessing Toolbar Options

 Toolbars rarely provide an exclusive way to do a particular task. Each of the tools you can access from the Standard and Formatting toolbars can also be accessed from the main menu or with keyboard shortcuts. For example, to copy data from a worksheet after you select it, you can click the Copy tool, select Edit | Copy from the main menu, or press Ctrl+C.

Toolbars do provide an easy-to-understand graphical interface, however, and the tool icons make the tools easy to access.

JUST A MINUTE

> The use of the mouse as described in this book is for a right-handed, two-button mouse. If you have configured your mouse for a left-handed person, just substitute the word *right* for *left* (and vice versa) when you are told to click a particular mouse button.

Accessing Menu Options

To access the main menu, you can use either your mouse or a key combination. Move the mouse pointer to the top of the screen, over the menu bar, and click one of the menu options with the left mouse button. The pull-down menu opens; you can move the mouse cursor through the menu choices. You can also use the arrow keys or the Tab key to move through the menu options. When the cursor is highlighting the menu option you want, press Enter or click the left mouse button to activate that command.

With most Windows 95 programs, you can use either the mouse or the keyboard to perform tasks such opening and closing a program, saving files, moving data around, and so forth.

Most of the instructions in this chapter focus on using the mouse to perform tasks because most users find this method to be the most intuitive. However, you can save wear and tear on your wrists—and maybe even gain speed—if you learn the keyboard shortcuts as well. For a list of keyboard shortcuts, open the Help menu and select Contents and Index; enter the word **shortcut** to see the shortcut keys entry and a list of the keyboard shortcuts you can learn for Excel. The section "Using Keyboard Shortcuts," later in this hour, offers additional insights into using keyboard shortcuts.

JUST A MINUTE

This book uses a shorthand way to refer to a particular menu choice: File | Save. This means that you should open the File pull-down menu from the main menu and select Save from the pull-down menu. Similarly, Insert | Break means that you select the Insert pull-down menu from the main menu and then choose Break. This terminology is used throughout this book.

Using the Right Mouse Button

One of Windows 95's useful innovations was to give increased functionality to the right mouse button. If you have some questions when you are looking around the toolbars or your worksheet, place the mouse cursor over an icon or symbol and press the right mouse button; a relevant menu pops up. When this menu pops up, you can scroll up and down through it using the mouse, the arrow keys, or the Tab key. When you want to select an option in the menu, you can press either the right or left button to choose it, or you can press Enter to choose the highlighted option.

Using Keyboard Shortcuts

As is true for many other Windows 95 programs, many commands within Microsoft Excel can be accessed with both the mouse and a key combination. Typically, these key combinations involve pressing the Alt key, the Ctrl key, or the Shift key and certain letter or function keys. The main menu lists common keyboard shortcuts for various common tasks. For example, if you select Edit | Copy from the main menu, you will see Ctrl+C listed on the same line as the Copy command. If you select File | Save from the main menu, you will see Ctrl+S listed on the same line as the Save command.

Ctrl+*Key* Combinations

Many of the keyboard shortcuts use the Ctrl key and some other key in combination. Some combinations are easy to commit to memory—such as Ctrl+N for new workbook and Ctrl+P for print. Some shortcuts lack an obvious connection between the letter and the function. For example, Ctrl+K inserts a hyperlink in the document.

When you see the key combination Ctrl+N, you first press and hold the Ctrl key and then press the N key (while still holding the Ctrl key). Then release both keys. (You don't press the + key as part of these shortcuts—that is just a symbol to indicate that the two keys are pressed at the same time. Nor do you press the Shift key to obtain the capital letter *N*—the uppercase character is used just to mimic the labels on the keyboard itself.) Table 3.2 shows some of the most commonly used Ctrl+*key* combinations.

Table 3.2. Ctrl+*key* shortcut combinations.

Ctrl+*key* Combination	Task
Ctrl+A	Save
Ctrl+B	Bold
Ctrl+C	Copy
Ctrl+D	Fill down
Ctrl+F	Find
Ctrl+G	Go To
Ctrl+H	Replace
Ctrl+I	Italic
Ctrl+K	Insert hyperlink
Ctrl+N	Open a new workbook
Ctrl+O	Open an existing workbook
Ctrl+P	Print
Ctrl+R	Fill right
Ctrl+S	Save (a workbook)
Ctrl+U	Underline
Ctrl+V	Paste
Ctrl+W	Quit
Ctrl+X	Cut (some text, such as data, a cell, or a group of cells)
Ctrl+Y	Repeat the last function
Ctrl+Z	Undo
Ctrl+1	Format cells
Ctrl+Del	Delete to the end of the line

Some of the Ctrl+*key* shortcuts are undocumented. For example, Ctrl+2 makes the highlighted text bold, just as Ctrl+B does.

Alt+*Key* Combinations

You can move through the items in the main menu with the aid of the Alt key. Just press Alt and use the left or right arrow key to open the various pull-down menus; press the up or down arrow key to move up and down these menus.

You can also access any option in the pull-down menus using the Alt key and the underlined letters in the menu options. Look at the main menu on your screen; the *F* in File is underlined, the *E* in Edit is underlined—as is the *V* in View, the *I* in Insert, the *O* in Format, the *T* in Tools, the *A* in Table, the *W* in Window, and the *H* in Help. That means you can access these menus by pressing Alt+F, Alt+E, Alt+V, Alt+I, Alt+O, Alt+T, Alt+A, Alt+W, and Alt+H, respectively. Once a pull-down menu is open, you can access a menu option by pressing the key for the underlined letter in the option you want to select. For example, if you press Alt+F to open the File menu, you can then press S to access the Save option on that menu.

What does a key combination like Alt+F+S mean?

☐ First, you press and hold the Alt key and then press F. The File menu opens. At this point, it doesn't matter whether you continue holding the Alt key or not; in either case, you can release the F key.

☐ Now press the S key to access the Save option on the File submenu.

If you act quickly, you can perform a key combination like Alt+F+S all in one motion (practice it). Look at the letters underlined on the pull-down menus to find other Alt+*key* combinations. For example, if you want to activate the Page Layout option on the View pull-down menu, press Alt+V+P (the View menu has the letter *V* underlined, and the Page Layout option has the letter *P* underlined). You can similarly devise other combinations.

TIME SAVER

> When you are working within a document, you can press Shift+F10 to bring up a context-sensitive shortcut menu, which contains a few commonly used commands. The shortcut menu you see depends on what you are currently doing in the program. You can also access the same shortcut menu by pressing the right mouse button.

Other Keyboard Shortcuts

You can access many of the tools in the toolbars by using the function keys, either alone or in combination with the Alt, Ctrl, and/or Shift keys. You can find a complete list of these shortcuts by searching for *keyboard shortcuts* with Office Assistant, as described later in this hour. The function keys are listed in Table 3.3.

Table 3.3. The actions of the function keys.

Key	Function
F1	Brings up Office Assistant
F2	Allows you to edit the active cell
F3	Pastes a name into a formula
F4	Repeats the action you just did
F5	GoTo (moves the insertion point to a cell or named reference that you specify)
F6	Moves to the next pane (if the window has been split into panes)
F7	Spell checks the document
F8	Extends a selection of cells (to where the cursor is located)
F9	Calculates the formulas in all worksheets in all open workbooks
F10	Activates the menu bar
F11	Creates a chart
F12	Equivalent to choosing File	Save As from the main menu

Opening or Creating a New Document from within Excel

What if you want to open a new workbook when you already have a workbook open? Select the File menu and then select New. Click Workbook to start a new file.

 A simpler way to start a new workbook is to click the tool in the Standard toolbar that looks like a dog-eared sheet of paper.

You can also start a new workbook by pressing Alt+F+N to open the File menu and select the New command. Alternatively, you can press Ctrl+N (as indicated to the right of the New command in the File pull-down menu).

Opening an Existing Excel Workbook

You do not have to open Excel before you open a document. If you access a workbook, Excel opens with that document displayed.

If you want to open a document you have used recently, you may be lucky enough to find it in the Start menu: Open the Start menu and choose Documents; then click the desired filename if it appears in the list.

3

Another way to open Excel with a particular document is to use the Windows Explorer, which is accessible from the Start menu. Once Windows Explorer is open, find the document in the directory structure and then double-click its icon.

If you know the folder in which you have saved a file, you will easily be able to find the file again. If you can't remember the folder in which you stored a file, see the section "Finding an Existing File."

When Excel is installed, a file called `samples.xls` is also installed. Its default location is `c:\Program Files\Microsoft Office\Office\Examples\samples.xls`. Navigate the directory structure to get to the file and then double-click its icon to open Excel and load that document.

Opening an Existing File from within Excel

If Excel is already open, you can still load an existing file into the program. To open an existing file from within Excel, select File from the main menu and then click Open. Alternatively, click the Open File tool in the Standard toolbar or press Ctrl+O or Alt+F+O. In response to any of these actions, the Open dialog box appears. Now select the name of the existing file you want to open. Remember that you can use the Open dialog box to change folders if you want to open a file from a different folder.

Finding an Existing File

If you aren't sure where a particular file is located on your system, Microsoft Excel includes a solution for that problem.

You can search through specific directories or drives for all the Excel files located in them. To do so, select File | Open. In the Open dialog box, click the Advanced button. When the Advanced Find dialog box appears, click the downward-pointing arrow next to the Look In option near the bottom of the dialog box to display a list similar to the one in Figure 3.6.

Figure 3.6.

Navigate the directory structure to find the desired directory.

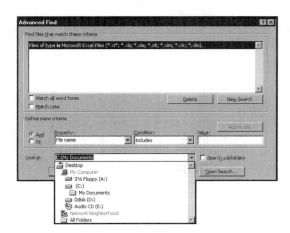

Browse through this list of the folders in your directory and drive structure to get the specific directory or drive you need. If you choose the All Folders option, Excel will search your entire system. If you choose a particular folder, make sure that you select the Search Subfolders checkbox if you want to search that folder's subdirectories as well.

Click the Find Now button; Excel searches the specified directories or drives. The results, of course, vary depending on what Excel files you have on your system and what directories or drives you choose to search. You see a list of the files in the various directories inside the Open dialog box. To open one of these files, double-click its icon.

Opening Excel with a Particular File

You can set up Microsoft Excel so that every time it opens, it loads a specific workbook. Perhaps you are working on a project and want to have the workbook for that particular project immediately accessible whenever you start Excel. Here are the steps to follow:

1. Go to Windows Explorer and find the desired workbook in the folders. For this example, locate `samples.xls` in the directory `C:\Program Files\Microsoft Office\Office\Examples\`.

2. Make a shortcut: Right-click the `samples.xls` file icon; a popup menu appears. Click the Create a Shortcut option; the shortcut icon appears.

3. Drag this shortcut icon to the Excel Start folder, located at `C:\Program Files\Microsoft Office\Office\XLSTART` (if you installed Excel in the standard way). Figure 3.7 shows the process in action.

The next time you open Excel, the `samples.xls` workbook also opens automatically.

Obviously, you should use the file you prefer to have loaded when you open Excel instead of `samples.xls`. If you no longer want Excel to start and load the particular file, just delete the shortcut from the XLSTART folder.

Figure 3.7.

Dragging a shortcut to the XLSTART *folder.*

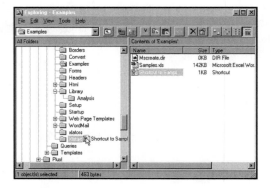

Understanding a Simple Workbook Example

Document management in Excel 97 is similar to that of many other Microsoft products adapted for the Windows 95 environment. An Excel workbook can be compared to a binder containing several (or many) sheets of paper. The workbook is the binder, and the worksheets are the sheets within the binder (by default, a workbook has three sheets). Just as you can move physical sheets of paper from one loose-leaf binder to another, you can move Excel worksheets from one workbook to another.

A *worksheet* is a grid that contains cells. In subsequent hours, you will find how you can add graphics and other stylistic features that eliminate the "grid" look of a worksheet.

When creating Excel workbooks, it is good practice to make the various worksheets within a single workbook relate somehow. However, that suggestion is for your convenience in organizing data, rather than a requirement. You can have a business profit-and-loss worksheet in the same workbook as your neighbor's home mortgage worksheet if you want. In subsequent hours, you will learn how to use data from one worksheet in another worksheet, whether that worksheet is in the same workbook or not.

Cells, Columns, and Rows in a Worksheet

Each unit within a worksheet is called a *cell*. On a typical screen, you can see about 150 cells at a time. A *row* is horizontal (that is, it goes across the screen from left to right), and a *column* is vertical (that is, it goes from top to bottom).

Excel labels the rows in a worksheet with numbers and the columns with uppercase letters. Rows are assigned numbers in sequential order, so there is no need for a more elaborate numbering system. You can have up to 65,536 rows in a spreadsheet. Columns are labeled A, B, C, and so on. If you have more than 26 columns, the alphabetical scheme continues by labeling subsequent columns AA, AB, AC, and so forth. If you exceed 52 columns, the alphabetical scheme continues with BA, BB, BC, and so forth. Continuing in this way, Excel allows you to have 256 columns.

A cell can contain either a label or a value. A *label* is typically a heading that indicates the category of data to which all the entries in that row or column belong (for example, in a profit-and-loss worksheet, cells may contain the labels January, February, March, and so on). A *value* can be in the form of text, dates, currency, and so forth. Hour 4, "Data Entry and Editing in Excel," describes the types of cell contents in greater detail.

Formulas are used to calculate results based on cell values. Formulas streamline and automate the worksheet and eliminate much of the potential for error. Formulas are discussed in detail in Hour 12, "Using Formulas in Excel."

Absolute Addressing and Ranges

If you want to refer to a specific cell, its address is given by its column letter and row number. In Figure 3.8, cell B3 is selected. This address is called an *absolute address* because no matter where you go in the worksheet, cell B3 is always in the same location—at the intersection of column B and row 3. By contrast, a *relative address* is a reference to a cell a particular distance from the current cell (for example, a cell that is two cells up from and one cell to the left of the current cell—regardless of what address the current cell has). Relative addresses come in handy when you are working with formulas and functions.

Figure 3.8.

Cell B3 is selected in this worksheet.

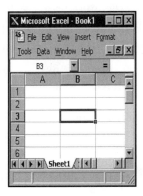

You will likely have occasion to refer to more than one cell at a time. A specific group of cells is called a *range*. If you want to refer to a range of cells in column C that includes rows 5 through 12, the usual way to refer to this range is C5:C12.

Of course, there are many variations in the way a range of cells can be represented in a worksheet. The following list gives some examples and the ways you refer to those ranges:

- ☐ If you want to refer to a range of cells within a single row (for example, row 9) that includes columns D through F, you write the range this way: D9:F9.
- ☐ If you want to refer to all the cells within columns M, N, and P, you write the range this way: M:P.
- ☐ If you want to refer to all the cells in row 6 through row 9, you write the range this way: 6:9.
- ☐ If you want to refer to all the cells within a single column, such as column E, you write the range this way: E:E.

Absolute references and relative references are discussed in greater detail in Hour 12 and Hour 13, "Using Functions in Excel."

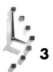

3

Resizing and Arranging Windows

You can resize both the worksheet window and the Excel window. You may want to resize the window by minimizing it (that is, reducing the window to an icon so that you can use the full screen for another purpose) or by maximizing it (that is, making the Excel window or the individual worksheet window take up all the space allowed by the screen so that you can see as much of your work as possible).

At some point in your computing odyssey, you will probably want to have two or more programs open, with both showing on-screen together. You may want to cut data from one application and past it in another, or you may want to play Solitaire while working on a spreadsheet. In any event, you can adjust the size of each program's window to make this possible.

Follow these steps to resize windows:

1. Look at the upper-right corner of your screen, where the Excel title bar and the worksheet's menu bar terminate. Notice the three little boxes in each of these bars: a fat underscore (the Minimize button), two overlapping sheets (the Restore Window button), and an × (the Close button). If your Excel window does not take up the full screen you will see the Maximize button (a single sheet) instead of the Restore Window button. The Excel program window has its set of three buttons that you can use to control the size of the Excel program window, and the worksheet window has a separate set of buttons.

2. Click the Excel program window's Minimize button (the fat underscore button in the title bar at the very top of the screen) to minimize the entire Excel program to an icon on the Windows 95 taskbar. The program is still running in your computer's memory, but you now have the entire screen in which you can do some other task.

   Click the Excel program icon in the task bar to restore the program window to its former size.

3. Click the worksheet window's Minimize button (the fat underscore button in the menu bar) to reduce the size of the worksheet window within the Excel window. You see a small horizontal bar with the name of the workbook at the bottom of the Excel window (see Figure 3.9).

4. Restore the worksheet window to occupy the full screen by clicking the Maximize button on the horizontal bar at the bottom of the screen.

5. Resize either the Excel program window or the worksheet window by moving the mouse pointer over one of the edges of the window. When the mouse pointer changes to a two-headed arrow, press and hold the left mouse button and drag the window to reduce or expand it to the size you want.

If you changed the size of the Excel program window, notice that the worksheet window is resized, too. If you make the Excel program window small enough, you will have enough room to open another application (for example, Microsoft Word or the Solitaire game); you can then resize the second application's window to fill the remaining space on-screen so that the two applications appear side by side for easy accessibility.

6. If you opened another application, close it now. Restore the Excel window to its former size by clicking the Restore Window button (the two overlapping pieces of paper).

Figure 3.9.

The horizontal bar at the bottom of the screen is actually a minimized workbook.

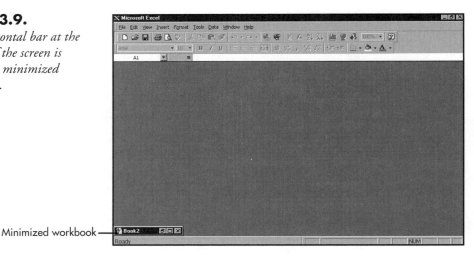

Minimized workbook ——

Saving Files

Once you've created an Excel workbook, you will probably want to save it so that you can access it the next time you use Excel. Excel has several ways to save a file. You don't have to remember all of them—just find a method that you like.

Choosing a Folder for Your Excel Files

The default folder in which Excel saves your documents is C:\My Documents. You can use that folder if you want. You can also create your own preferred folder within Windows Explorer, or you can save your documents in a folder you have already created.

Saving a File with File | Save

If you are working with a new document that you want to save, open the File menu and select Save. Alternatively, press Ctrl+S or Alt+F+S, or click the floppy disk tool in the Standard toolbar. The Save As dialog box appears.

3

If you want to save a new document with the default name chosen by Excel, such as Book1.xls, just click the Save button in the dialog box. If you want to change the name to something more meaningful, position the mouse cursor in the File Name box. Highlight the current name, press the Del key on your keyboard to clear the text box, type the name you want to give the file, and then click Save.

 If the document you are working with has been saved before (that is, if it has already been assigned a name or the default name has been accepted), the document saves automatically when you select the File | Save menu option, press Ctrl+S or Alt+F+S, or click the Save toolbar button. If you want to save your document under a different name, choose File | Save As, as described in the following section.

To save your documents in a different format than Excel 97, select File | Save As from the main menu to display the Save As dialog box. Choose from the different options available in the Save As Type drop-down list (for example, Microsoft Excel 5.0/95 Workbook). If you are sharing your Excel 97 files with people who use a Windows 3.1 version of Excel, for example, you must save your files in a format other than Excel 97. You can also save your Excel file in a format compatible with another spreadsheet program, such as Lotus 1-2-3. Hour 17, "Exploring Excel's Utilities and Add-Ins," discusses a way to convert batches of files to and from various file formats.

Caution

With Windows 95, you can name your files with long filenames—up to 256 characters. You can be as descriptive as you want within those bounds. However, because you may be sharing your files with people who use Windows 3.1, you may want to save your files with filenames in the standard Windows 3.1 format: up to 8 characters for the filename, and up to 3 characters for the extension.

Saving a File with File | Save As

If you have saved your document already and want to save it again under a different name, select File | Save As from the menu or press Alt+F+A. In the File Name text box, replace the current filename with the new filename and click Save. (If you decide you don't want a different name after all, just click Save without changing the name.) Now you have two versions of the document: one with the old filename and one with the filename you just specified.

Creating Backups

Keeping backups of your files is essential if your data is of any value. You can save yourself a great deal of stress and worry by creating backups of your work at regular intervals.

You can save backups manually. Suppose that you want to keep a backup copy of your workbook on a floppy disk. Once you've saved the file with its usual filename using the File | Save command, use the File | Save As command to save the file to the floppy disk (you can also save the file to another drive or to another folder on the same drive). Having an organized backup system in place is essential for any individual or company with important data.

Closing a File with File | Close

If you want to close your workbook without quitting Excel, select File | Close. If you haven't made any changes since you opened the file or since you last saved it, the workbook closes but Excel remains running. If you have made changes since you last saved the workbook, the confirmation dialog box appears. Select Yes if you want to save changes, No if you do not, and Cancel if you want to return to the workbook without either saving or closing it.

Saving a File Automatically

If you've used computers for any length of time, you have probably had the sad experience of losing hours of work when someone steps on the extension cord, the system locks up, or you otherwise experience bad luck. Using manual backups, as described in the preceding section, certainly helps. Excel's AutoSave feature, which is also present in other Microsoft Office applications, can help alleviate the heartbreak of lost data because this feature forces Excel to save your work every few minutes.

You can read about installing various Excel components such as AutoSave in Hour 2, "Installing Excel 97."

If AutoSave is installed for Excel, you will see the AutoSave option on the Tools menu. Select the AutoSave option to display the AutoSave dialog box. Specify how many minutes you want Excel to wait between automatic saves and specify whether you want to be prompted before a save is made. If you specify that Excel should save your work every 10 minutes, you will probably never lose more than 10 minutes of work. If you specify a time of every 5 minutes, you will probably never lose more than 5 minutes work, and so forth. You must balance the amount of work you stand to lose against the very minor interruption caused by the Save feature.

Saving a Workspace

You can save a *workspace configuration*. This means that if you have opened a workbook or group of workbooks and made configuration changes, you can save these changes for the next time you open Excel. Excel users often develop strong preferences for certain window sizes and other configuration changes they have made, and it's only natural to want to get those back again without effort.

To save a workspace, select File | Save Workspace from the main Excel menu. Enter an appropriate name for your workspace and change the folder if you want to save the workspace

3

file in a different location. Any filename ending with .xlw is a workspace file. A workspace file doesn't actually save the data files themselves—just your settings. Make sure that you save all your workbooks as usual.

To access this workspace the next time you use Excel, just open the workspace file as you would any other file.

If you open a workbook that is used in a workspace file in the usual way, the workbook shows no sign of being part of the workspace file. Saving a workspace does not affect the workbooks involved, and working with the workbooks does not affect the workspace.

Getting Help within Excel

There are at least two ways to access Excel's online help: with Office Assistant or with the traditional Help menu. You can also access the Microsoft Excel Web site from within Excel, and you can use a special pointer to tell you what the different icons and symbols mean.

Getting Help with Office Assistant

Office Assistant is new to Office 97. It can provide both verbal and written assistance when you are working on various tasks. It takes the guise of a charming and ever-patient cartoon character.

To invoke Office Assistant, you can do one of several things:

☐ Click the ? icon at the right end of the Standard toolbar.

☐ Press F1.

☐ Select Help from the main menu and then select Microsoft Excel Help.

When Office Assistant is activated by any of these means, you see the figure and menu shown in Figure 3.10.

Figure 3.10.

Office Assistant at work.

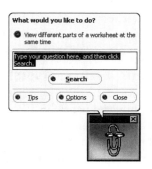

To move the Office Assistant around the screen, drag it with the mouse and drop it at the desired location. The Office Assistant moves out of your way when you are typing, but if you find its presence irritating, you can close it by clicking the × symbol in the upper-right corner of the cartoon's box.

If Office Assistant's main menu has closed, you can reopen it by left-clicking anywhere in the cartoon's box.

To change the appearance or the behavior of Office Assistant, right-click the Office Assistant's cartoon box to display a popup menu that allows you to make selections regarding these behaviors.

To have Office Assistant help you with a specific topic, enter an ordinary sentence, just as if you were talking to an actual human being. Try entering the following question: **How do you open a workbook?** Press the Enter key or click the Search button to see the response shown in Figure 3.11. Click the round button next to the response that best matches your request to display details about that topic. Alternatively, click the See More arrow to view additional response options.

Figure 3.11.

Office Assistant answers.

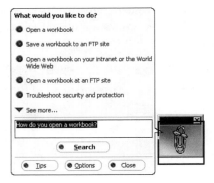

This feature is not perfect, and you may get some results that aren't quite accurate or just what you want with some of the questions. Try rephrasing the question or just use the key words or phrases you want information about.

Customizing Office Assistant

You can customize the form of your Office Assistant. The default Office Assistant is *Clippity*—an animated paperclip. To choose another form, select Options from the Office Assistant menu; the options dialog box appears. Click the Gallery tab and then page through a variety of different forms for your little friend. You can select an Office Assistant character that resembles Einstein, Shakespeare, Mother Nature, or one of several other humorous "personalities." Each character has its own individual sounds and personality, but all give the same information.

3

In addition to changing its appearance, you can customize the functions and behavior of your Office Assistant. To change these aspects of the Office Assistant, select Options from the main Office Assistant menu; the Options dialog box appears. Select the Options tab in the dialog box.

From the Options tab, you can choose whether or not Office Assistant will make those charming sounds, whether or not you want to see a Tip of the Day, and several other things. Just check or uncheck the desired boxes by clicking them and then click OK. If you specified that Office Assistant is to give you a Tip of the Day, the tip box will be right there on your screen when you start Excel and will stay there until you close it.

Getting Help with the Help Menu

If you prefer to use the usual Help you are familiar with from earlier versions of Microsoft Office, just select Help from the main menu.

The Help | Contents and Index Option

For wide-ranging assistance with problems you encounter when working with Excel, select Help | Contents and Index or press Alt+H+C. The dialog box shown in Figure 3.12 appears. Select the Contents tab to view an organized tutorial you can use to get up and running with all of Excel's many features. Working through the tutorial is especially useful if you are a beginner. You can also read some general information about Excel.

Figure 3.12.

The Contents and Index dialog box.

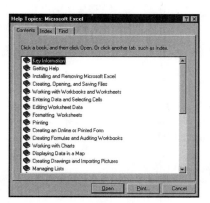

If the Index tab doesn't appear automatically when the Contents and Index dialog box opens, click the Index tab. In the text box, begin to type the word for which you want information. As you type, the Index moves to the correct alphabetical section. For example, if you begin by typing the letter **a**, the Index moves to the beginning of the entries starting with *A*. As you continue typing the word you want help for, the Index continues to narrow the choices presented to you until you find the index term you are looking for. You can also scroll up and down through the entries using the mouse or the arrow keys.

To search through the Help system for a particular word, click the Find tab in the Contents and Index dialog box. Microsoft Excel generates a database of all the words in the help files, and you can then do a search. If this is the first time you have used Find, you see a dialog box that offers several options for setting up the database. If you choose the Maximize Search Capabilities option, Excel creates a Find database file that takes up a lot of space on your hard drive. Choose the Customize Search Capabilities option if you want to search only certain help files. The recommended choice is Minimize Database Size because this option allows you to search effectively through all the files without creating a huge search file on your hard disk. Once you've made your database configuration choice, click Next and follow the prompts.

The Help | What's This Option

The What's This item on the Help menu is a pointer that can give you a brief description of every component on the screen. You can also activate this special pointer by pressing the Shift+F1 key combination. Use this special mouse pointer to point to various icons and components of the toolbars; click the ones you want to know more about. A short popup comment appears.

TIME SAVER

Every dialog box has an easy way to access the What's This pointer. Click the ? button in the upper-right corner of the dialog box and use the pointer to click any item you want additional information about.

The Help | Microsoft on the Web Option

If you have an Internet connection, you can easily jump to the Microsoft Office World Wide Web site from within Excel. Go to the Help menu and select Microsoft on the Web or press Alt+H+W. Select the category about which you want information from the cascading menu, and your default browser (Netscape Navigator or Internet Explorer) will open up and go to the site specified.

- ☐ Choose the Free Stuff option from the cascading menu to view a page on which Microsoft offers a number of add-ons and templates (such as a business planner, car-lease advisor, loan manager, and several others) you can download for free to add more power to Excel.

- ☐ The Product News option, as you might expect, tells you about Excel.

- ☐ The Frequently Asked Questions option provides answers to common questions.

- ☐ The Online Support option leads to an area where you can enter search queries about Excel and other Microsoft programs. This option and the Frequently Asked Question option supplement the online help available within Microsoft Excel.

The other entries on the Microsoft on the Web submenu are self-explanatory.

The Help | Lotus 1-2-3 Help Option

Choosing the Lotus 1-2-3 option from the Help menu displays a dialog box especially designed to help 1-2-3 users adapt to Excel. Microsoft is very interested in helping Lotus loyalists become happy Excel users and so has introduced this dialog box as an easy way to compare equivalent commands in the two programs.

Select the Lotus menu you want to learn about from the list at the left side of the dialog box. Click the menu name to see another list of the corresponding submenu's options. Continue selecting submenu options until you find the Lotus 1-2-3 command you are looking for. Click the Instructions button to see written information about how to perform that command in Excel. Click the Demo button to see an animation indicating the menus you have to access to perform the command in Excel.

The Help | About Microsoft Excel Option

When you select the About Microsoft Excel option from the Help menu, you get a dialog box like the one shown in Figure 3.13.

Figure 3.13.

About Microsoft Excel.

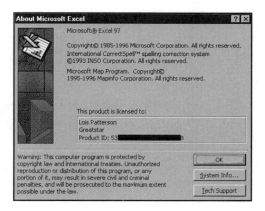

When you install your version of Microsoft Office or Microsoft Excel, you get your own Product-ID number. If you ever have to contact Microsoft technical support, you must give the technician this number.

Click the Tech Support button to display a list of the different ways you can access Excel help. Microsoft has support forums on America Online, CompuServe, and other providers, as well as telephone support.

Click the System Info button to see information about your particular computer system. The dialog box you see depends on your particular system configuration, but a typical one is shown in Figure 3.14. This box tells you how much memory you have free and other details about your system.

Figure 3.14.

The System Information
dialog box.

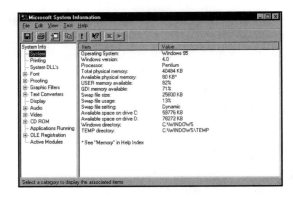

Exiting Excel

A graceful exit is always a good idea—particularly for Windows 95 programs. You have
several ways to quit Excel:

- [ ] Select File | Exit
- [ ] Press Ctrl+W
- [ ] Press Alt+F+X
- [ ] Press Alt+F4

 [ ] Click the Close button (the × button) in the upper-right corner of the title bar

If you saved the files on which you were working and haven't made any further changes, you
exit from Excel without further prompting.

If you have made changes to your documents and haven't saved the files yet, you see a dialog
box asking whether you want to save those changes. Select Yes if you want to save the changes
in the document and then continue the Exit process. Select No if you want to exit without
saving changes to your documents. Select Cancel if you just want to return to the program.
Make sure that you do not click No if you really do want to save your changes; doing so causes
all your work to be lost. It's all too easy to have a slippery trigger finger.

Summary

Microsoft Excel 97 shares many features of its interface with other Windows 95 programs,
and especially with other Office 97 programs. If you've used one Microsoft Office product,
you will readily find your way around Excel.

In this hour, you learned how to open Microsoft Excel and how to create a new workbook. You learned how to open an existing workbook and save workbooks to which you have made changes. You also learned how to use the online help available with Excel.

Hour 4, "Data Entry and Editing in Excel," describes how you actually enter the data and format the cells of a worksheet. Hour 5, "Navigating and Manipulating Excel Documents," discusses in greater detail how to manipulate workbooks and worksheets.

Workshop

Term Review

cell   The basic unit of an Excel worksheet. A cell is a single block in the grid.

column   A vertical group of cells, one cell wide, extending the length of the worksheet.

custom toolbar   A toolbar specially created by the user.

keyboard shortcut   A one-key, two-key, or three-key combination for performing a task; used instead of accessing the menu system with the mouse.

main menu bar   The toolbar at the very top of the Excel worksheet; it begins at the left edge with the Excel symbol and continues across the screen to the Help menu option. The Excel symbol and each of the menu names have a corresponding pull-down menu.

Office Assistant   An animated character that can provide assistance with all the features of Excel. You can turn it on or off by pressing F1.

range   A group of contiguous cells.

row   A horizontal group of cells, one cell long, extending the width of the worksheet.

toolbar   A bar, often the length of the Excel window, that contains various tools. You click the tools to perform certain tasks. You can add or remove toolbars by choosing View | Toolbars from the main menu.

workbook   A single Excel file that can contain one or more worksheets; it can also contain charts, macros, and other objects.

worksheet   Another term for *spreadsheet*. By default, a new workbook in Excel has three worksheets in it.

Q&A

Q Can you perform the same task in different ways?

A Yes. Most tasks in Excel can be done in at least two of the following ways: by selecting options from the main menu, by pressing a keyboard shortcut, or by clicking an icon or tool.

Q How is Excel similar to other Windows 95 programs?

A It has a similar main menu bar to other Windows 95 programs. The Restore, Minimize, Maximize, and Close window buttons are common to all the programs.

Q What can Office Assistant do?

A If you press F1, you see Office Assistant, a cute little cartoon figure that can help you find the answers to any Excel problem you may have.

Hour 4

Data Entry and Editing in Excel

One of the features that makes Excel so powerful is its ability to distinguish between different types of data. Excel can tell—with a fair degree of accuracy—whether you are entering dates, money amounts, times, or any one of several other formats, and Excel has default formatting in place for each of these possibilities. You can always change the default if you prefer to do so, and Excel provides a great deal of latitude to the user to change the appearance and behavior of the cells and the data contained within the cells.

The cells of a worksheet contain either values or formulas. The *values* can be text, numbers, or both. *Formulas* perform calculations based on the values of other cells; this topic is discussed in greater detail in Hour 12, "Using Formulas in Excel."

Probably the best way to work through this hour is to start by opening Excel to a default workbook. Experiment with the possibilities by entering different types of data and formatting them in the various ways described throughout this hour.

Basic Cell Entry

When working in Excel, one cell in the worksheet is usually highlighted at all times. The address of this cell is listed in the name box in the upper-left corner of the screen, just above the column letter A.

To enter data, select the cell you want by clicking it with the left mouse button. Type the data—numbers, text, or both. When you are done typing, press Enter, click the green checkmark (look for it on the line above the column letters at the top of the screen), or use the arrow keys to move to the next cell.

JUST A MINUTE

> Cells that contain formulas are discussed in Hour 12 and Hour 14, "More Data Manipulation."

How you organize your worksheet is up to you. People commonly put some identifying information—such as the company name or the name of the project—at the top of the worksheet. In general, you will have text values at the top and along the left side of the worksheet to identify the data below and to the right. Figure 4.1 shows a basic spreadsheet that does not begin to capture the complexity of what you can do with Excel. As mentioned in Hour 1, "Introduction to Excel 97," you can use Excel for many more complicated tasks than just a simple ledger. You don't have to follow the format shown in Figure 4.1—and you probably will not.

Figure 4.1.

An example of a simple spreadsheet.

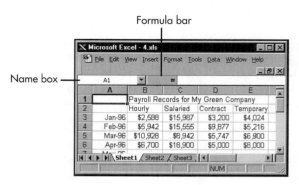

Here are some basic data entry and navigation tips:

☐ To jump to another cell in a worksheet, position the cursor in the name box at the top left of the worksheet window, type the new cell's address, and press Enter to move to that cell.

4

☐ To select an entire row of cells, click the appropriate number along the side of the worksheet. To select an entire column, click the appropriate letter along the top of the worksheet.

☐ To cancel a selection of a cell or group of cells, click elsewhere in the worksheet.

☐ To highlight a rectangular group of cells, click the cell in one of the corners of the rectangle you want to highlight. Hold the left mouse button and drag the mouse pointer diagonally to the opposite corner of the desired rectangle of cells. Release the mouse button when all the cells are highlighted.

☐ To change the data in a cell, click the cell and position your cursor at the point where you want to start typing the new data. Type the new data. In Insert mode, the old data remains in place. In Typeover mode, the old data is replaced if you position the cursor to type over the data. To toggle between Insert and Typeover mode, press the Ins key.

☐ You can clear the contents of a cell or group of cells in a few easy motions. You can highlight the cell or group of cells and then press the Del key. Alternatively, you can select the cells, right-click within the worksheet, and select Clear Contents from the popup menu that appears.

Types of Data

Your data can have text values or numeric values. *Text values* are just that: anything you can type from the keyboard—characters, numbers, and some symbols. The *numeric values* can be currency, times, dates, and many others, as described in the section "Numeric Values," later in this hour. For both text and numeric values, you can control the fonts, the alignment, the colors, the background patterns, and more.

Text Values

Text values are straightforward to enter and can include both text and numbers. In Part III of this book, "Excel and Interactive Data," you learn various ways to manipulate text values, but the actual data entry process is simple.

Data that consists of letters, punctuation, and other symbols is automatically recognized as text. If you combine letters and numbers in a single cell entry, the combined entry is recognized as a text entry.

To enter text in a cell, select the cell and start typing. Press Enter when you are done or click the green checkmark on the formula bar.

If you want a line of text wrap within its cell, press Alt+Enter where you want the hard carriage return to appear in the line of text.

You can also format as text numbers by themselves (for example, addresses or telephone numbers). You want to format number as text when you do not want to inadvertently perform mathematical calculations on those numbers. (What significance does multiplying one telephone number by another have?) The section "Applying Formats to Numeric Values," later in this chapter, explains how to do just that.

In general, to apply a format to data, highlight the cells to which you want to apply the format. Choose Format | Cells from the main menu and then select the various formats you want to apply to the selected cells.

TIME SAVER

> In Excel, text is left aligned by default; numerical values are right aligned by default. If you've entered some data, you can tell which category Excel has placed it in by looking to see how it is aligned.

Numeric Values

A numeric value can contain any of the following characters:

```
0   1   2   3   4   5   6   7   8   9   +   -   (   )   ,   /   $   %   .   E   e
```

You can also use a single space when entering fractions, times, or dates.

Excel has defined formats for each of the types of numeric values listed in Table 4.1. These number formats differ in how the numbers are aligned, whether or not there are accompanying symbols and how they are placed, and other features.

You can also apply the formats you want to cells *before* you enter the data. Then, no matter how you enter the data, the data is converted to the selected format.

Table 4.1. Numeric formatting.

Format Name	Description
General	For any numbers that have no specific characteristics.
Number	For numbers that have a specific number of decimal places.
Currency	For general monetary values.
Accounting	For monetary values that you want to align at the decimal point.
Date	For date values.
Time	For time values.

4

Format Name	Description
Percentage	For percentages, followed by the percent (%) symbol.
Fraction	For fractions.
Scientific	For scientific (exponential) notation.
Text	For numbers you want to treat as text (for example, the numbers you use to identify students in an educational setting).
Special	Includes ZIP code, phone number, and Social Security number formats.
Custom	For formats you create yourself.

Each of these different formats is described in detail in the following sections. Note that you can apply any of these format options to a cell or group of cells before or after you enter data in the cells.

TIME SAVER

You can format numbers as text by typing an apostrophe (') in front of the numbers. For example, typing '15 results in the characters 15 inside the cell, left-aligned.

4

Applying Formats to Numeric Values

You apply a format to a numeric value in much the same way, regardless of which format you are applying. You can apply a format either before or after you enter data into a cell. If you apply a format *before* entering data into a cell, the data (if it is of the correct type) is automatically changed into that format. Similarly, if you apply a format *after* entering the data, the data is automatically changed to that format.

Suppose that you want to format some cells in Currency format; you want the Canadian dollar to be the currency symbol, and you want the data to be formatted to two decimal places. Here are the steps you would follow:

1. Select the cell or cells you want to format.

2. Choose Format | Cells from the main menu to display the Format Cells dialog box.

3. Click the Number tab.

4. Make your formatting selections:

☐ Select Currency from the Category list.

☐ To display the data with two decimal places, select 2 from the Decimal Places list.

☐ To change the currency symbol, use the drop-down list and select $(English) Canadian.

5. Click OK when done.

Any data in the selected cells is changed to Canadian currency format. Any data you enter in those cells in the future is also changed to Canadian currency format.

In general, to format a cell or cells, you first select the range. Then you choose Format | Cells from the main menu, and click the Number tab. You can make your choice from the Category list, from the Decimal Place option (if applicable), and from the Type drop-down list.

The General Format

The General format, as its name implies, is for general numbers that don't fall into any of the other categories. No formatting is applied to the number, and its value is not affected in any way. You get exactly what you enter in the cell.

The Number Format

The Number format differs from the General format in that numbers are rounded off to the specified number of decimal places; zeroes are added when necessary.

If a number is rounded, it appears as rounded on the worksheet display but it still has its original form in memory. That means that if you do calculations with the rounded numbers, the full number is used in the calculation.

For example, if you enter the numbers 3.4 and 1.4 in two cells and round them to whole numbers, the cells display 3 and 1. If you add these cells together, however, the actual values add up to 4.8 (rounded up to 5). When you look at the numbers displayed in the cells, however, you expect them to add up to 4. (You learn how to add cells together in Hour 12) You can see the original number values again by reformatting the cells so that they display more decimal places.

The Currency Format

The Currency format is for general monetary values. The values are right aligned in the cell, but they are not also left aligned as they are with the Accounting format, described next.

You can choose the currency symbol appropriate for your data if you select the Currency format. A variety of possibilities are represented, with the default being the U.S. dollar sign ($).

The default currency format uses the dollar sign and a comma as separator. If a cell is formatted in Currency format with no decimal places to be displayed, and you enter the number 1234, the cell displays the number with this formatting: $1,234.

4

The Accounting Format

Numeric values are right aligned in their cells by default. However, the Accounting format causes the values in the cells to be aligned at the decimal point. This is perfect for dealing with sums of money that range from large to small.

Figure 4.2 shows the difference between the Currency and Accounting formats. With the Accounting format, the cells are both left aligned and right aligned (notice that the currency symbol is moved to the leftmost position and that the figures are aligned at the implied decimal point). With the Currency format, the numbers are simply right aligned (the default Currency format provides the dollar sign and the comma within the number).

Figure 4.2.

The Currency and Accounting formats.

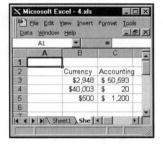

The Date Format

Excel automatically recognizes most formats when you enter dates. Whether you enter 3/13/97 or 13/3/97 or March 13, 1997 or 13-Mar-97 or one of several other formats, Excel automatically recognizes what you enter as a date and reformats it to the default setting. Excel does not require the year to interpret an entry as a date. 5-29 and 5/29 are treated as equivalent to May 29.

JUST A MINUTE

The default setting for dates—as well as other settings such as currency, time, numbers and so forth—can be accessed from the Control Panel. Choose Settings from the Start menu, and select Control Panel. Click the Regional Settings tab in the dialog box that appears. For most readers of this book, the appropriate setting is English (United States). You can change all the settings at once by choosing the language and country you prefer, or you can change particular formats from the menu. The default setting used in this book is English (United States).

If you've entered dates and want to change their appearance, select the cell or cells that contain the dates, and choose Format|Cells to display the Format Cells dialog box. Click the

Numbers tab and select the Date option from the Category list to display the list of possible
formats shown in Figure 4.3. Select your preferred format and click OK.

Figure 4.3.

*The Date format
possibilities.*

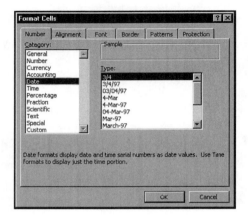

The Time Format

The thing to remember about the Time format is that you can use either a 12-hour clock or
a 24-hour clock. The default is a 24-hour clock. If you enter 1:32, Excel assumes that you
mean 1:32 A.M., not 1:32 P.M. If you want to enter 1:32 PM in a 24-hour clock, you must
include a p or PM after the time. Otherwise, enter 13:32 in the 24-hour clock system.

You can also include times in the hh-min-sec format, like this: 23:59:59 (this time is one
second before midnight). Similarly, you can enter 9:02:15p or 9:02:15 PM.

You can see the various time formats available for you to choose from when you access the
Format I Cells dialog box and select Time from the Categories list, as shown in Figure 4.4.

Figure 4.4.

*The Time Format
possibilities.*

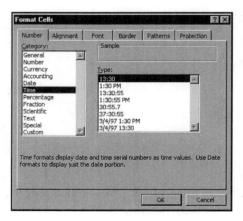

4

JUST A MINUTE

You can create your own custom time, date, and other formats suitable for your particular needs. For example, if you are preparing spreadsheets to calculate data related to employees who work a 40-hour week, you can create a time format based on that criterion. Preparing custom number formats is discussed in detail in Hour 14.

You can enter data that includes both a date and time within a single cell. Separate the date and time by a single space. You can use your preferred format for either when you enter the data, and Excel reformats it to the default setting. You can change the format of the date and time if you want by using the Format | Cells dialog box.

TIME SAVER

If you don't like the look of gridlines in your worksheet or find them confusing when you are entering data, open the Tools | Options menu and select View. Deselect the Gridlines box under Window Options and click OK. You can also customize the appearance of your workbook with the other options available in the View dialog box.

4

The Percentage Format

There are two ways you can enter percentages in Excel. You can enter percentages directly by typing 50%, 75%, and so forth. You can also enter percentages as fractions or decimals and then format the cells with the Percentage format. The Percentage format allows you to specify the number of decimal places you want. The Percentage format multiplies the number you enter by 100 and adds the % sign.

For example, if you entered the number 1 1/4 and then format the cell with the Percentage format with no decimal places, the cell displays 125%. If you enter 0.3355 and format the cell as a Percentage with 2 decimal places, the cell displays 33.55%.

You can easily convert numbers formatted as percentages into fractions, just as you can convert numbers formatted as fractions into percentages. Select the group of cells currently formatted with the percent format, select Format | Cells, select the Number tab, and select the Fraction item from the Category list, as described in the following section.

The Fraction Format

The Fraction format takes numbers that include a slash (/) and treats them as fractions.

You can enter fractions like this: 5 3/8. Leave a single space between the whole number and the fraction. Excel treats fractions such as 1/4 (fractions with no whole-number component) as a date. To get around this problem, enter the fraction with a 0 preceding it to format it correctly: 0 1/4. When you press Enter or otherwise switch to another cell, the 0 disappears.

You can convert numbers entered in decimal format to fractions. For example, if you enter 5.1 in a cell and then format the cell with the Fraction format, 5 1/10 is displayed.

Fraction format allows you to choose how many digits there will be in the denominator by selecting the appropriate number from the Type menu on the Fraction tab. If your fraction doesn't fit in the cell, Excel rounds it for you. For example, if you enter the fraction 1 11/25 and allow 1 digit in the denominator, 1 4/9 is displayed.

The Scientific Format (Exponents)

Scientists use exponents as a convenient way to express very large or very small numbers. To write a number such as 800,000, you can enter 8E5. That is just a different way of writing 8×10^5. You can also use a lowercase e if you prefer: 8e5. To write a number such as 0.0000908, enter 9.08E-5. If you choose to do so, you can also enter the same number as 90.8E-6 (or some other combination that results in the same number); the Scientific format converts the value you enter to standard scientific notation. The number before the E is always less than 10 in standard scientific notation.

You can convert numbers written in the ordinary way to scientific notation by assigning the Scientific format to the cell.

COFFEE BREAK

Fixed Decimal Places and Negative Numbers

If you are entering a series of numbers that have the same number of decimal places, you can facilitate the data entry process. First, format the cells in which you are going to enter those numbers and then enter the numbers without bothering to insert the decimal point. Here's how: Choose Tools | Options and select the Edit tab in the dialog box. Choose Fixed Decimal and select the number of decimal places you know your numbers have. Click OK.

If you specify 2 decimal places and want to enter the number 531.25, you do not have to pause to enter the period. Just type 53125 and Excel inserts the decimal place correctly. If you type 4, these preformatted cells interpret the value as 0.04.

You can enter negative numbers in cells formatted with any format except Date, Time, and Special. To enter negative numbers, just precede the digits with the minus sign (-) or enter the number in parentheses: (32).

The Text Format

In Excel, you can treat numeric data as text. The worksheet in Figure 4.5 shows rental payment records for the apartments in an apartment complex. Notice the apartment numbers in column A; you are not going to perform any mathematical operations on those numbers. For all intents and purposes, you want to treat the apartment numbers as text.

Highlight the group of cells you want to format as Text, select Format|Cells, select the Numbers tab in the dialog box, and choose Text from the Category list.

Figure 4.5.

The highlighted apartment numbers are to be treated as text.

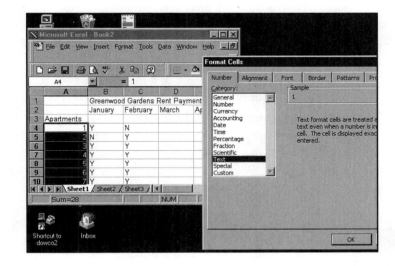

The Special Format

The Special format includes several specific types of numbers. Four options appear in the Type list for the Special format:

- ☐ Zip Code (the standard 5-digit version)
- ☐ Zip Code + 4 (the standard 5-digit + 4-digit version)
- ☐ Phone number (can include the area code or not)
- ☐ Social Security number

The Custom Format

The Custom format includes a variety of different types of formats for different types of numbers. There are date/time formats, percentage formats, and others. If you have a specific requirement for formatting, you may be able to find it in the Custom format list.

Using Automated Tools for Data Entry

Excel has two tools that speed up the data entry process: AutoFill and AutoComplete. Both work by intelligently guessing what your next entries will be, based on what you have entered in other cells. Both features are turned on by default; if you don't want to use these features, you can disable them.

The AutoFill Tool

If you have a cell entry that you want to repeat, the AutoFill feature can save you a lot of typing. Highlight the cell that contains the data you want to repeat and put the mouse cursor on the lower-right border of the cell. A + symbol appears at the cursor point. Drag the cursor horizontally if you want to fill cells across a row. Drag the cursor vertically if you want to fill a column of cells.

If you want to disable the AutoFill feature, select Tools | Options, click the Edit tab in the dialog box, deselect the Allow Cell Drag and Drop checkbox, and click OK.

Using AutoFill to Complete a Series

The AutoFill tool is smart enough to recognize certain series and complete them for you. Suppose that you want to enter text labels for each of the 12 months of 1997. All you have to do is enter the first two: Jan97 and Feb97. AutoFill can recognize that you want to list the months in order and will complete the series for you.

To use AutoFill in this situation, type the first two entries in adjacent cells and highlight both cells. Place the mouse cursor on the bottom-right corner of the range and drag the cursor across or down for as many cells as you require month labels. AutoFill continues the series as long as you continue to drag the cursor over the cells. If you continue to drag the tool for more than 12 cells, you get entries such as Jan98, Feb98, and so forth. AutoFill is very "talented" at filling out series.

Similarly, you can use AutoFill to complete sequences of numbers. In Figure 4.6, the second number is 32 less than the first number. If you select these two cells and drag them down seven cells, you get a sequence of negative numbers. If the sequence stops where the cursor is in the figure, the last entry will be -192.

Figure 4.6.

AutoFill can recognize sequences of numbers and complete the sequence for you.

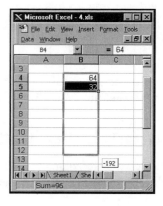

When you use AutoFill, you can drag the cursor left, right, up, or down. Although you cannot use AutoFill to fill columns and rows at the same time, you can do them separately.

Here are some examples of sequences that the AutoFill feature can recognize (you actually only need two entries to use AutoFill, but I've shown three entries here so that you can get a better idea of what the sequence looks like):

```
Monday, Thursday, Sunday, . . .
T1, T2, T3, . . .
25,30,35, . . .
12:20, 12:40, 1:00, . . .
01 December 1996, 02 December 1996, 03 December 1996, . . .
```

AutoFill can recognize and fill only those sequences in which the units are a fixed distance apart. AutoFill cannot recognize geometric sequences like 1, 3, 9, 27 or sequences based on various esoteric criteria such as prime numbers or stock market fluctuations. If you are using AutoFill for dates, the distances can be in terms of days, weeks, months, or years. The development of custom-fill series that use more sophisticated formulas to create sequences is discussed in Hour 14.

The AutoComplete Tool

Excel can guess not only what type of data you are entering, it can even sometimes guess what you are going to enter next. Excel can recognize if you are typing the same entry repeatedly within a row or column—regardless of whether the entry is text or text and numbers together. Click a cell in your worksheet and type Andromeda (or whatever word you want) in two consecutive cells in a row or column. When you start the second entry in the row or column by typing the letter A, the word Andromeda fills the cell instantaneously.

AutoComplete can be irritating when it doesn't type what you want. To turn off the AutoComplete feature, open the Tools | Option menu and choose the Edit tab. Deselect the Enable AutoComplete for Cell Values checkbox and click OK. You can also undo AutoComplete for single or multiple entries by selecting Edit | Undo or pressing Ctrl+Z and repeating as necessary.

Using Automatic Correction Tools

Just as Excel can automate the process of data entry, it can also automate the process of data correction. Excel provides the Undo, AutoCorrect, spell check, and find and replace features to help correct errors as you are entering data or after you have completed the data entry process. All the correction tools described in the following sections are used in Microsoft Word as well.

The Undo Feature

Inevitably, you will type some data, perform a calculation, or do some action in Excel that you know immediately is incorrect. Fortunately, help is close at hand. As do most Microsoft applications, Excel comes with an Undo feature.

With previous versions of Excel, you could undo only a single action. Excel 97 allows you to undo multiple actions—and you can also "redo" single or multiple actions if you inadvertently reverse changes you meant to keep.

If you want to undo, or cancel, your last entry or action, just press Ctrl+Z or select Edit | Undo from the main menu. Repeat the Undo command until you are back to where you wanted to be.

If you want to redo what you have undone, press Ctrl+Y and repeat if necessary.

The AutoCorrect Tool

AutoCorrect can assist you greatly and automatically correct simple errors. When you start Excel, this feature is available with certain default settings. AutoCorrect is very helpful for typo-prone typists—and aren't we all? To change the settings for the AutoCorrect feature, choose Tools | AutoCorrect from the main menu. AutoCorrect's default options are shown in Figure 4.7.

Figure 4.7.

The default AutoCorrect options.

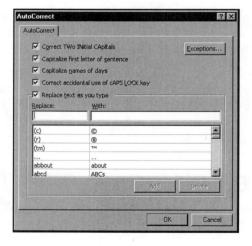

Most of AutoCorrect's default options work well most of the time, but you may prefer to turn off some of them, depending on the type of data you are entering. I find the Replace Text as You Type option irritating, so I deselect that checkbox. Try different options and see what works for you.

4

You can also click the Exceptions button in the AutoCorrect dialog box to customize AutoCorrect to your needs. For example, you can use this button to create specific capitalization rules.

You can use AutoCorrect to convert shorthand references to the complete term to save yourself from typing long words or phrases. For example, if you want the word Microsoft to appear every time you type ms, just type **ms** in the Replace box, type **Microsoft** in the With box, and click Add. Another handy use of this replace feature is if you are prone to particular typing errors; you can enter the erroneous version in the Replace box (for example, teh) and the correct term in the With box (for example, the). Now, every time you type **teh**, Excel replaces it with the.

The Spell Check Feature

The spell check feature is part of the Office 97 package, so you can use it with all applications. When you invoke the spell check feature, it checks your spelling and allows you to correct errors. The spell check does not have a complete dictionary, of course, and it cannot recognize many proper names, as well as idiosyncratic abbreviations and spellings. However, as with almost all Excel features, you can customize the spell check tool to suit your needs. If you use a particular word or spelling throughout your document and don't want the spell check tool to flag it every time it comes across that term, just select Ignore All from the Spell Check dialog box. You can also click the Add button to add a particular word in the dictionary that the spell check uses to check your text.

To invoke the spell check tool, press F7 or select Tools | Spell Check from the main menu.

The Find and Replace Features

You can quickly locate particular data within your worksheet by using the Find feature. Select Edit | Find or press Ctrl+F to display the Find dialog box. You can choose to search your worksheet by rows or by columns, and you can search formulas, values, or text comments for particular data. The Find feature is particularly useful when you have a large worksheet—one that extends beyond the bounds of a single screen.

You can also replace certain data entries with other data in a somewhat automated manner. Press Ctrl+H or select Edit | Replace from the main menu to display the Replace dialog box. Once again, you have several options: You can make the search case sensitive if you want, and you can search by rows or by columns.

Other Formatting Options

The Format | Cells dialog box offers many options for formatting your data. For example, you can control the alignment of the cell contents, the fonts used to display the data, the color of the data characters, and backgrounds. Each of these options is described in the following sections.

Aligning Cell Contents

To align data within cells, first select the data you want to format. Select Format|Cells to display the Format Cells dialog box and then select the Alignment tab.

You can choose from the various alignment options. The default horizontal alignment for text is left alignment. The default alignment for numbers is right alignment. You can change the alignment for the range of selected cells to any of the following:

Horizontal Alignment Option	Description
General	The default.
Left (Indent)	Indents the data to the left (use with numerical data that is right aligned).
Center	Centers the data.
Right	Indents the data to the right (use with data, such as text, that is left aligned by default).
Fill	Takes the characters in the cell and repeats them within the cell until the entire cell is filled up.
Justify Across Selection	Justifies the data in a selection of cells.

The default choice for vertical alignment for both text and numbers is Bottom. That means that, regardless of how big or tall the cell becomes, the last line of the data in the cell is at the bottom of the cell. Once again, you have a variety of options:

Vertical Alignment Option	Description
Bottom	The data aligns against the bottom of the cell.
Top	The data aligns against the top of the cell.
Center	The data is centered in the cell.
Justify	The data is justified within the cell (that is, it is spaced within the cell, like text in a newspaper column).

Changing the Orientation of Data

You can cause your data to appear tilted within its cell. First select the cell that contains the data for which you want to change the orientation. Open the Format Cells dialog box and look at the semicircle at the right side of the dialog box. Drag the Text line to the position on the semicircle at which you want to tilt the contents of your cell (see Figure 4.8). Alternatively, you can use the spin buttons underneath the semicircle panel to choose the angle of inclination.

4

Figure 4.8.

Adjusting the orientation of selected cells.

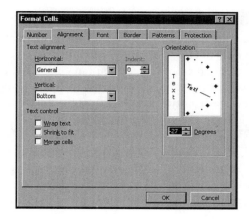

Changing Fonts

Using different fonts for different kinds of data is one way to put some variety and visual appeal into your worksheet. As you do with all the other formatting options, first highlight the cells you want to format with a particular font. The cells can contain data or be empty. Right-click the highlighted range to display the popup menu and choose Format Cells; alternatively, select Format | Cells from the main menu to display the Format Cells dialog box. Click the Font tab.

You can change any characteristic of the font you are using:

☐ **Font (font face).** Any of the variety of TrueType fonts you have installed on your computer. The most commonly used fonts are Arial, Courier, and Times New Roman.

☐ **Font style.** Regular, Italic, Bold, and Bold Italic.

☐ **Size.** How big the characters are (measured in points).

☐ **Underline.** None, Single, Double, Single Accounting, and Double Accounting.

☐ **Color.** One of 56 choices.

☐ **Effects.** Special treatments you can apply to the font (strikethrough, superscript, or subscript).

To see how a particular font looks, just look in the Preview window in the Format Cells dialog box.

Although Excel gives you the option to include literally dozens of different fonts in a worksheet, doing so is not generally a good idea. Keep basic design principles in mind—the simpler, the better.

Adding Cell Borders

Using the border feature is a good way to delineate data and make it more attractive. Select the group of cells you want to enhance with a border, display the Format Cells dialog box, and choose the Border tab. You can choose to have borders appear on the right, left, top, bottom, or any combination of these options for the selected range of cells. You can also choose the line style and color used for the border.

Setting Up Background Patterns

To further enhance your worksheet, you can choose a color and patterned background for a cell or group of cells. You may want to do this to highlight a particular group of cells or just to provide some subtle interest in the worksheet. Select the cells you want to treat with a particular pattern or background color, display the Format Cells dialog box, and select the Patterns tab.

Choose the color you want for your cell and click the Patterns drop-down list. You can choose from an assortment of different dotted, checkered, or striped patterns. There are 56 colors available. Figure 4.9 shows how different colored patterns, fonts, and borders can break up the monotony of a typical black-and-white worksheet. Even though you can't appreciate my psychedelic color scheme, you *can* see the different shadings!

Figure 4.9.

A worksheet showing some formatting features.

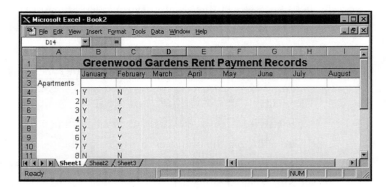

Taking a *little* effort to make your worksheets more attractive is not a waste of time (although taking a *lot* of effort to do so may or may not be). If the different regions of a worksheet are separated from each other by text and color cues, you are less likely to make errors when entering data, and anyone who has to use your files at a later date will find his or her work easier.

Setting Column and Row Sizes

You can control the appearance of your spreadsheet to a large extent by how you set up the rows and columns. As usual, Excel allows you a lot of freedom, as described in the following sections.

Changing the Height of a Row or Rows

Why would you want to change the height of rows? Suppose that you want to use a larger or smaller font than the default, you like the look of white space, or you want to have more than one line of text in a cell. The height of a cell is based on font size. If you have a row height of 10, for example, a character in a 10-point font fits exactly in the cell. If you use a font that is larger than the height of the cell, part of the text is hidden from view (although the data will still be there).

Highlight the row whose height you want to change. You can click the row number to highlight the entire row, or you can select a single cell in the row you want to change. Select Format | Row and then choose Height. Type the desired height of the row. You will probably have to experiment to get the right height for your cells.

To reduce or expand the height of a row with your mouse, place the mouse cursor at the edge of the row number, as shown in Figure 4.10. Once the cross with the vertical arrows appears, you can drag the row boundary up or down to either increase or decrease the height.

Figure 4.10.

Reducing or expanding the row height with the mouse.

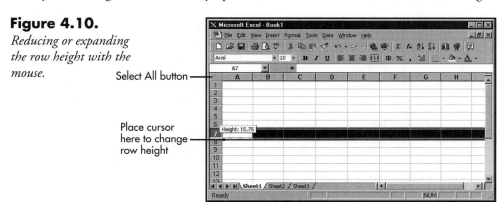

Select All button

Place cursor here to change row height

To change a group of rows to the same height, highlight all of them. Then select Format | Row and choose Height; specify the desired height, as just described.

If you want, you can change the height of all the rows in the worksheet. First, click the empty gray box in the upper-left corner of the worksheet window (where the column labels and the row numbers intersect); this box is known as the Select All button. All the cells in the worksheet are highlighted. Then select Format | Row and choose Height; specify the desired height, as just described.

Fitting the Rows to Size

You may have entries in a row that occupy different heights, particularly if some of the entries consist of wrapped text. Parts of some of the entries may be obscured. To automatically fit the height of a row to its entries, first select the row. Choose Format | Row from the main menu and select the AutoFit option. Alternatively, you can select the row and then double-click the boundary line underneath the row label (the gray number). If you later reduce or increase the height of some cells by wrapping data within them or deleting data, the rows automatically shrink or expand to fit the height of the text or values in the cells.

Changing the Width of a Column

Just as you can set the height of a row, you can set the width of a column. To set the column width with the mouse, place the mouse cursor near the letter of the column you want to widen. Move the mouse pointer over the border until you see the cross symbol with the horizontal arrows. Drag the mouse pointer until the column is the desired width.

As an alternative to the mouse method, you can select the column or a cell in the column and choose Format | Column from the main to display the Column Width dialog box. Enter the new column width and click OK.

Fitting the Columns to Size

Within a single column, some of the cell entries are short and others are lengthy. You can make the width of the cells in a column fit the lengthiest entry in the column. To do so, first select the column. Then choose Format | Column from the main menu and choose AutoFit Selection. The column expands to the width of the widest cell.

Summary

Excel has two basic types of data: text values and numeric values. You have a great deal of control over the appearance of the cells in an Excel worksheet, and you have a variety of formatting options. Excel has a number of tools that automate, to some extent, the data entry and data correction processes. Excel frequently can guess the type of data you are entering and adjust formatting accordingly. Excel can recognize many common errors and correct them instantly. As you have learned in this past hour, there are many ways you can control the appearance of the cells and the spreadsheet as a whole.

Workshop

Term Review

alignment   The positioning of data within a cell. You can horizontally align data to the left, the right, or the center; you can vertically align data to the top, the bottom, or the center.

column   A vertical group of cells, one cell wide. Each column is identified by a letter.

data   The contents of the cell. Data can be numeric or text; you can format the data in a cell based on the specific type of data it is.

row   A horizontal group of cells, one cell high. Each row is identified by a number.

Q&A

Q Why is it important that cells have the correct format?

A If you are doing calculations with the numbers or manipulations with text as described in Hour 12, "Using Formulas in Excel," and Hour 13, "Using Functions in Excel," the numbers must be in the correct format.

Q What are the four automated tools Excel offers to the user?

A AutoFill, which automatically fills out a data entry pattern.

AutoComplete, which automatically recognizes the beginnings of words and fills in the rest without the user typing it.

AutoCorrect, which automatically corrects spelling errors.

AutoFormat, which automatically formats cells according to a prescribed pattern.

Exercise

Here's a simple exercise to test your knowledge.

Jane wants to keep records of how many of different types of products she is selling at her bakery. She sells cinnamon bagels, onion bagels, and plain bagels. She also sells cinnamon rolls, Parker rolls, and plain rolls. Try re-creating the chart shown in Figure 4.11.

Figure 4.11.

A worksheet to test your data entry knowledge.

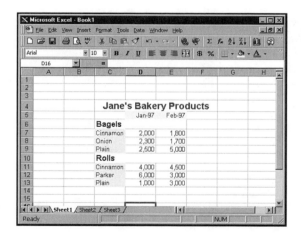

1. Open Excel; a workbook opens automatically.
2. Type the text and numbers shown in Figure 4.12 into the worksheet (you will correct the formatting of the headings in the next step). Excel automatically formats the cells according to the type of data you enter.

3. Select the text heading `Bagels` and the two adjacent cells. Click the Merge and Center tool on the Formatting toolbar. Select Format | Cells to display the Format Cells dialog box, click the Alignment tab, and change the alignment to General.

4. Repeat step 3 for the `Rolls` heading.

 5. For the heading `Jane's Bakery Products`, use the Merge and Center tool so that the heading covers four columns.

6. Some of the data is not entirely visible within the cells. Use the AutoFit tool to adjust the width of the columns: Select the column you want to adjust; in this example, the column that lists the products must be widened (column C) . Select Format | Column | AutoFit Selection.

4

Hour 5

Navigating and Manipulating Excel Documents

In the last hour, you learned how to do basic data entry and use automated data entry and correction tools. In this hour, you learn more ways to manipulate cells and worksheets and to customize Excel to your preferences and requirements. It's not necessary to absorb all this information at once. Start working with Excel and learn the various features as you need them. Still, it's a good idea to know what's available because Excel has features you are not likely to even think about if you don't know they are there.

Manipulating Cells, Rows, Columns, and Ranges

Office 97 applications use a device called the *Clipboard* for transferring data between different documents and applications. The Clipboard "holds" the data you place there. You can cut or copy data from one document, place it on the Clipboard, and then transfer that data by pasting it in another location. That location can be within the same document or in another document—and the other document can be in the same application or in a different application.

When creating documents, it is a great help to be able to move data around. You can change your perspective by changing the placement of the data.

Copying and Pasting a Cell or Range

Being able to easily move data from one location to another has been key to the success of Windows. You can use either a mouse or the keyboard—or a combination of both—to copy a cell or cells from one location to another in Excel. The technique is similar to that of other Windows 95 programs.

Using the Mouse to Copy and Paste

To use the mouse or the keyboard, that is the question. Users quickly develop their own preferences. Frequent users switch between the two methods to save wear and tear on their hands and wrists.

Here's how to copy and paste groups of cells using just the mouse:

1. Select the desired cells with the mouse. To do this, move the pointer to the upper-left cell of the block you want to define. Press and hold the left mouse button and drag the pointer to the lower-right corner of the block of cells. Release the mouse button.

2. Move the mouse pointer to the border of the region you have just selected so that the usual cross symbol changes into an arrow.

3. Keeping the mouse pointer along the border, press and hold the Ctrl key so that a tiny plus sign appears next to the mouse pointer (see Figure 5.1).

4. Press and hold the left mouse button and drag the cells to the new location. You can see the outline of the box as you move it around to help you determine its correct position.

5. Release the Ctrl key and the mouse button. You will now have the same data in two different places.

5

Figure 5.1.

Preparing to copy a group of cells.

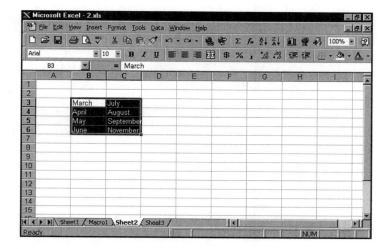

Copying and Pasting Cells with the Keyboard

Here's how to copy and paste groups of cells using just the keyboard:

1. Use the arrow keys to move the cursor to the upper-left corner of the rectangular group of cells you want to highlight.

2. Press and hold the Shift key and use the arrow keys to move the cursor to the lower-right corner of the group of cells you want to highlight.

3. Press Alt+E+C to invoke the Copy option (alternatively, press Ctrl+C or choose Edit | Copy from the main menu for the same effect).

4. Use the arrow keys to move the cursor to the upper-left corner of the region in which you want to paste a copy of the cells you just highlighted and press Enter (or choose Edit | Paste from the main menu). A copy of the cells you initially highlighted appears in the new location.

You can use any combination of mouse and keyboard you want.

Cutting and Pasting a Cell or Cells

The procedure for cutting data from one area of the worksheet and pasting it in a new location is quite similar to that for copying a cell or cells.

Follow these steps to cut and paste using the mouse:

1. Select the cells you want to cut with the mouse or the keyboard, as described in the previous sections.

2. Place the mouse pointer along the highlighted border so that the pointer changes to an arrow.

5

3. Press and hold the left mouse button and drag the cells to their new location. Once again, use the outline of the box as a guide to help you position the cells in their new location.

4. When the mouse pointer is in the upper-left corner of the area in which you want the cells to appear, release the mouse button.

Here's how to cut a cell or a group of cells with the keyboard:

1. Select the group of cells you want to move using the Shift key and the arrow keys.

2. Press Alt+E+T or Ctrl+X to cut the group of highlighted cells. A dashed border appears around the highlighted cells, as shown in Figure 5.2.

3. Use the arrow keys to move the cursor to the upper-left corner of the new location for the cells.

4. Press Alt+E+P or Ctrl+V to paste the cells in this new location.

Figure 5.2.

Note the dashed border around cells to be cut.

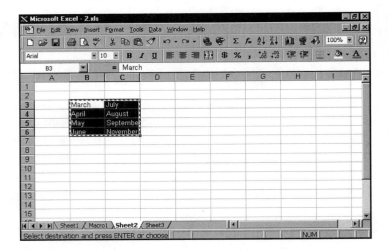

Clearing the Contents of a Cell or Range

To clear the contents of a cell or range, select the desired cells. Right-click the highlighted area to make the popup menu appear. Then select Clear Contents from the popup menu.

CAUTION

Deleting a cell or group of cells is different than clearing them. When you *delete* a cell or cells, the other cells in the worksheet readjust their positions to fit the "hole" created by the missing cells. When you *clear* a cell or group of cells, all the other cells remain the same because you have simply cleared the data and left the cells themselves alone.

5

Deleting a Cell or Group of Cells

To actually delete a group of cells, first select the cell or group of cells you want to delete. Right-click, and a menu will pop up. Choose Delete from this menu and click.

Inserting a Row or Column

To insert a new, blank row or column into a worksheet, place the cursor where you want the row or column to be inserted. You can position the cursor in any cell in the row or column. Choose Insert | Rows or Insert | Columns from the main menu. A row is inserted *above* the current row. A column is inserted *to the left of* the current column.

Inserting Cells

You can insert cells or a group of cells by using the Insert | Cells command. If you choose Shift Cells Right or Shift Cells Down from the Insert Cells dialog box, the highlighted cell or cells are dislocated without the effect of inserting a full row or column.

In Figure 5.3, the four cells F4, G4, H4, and I4 were originally in the highlighted region (cells B4, C4, D4, and E4). We selected Insert | Cells and then chose Shift Cells Right from the Insert Cells dialog box. All four cells moved four cells to the right. Had only one cell been highlighted, and this same command invoked, the cells would have moved only one place.

You can also select the spot at which you want to insert blank cells and right-click to see a popup menu. Choose Insert to display the same Insert Cells dialog box just described.

Figure 5.3.
Shifting cells to the right.

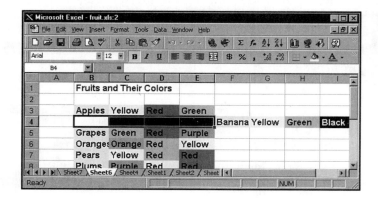

Increasing or Decreasing the Indentation of Cell Contents

You can control the amount of indentation in a cell. You usually indent data in a cell for aesthetic reasons and to make the data easier to follow and understand.

If you want to indent cells containing text or numeric values, you can choose Format | Cells and then select Alignment from the dialog box. You learned how to align the contents of cells in Hour 4, "Data Entry and Editing in Excel."

You can also change the indentation by clicking either the Decrease Indent or the Increase Indent tool from the Formatting toolbar.

 If you want to indent text within a particular cell or group of cells using the Formatting toolbar, you can do so. First, highlight the cell or cells you want to format and then click the Increase Indent icon on the Formatting toolbar. The block of text indents to the right a small amount. Continue clicking this icon to further indent the text, a little at a time.

 If you indented the text too far, you can use another toolbar icon to bump it back to the left. First, highlight the cell or cells you want to format and then click the Decrease Indent icon on the Formatting toolbar. The text bumps back to the left a small amount. Continue clicking this icon to bring the text closer to left alignment.

Picking from the List

Excel includes yet another way to speed data entry. Suppose that you are entering data in a row or column, and the various entries repeat themselves throughout the row or column, but not in a consistent pattern (see Figure 5.4). With Pick from List, you can enter each of the possibilities in the row or column, and then select the appropriate entry from a drop-down menu. Select a cell, right-click it to display the popup menu, and choose Pick from List. The items shown are the other entries from the same row; you can choose one of these entries if it is appropriate for the current cell.

Figure 5.4.

Pick from List entries.

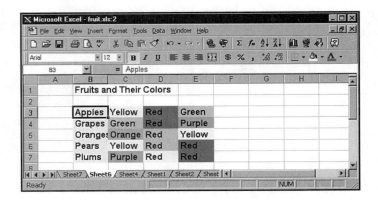

Using AutoFit with Rows and Columns

You can set your rows and columns so that they automatically expand or contract in height and width to accommodate the data they happen to contain. Select the row or column you want to adjust, choose either Format | Rows or Format | Columns, and select AutoFit from

5

the submenu. Now, regardless of how much data you enter into a cell in that row or column, the column will widen or the row will become taller to accommodate the data.

Setting a Standard Width for Columns

If you don't want the default column width of 8.43 for your worksheet, select Format | Column | Standard Width and enter a new value. For more information about selecting column widths and row heights, see Hour 4.

TIME SAVER

> How is column width measured? If you specify a column width of 8, that means that 8 digits in the standard font can fit within the cell. The "standard font" is the one used for the Normal style. Thus, if the Normal font is 10-point Arial, and the column width is 8, you can fit 8 digits in the 10-point Arial font inside the cell.

Moving or Copying the Content of a Cell

You don't have to cut or copy an actual cell to cut or copy its content. Follow these steps to cut or copy the contents of the cells while leaving the actual cells themselves alone:

1. Double-click the cell whose contents you want to access.
2. Place the cursor inside the cell and highlight the content you want to move or copy. You don't have to highlight the entire contents of the cell; you can highlight any portion of it that you want.
3. Cut the data by selecting Edit | Cut from the main menu or copy the data by selecting Edit | Copy from the main menu.
4. Select the cell to which you want to copy the data. You can place the cursor anywhere in the cell if you want the copied data to be positioned in the middle or at the end of the cell.
5. Select Edit | Paste from the main menu to copy the data into the cell.

Merging Cells

If you want to merge two or more cells, first select the range of cells you want to merge. Only the data in the upper-left cell is kept for the resulting new cell. If you want the upper-left cell to contain *all* the data from the cells in the selected range, you must first copy the contents of the various cells into that upper-left cell (as described in the preceding section) before you merge the cells together. When you merge cells, all the selected cells combine into a single large cell. Merging cells is a good idea, for example, if you want to put a single descriptive header above a labeled row of cells.

5

Select the range of cells you want to merge. Click the Merge and Center tool on the Formatting toolbar to merge the cells and center the contents horizontally. The vertical alignment remains the same.

Switching Columns to Rows and Rows to Columns

In Excel, you can transpose rows and columns. This capability can come in handy if you decide that your data may look better with a different orientation. To switch the positioning of data in columns to data in rows (or vice versa), select the cells you want to move and press Ctrl+C to copy them (alternatively, select Edit | Copy or right-click the selected cells and select Copy from the popup menu). Move the cursor to the upper-left corner of the area in which you want to paste the cells. Choose Edit | Paste Special from the menu and select Transpose.

Hiding and Displaying Rows and Columns

Your worksheets may grow to include lots of data in rows and columns that extend across more than a single screen. You can hide rows or columns of data in your worksheet if they are irrelevant to the work you are currently doing or if their appearance in the worksheet is distracting and hogs valuable screen space. Even after you hide a row or column, you should understand that the data is not gone (the column letters and the row numbers are interrupted to remind you that entire chunks of data are not on display); of course, you can always redisplay the hidden columns or rows to see your data again.

First, select the row or column you want to hide. You can select the entire row or column by clicking the row number or the column letter, or you can simply position the cursor in any cell in the row or the column you want to hide. Then select Format | Row | Hide if you want to hide a row; select Format | Column | Hide if you want to hide a column.

To display a hidden row, select a range of cells that includes at least one cell in the row above and one cell in the row below the hidden row. Then select Format | Row | Unhide. To tell which row or rows have been hidden, look for the missing row numbers along the left side of the screen.

To display a hidden column, select a range of cells that includes at least one cell to the left and one cell to the right of the hidden column. Then choose Format | Column | Unhide. To tell which column or columns have been hidden, look for the missing column letters along the top of the screen.

Manipulating Worksheets

You can delete, insert, copy, move, hide, and display worksheets and workbooks as readily as you can do these operations with cells and ranges.

5

Hiding and Displaying Workbooks

If you want to hide a workbook, select the Window menu and choose Hide (or press Alt+W+H). The workbook disappears from view. Although you can still reference and manipulate data in a hidden workbook, as described in Part III, "Excel and Interactive Data," you (and other users) cannot see the workbook.

It's easy to display the workbook again. Select the Window menu and choose Unhide (or press Alt+W+U). If more than one workbook has been hidden, Excel displays a menu from which you can select the workbook you want to display again.

Why would you want to hide a workbook? The usual reason is that it helps keep the screen uncluttered when you are working with lots of data.

Hiding and Displaying Worksheets

To hide a single worksheet within a workbook, first make that worksheet active by clicking the appropriate sheet tab. You can hide only the sheet you are currently working with, that is, the *active worksheet*. Once the sheet you want to hide is active, choose Format | Sheet and then choose Hide from the submenu.

To display the hidden worksheet again, select Format | Sheet and then select Unhide from the submenu. Select the sheet you want to display and press OK.

Inserting and Deleting Worksheets

The default number of worksheets in a workbook is three, but you can add or delete worksheets as you please.

To delete a worksheet, first make it active by clicking its tab if it is not already active. Select the Edit menu and choose Delete Sheet. All the data on that worksheet is lost.

To delete worksheets adjacent to each other, press and hold the Shift key and click the tab of the first one you want to delete. Continue holding Shift while clicking the tabs of the other worksheets you want to delete. Release the Shift key and select Edit | Delete Sheet or press Alt+E+D. If you want to delete worksheets that are not adjacent to each other, press and hold the Ctrl key as you click the tabs of the worksheets you want to delete.

To insert a new, blank worksheet into the current workbook, select Insert | Worksheet from the main menu. A new worksheet is added to the "bottom" of your stack of worksheets. The new worksheet has a name such as Sheet4, or whatever sheet number is next in the workbook. Of course, you can change the name if you want.

Naming Worksheets

The default names for the sheets in a workbook are Sheet1, Sheet2, Sheet3, and so forth. These are pretty boring names and are unlikely to reflect what you are actually doing with your data.

Suppose that you have monthly company reports for the last third of 1996 and that you also have a summary worksheet that provides a table of contents and a commentary—for a total of five worksheets. You could rename these worksheets (for example, Summary, Sep96, Oct96, Nov96, and Dec96). Choose any names that are meaningful to you—or to anyone who might use your work. (Programmers, writers, and others are notorious for inventing their own classifying systems that make no sense to their successors, so keep in mind that you probably don't know who might need your data at some point.)

To rename a worksheet, click its tab. The worksheet name is highlighted, as shown in Figure 5.5. Type the new name to replace the old name.

Figure 5.5.
Highlighting a worksheet name before renaming it.

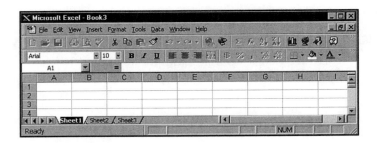

Scrolling and Tabbing through a Workbook

When you are working in a worksheet, you cannot see all its rows and columns at once. There are simply too many. However, you can use the scrollbars to get to where you want to go within the worksheet.

Suppose that you want to see the data located in Cell Z29. Click the right-pointing arrow on the horizontal scrollbar to move to the right as far as necessary. Click the corresponding arrow on the left end of the scrollbar to move to the left. To move vertically, click the up and down arrows on the vertical scrollbar.

As mentioned in Hour 4, you can also type the address of the cell to which you want to jump in the name box and press Enter. (The name box is located just above the column labels, at the left side of the screen.) To move from one worksheet to another, just click the tab of the one you want to make active.

Moving Worksheets

You can easily change the position of a worksheet within the same workbook by dragging it with the mouse. Place the mouse pointer on the tab of the worksheet you want to move. As you drag the tab along or between the other worksheet tabs to its new location, an icon shaped like a sheet of paper appears. Drop the icon where you want the worksheet to be in respect to the other worksheets.

5

You can also move worksheets by using the menu. First, select the tab of the sheet you want to move. Then choose Edit | Move or Copy Sheet. The Move or Copy dialog box appears (see Figure 5.6). In the dialog box, choose the preferred destination for the selected worksheet. Notice that you can select the Create a Copy checkbox if you want to create a copy of the selected sheet at this new location.

Figure 5.6.

The dialog box for moving or copying a worksheet.

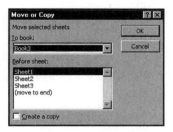

Moving or Copying Multiple Sheets at Once

You can select two or more worksheets for copying or moving at one time.

If the sheets are adjacent to each other:

> Press and hold the Shift key, click the tab for the first sheet you want to copy or move, and then click the remaining tabs for the other sheets. Release the Shift key. Drag the sheets to their new location or use the Edit | Move or Copy Sheet menu option.

If the sheets are not adjacent to each other:

> Press and hold the Ctrl key, click the tab for the first sheet you want to copy or move, and then click the remaining tabs for the other sheets. Release the Ctrl key. Drag the sheets to their new location or use the Edit | Move or Copy Sheet menu option.

Opening Multiple Workbooks

You can have multiple workbooks open at once. Just leave the current workbook open and then either create a new one or open an existing one. You can open as many workbooks as your system can support (opening additional workbooks takes up a lot of memory). To move between open workbooks, press Ctrl+F6 to "page" between the various workbooks.

Using the Window Menu

If you have more than one workbook open, you can use several options on the Window menu to display the workbooks in different ways.

Arranging Workbooks

To arrange the various workbooks you have opened on your Excel screen, select Window | Arrange to display the Arrange Windows dialog box (see Figure 5.7). Select one of the options and click OK.

Here are descriptions of the options available in the Arrange Windows dialog box:

Arrange Option	Description
Tiled	The various workbooks are displayed on the screen like tiles; the arrangement differs depending on the number of open workbooks.
Horizontal	The workbooks are displayed in horizontal strips, adjacent to each other.
Vertical	The workbooks are displayed in vertical strips, one on top of the other.
Cascade	The workbooks are displayed diagonally, with only a little of the workbooks underneath displayed and most of the top workbook displayed.

Figure 5.7.

The Arrange Windows dialog box.

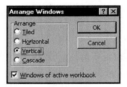

If you want to arrange the work*sheets* within a single workbook, you can use the Arrange Windows dialog box as well. Choose your preferred arrangement, whether that be tiled, horizontal, vertical, or cascade. Select the Windows of Active Workbook checkbox and click OK. Now select Window | New Window from the main menu; another copy of the workbook appears. Select the sheet you want to work on. Repeat the preceding step as necessary until all the different worksheets you want to work with are visible.

By using this feature in this way, you can see more than one sheet of the active workbook at the same time.

Splitting Windows

If you are working on a complex worksheet, any visual cues that help separate the information you are working with can be very helpful. Excel provides a feature that divides a single worksheet into separate windows, each of which you can use to manipulate the worksheet without affecting the views in the other windows.

5

Select Window | Split to display bars across your worksheet (see Figure 5.8). The bars are intersecting horizontal and vertical lines that divide the worksheet into four separate panes. These bars do not affect the content of your worksheet, but they can help keep the different components separate. Note that you can drag the bars to different locations on the screen as necessary.

Figure 5.8.

Splitting a worksheet.

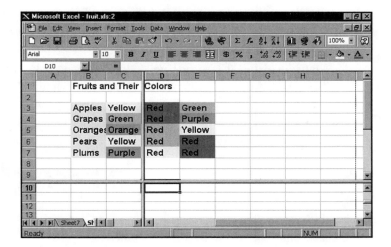

Understanding File Properties

A filename, even if it's the maximum 256 characters long, cannot give all the information about a file you may want. You can find out about your file (or someone else's) by selecting Properties from the File menu. The Properties dialog box appears; click the Summary tab to display the page shown in Figure 5.9.

The Author box shows the name that was entered when the Excel program was installed. Change it to the name of the person who actually created the document (your own name), if need be. You can fill in any of the other details as you see fit; press OK when finished. The following chart lists the other options you can specify.

Property	Description
Title	Choose a descriptive title for your document. A title can help you later when you are looking through a bunch of files and can't recall which one you want.
Subject	Enter the subject of your document if you want.
Author	Enter your name; the default is the name of the person specified in the initial installation process.
Manager	Enter the name of your manager, if you want.

Property	Description
Company	Enter the name of your company.
Category	This option is self-explanatory.
Keywords	Enter a keyword or keywords to help when you are doing a search through your files at a later date. Think of descriptive words that you or someone else would likely use to find this file.
Comments	Enter any comments about the file that don't fall neatly into any of the other options.
Hyperlink base	Enter the base URL for all hyperlinks in the document (this concept is discussed in Hour 20, "Excel and the World Wide Web").

You can select the Save Preview Picture checkbox if you want to be able to view the first page of the file when previewing it from the Open dialog box. Checking this option increases the size of the file, however.

Figure 5.9.

The Summary tab of the Properties dialog box contains useful information about a file.

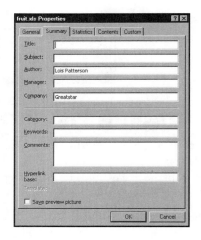

The General tab of the Properties dialog box provides information about the file, such as file size, location, filename, dates of creation, modification, and access, as well as particular attributes.

The Statistics tab of the Properties dialog box can track changes in the file by listing the dates of creation, modification, and access, as well as implementing a tracking system for revisions made (if you have chosen to track revisions).

The Contents tab lists the names of the worksheets contained within the workbook file.

The Custom tab of the Properties dialog box helps you keep track of different people working on a single file—if that situation applies to you.

5

E-Mailing a File

If you have Microsoft Exchange, you can e-mail an Excel file from within Excel, whether the e-mail is sent over the Internet or over a corporate network. Choose File | Send To | Mail Recipient and follow the prompts to send a workbook to another person.

Routing files over a network is discussed in Hour 21, "Sharing Workbooks and Consolidating Data."

JUST A MINUTE

> Of course, if you don't have Microsoft Exchange, you can open any e-mail program that supports attachments and send your Excel file to another recipient that way.

Don't forget the homely floppy disk. This is still a practical method of transporting files around. You can copy your files to the floppy disk and then take the floppy disk wherever you need to go, whether it's to an adjacent computer or a computer across the country.

To copy a file to a floppy disk, insert the disk in your floppy drive. Go to Windows Explorer and find the file you want to copy in the directory structure. Highlight the file icon, right-click it, and select Copy from the popup menu. From the All Folders drop-down list in the upper-left corner of Windows Explorer, choose the A or B drive, depending on which is installed as your floppy drive. Windows copies the selected file to the indicated floppy disk.

Changing the Appearance of the Screen

You can change the appearance of your screen by using the View menu. You can show toolbars or not, see where the page breaks are, and make the worksheet occupy the entire screen.

The default choice is Normal, which is the look for most of the screens shown in this book. In this view, you see the scrollbars at the bottom, the title bar at the top, the Windows 95 toolbar at the bottom, and as many toolbars as you have chosen to display.

The Full Screen option eliminates all toolbars and scrollbars from your screen so that as much space as possible is devoted to the worksheet itself. Note that the Windows 95 taskbar also disappears. To select this option, choose View | Full Screen.

TIME SAVER

> If you want to see as much of your worksheet as possible, crank up your screen resolution as high as you can. Choose Settings | Control Panel from the Windows 95 Start menu and double-click the Display icon. Choose the Settings tab and move the indicator for Desktop Area to More.

You can see where the page breaks are by choosing View | Page Break Preview from the main menu. In Hour 11, "Printing Excel Documents," you learn more about the page-break feature.

Headers and Footers

With the View menu, you can also add headers and footers to your Excel spreadsheets. Headers and footers do not show up on the screen, but if you print the worksheet, they appear. A typical header or footer lists the page number and information such as the date, author's name, company name, filename, and so forth. You can decide for yourself what information you want your header or footer to contain, and whether you want neither, either, or both. A *header*, of course, is information that appears at the top of a page, separate from the main data. A *footer* is information that appears at the bottom of a page, separate from the main data.

To create a header or footer, choose View | Header and Footer to display a dialog box (see Figure 5.10).

To use an already-created header, click the down arrow next to the Header combo box to see the drop-down list of header options. You can choose any of the possibilities listed in the menu for your header or footer, such as the page number, filename, author's name, and so forth. Click OK when you have made your choice.

Similarly, to use an already-created footer, click the Footer combo box to see the drop-down list of footer options. You can choose any of the listed possibilities. Click OK when you are done.

Figure 5.10.

Selecting options to create a header.

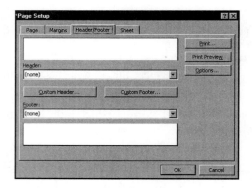

You can also create your own custom header or footer by clicking the Custom Header or Custom Footer option.

If you click Custom Header, the Header dialog box appears; if you click Custom Footer, the Footer dialog box appears. Each of the buttons on these dialog boxes has a purpose. Choose the correct information for each section of the box, using the buttons if you want to change a font, insert the date, time, filename, page number, or total number of pages. Click OK when done. Remember that you can have both a header and a footer in your document if you want.

Figure 5.11 shows a custom header in progress. My name appears in the left section. I clicked the filename button to position the entry in the center section. I clicked the page number button to display the entry in the right section, typed the word **of**, and then clicked the total page button. Then I highlighted the entry in each section with the mouse and clicked the font button (represented by the stylized *A*) to make the text in the header bold. Here is what the final header looks like when the spreadsheet is printed (with the appropriate total number of pages and correct page number substituted):

```
Lois Patterson    book3.xls    Page 1 of 12
```

Footers are prepared in a similar manner.

Figure 5.11.

Preparing a custom header.

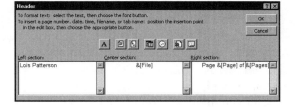

Zooming in on a Worksheet

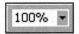

To zoom in on the worksheet screen, just click the box with the percentages (located at the right side of the Standard toolbar). Alternatively, select View | Zoom from the main menu.

Choose the size at which you prefer to view the screen. If you have a huge spreadsheet, the zoom feature allows you to see more of the cells at once by reducing their apparent size. The zoom percentage ranges between 10 percent and 400 percent, meaning that you can see the spreadsheet at one-tenth its actual size and up to four times its actual size—a 40-fold difference. Note that you may also be able to change the resolution of your screen to increase or decrease the amount of information on your screen; you can also remove toolbars and scrollbars from view, as explained in the preceding section, "Changing the Appearance of the Screen."

Configuring Excel's Options

Select Tools | Options to display the Options dialog box, which you can use to configure a number of characteristics regarding how Excel looks and behaves.

The View Tab

Select the View tab of the Options dialog box to see the page shown in Figure 5.12. This page gives you many different options about what is or is not visible on your screen. Check and uncheck the boxes according to your preferences. Some of the options—such as those regarding comments, formulas, and objects—are discussed in greater detail in later chapters.

Figure 5.12.

The View tab of the Options dialog box.

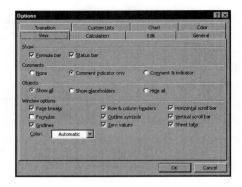

The General Tab

The General tab of the Options dialog box offers lots of different options for configuring Excel. You can choose a different default font for your Excel documents, change the addressing system, change the default directory for saving documents, and numerous other features.

The Edit Tab

The Edit tab of the Options dialog box allows you to control the behavior of cells and customize that behavior to your liking.

You can control whether you can edit within the cell itself, whether you can drag and drop cells, whether or not adjacent cells become active after you finish editing the previous cell, whether AutoComplete is enabled, and more.

The Transition Tab

Excel 97 is designed to aid the user who is accustomed to other spreadsheet programs or who has to continue to use other spreadsheet programs. By default, you save your workbooks in Excel 97 format, but you can choose a different default. To change this option, click the Transition tab in the Options dialog box.

Select the preferred format for your files by choosing from the Save Excel Files As drop-down list.

Looking Up Reference Material

You can use the Lookup Reference tool to look up a particular word or phrase from Microsoft Bookshelf or other reference materials you have installed. Choose Tools | Lookup Reference and perform a search as necessary. Don't forget that you can also start a Web search from within Excel by going to the Help menu and selecting Microsoft from the Web | Search the Web submenu.

5

Creating Customized Toolbars

You can create your own customized toolbar that you can then display in combination with the other toolbars or by itself. To create your own toolbar, choose Tools | Customize to display the Customize dialog box and select the Toolbars tab. Choose New and enter the name for your new toolbar. A blank toolbar appears next to the dialog box. Once the toolbar appears, choose the Commands tab in the Customize dialog box. Drag the commands, as shown in Figure 5.13, to your new toolbar. When you are finished adding commands to the toolbar, click Close.

Figure 5.13.

Making a custom toolbar.

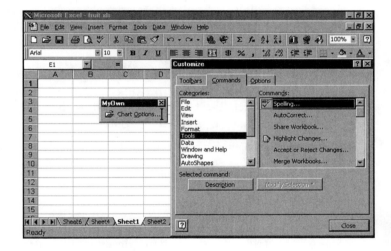

If you put a command that does not have an icon onto your toolbar, no picture icon is displayed but you do see a text button.

If you want to delete a toolbar, open the Toolbars tab of the Customize dialog box, select the name of the toolbar you want to delete, and click Delete. You can delete only the toolbars you have created yourself.

Tracking Changes

It's common for several people to work on a single workbook. Excel lets you keep track of who has done what work, and what changes can be made. This means that any revisions do not necessarily have to overwrite the original work, and that you can restore the original file at any time if necessary.

To keep track of changes made to a document by you and others, select Tools | Track Changes from the menu. Select the Track Changes While Editing checkbox and select your preferences from the When, Who, and Where drop-down list boxes. If you select the Track

Changes While Editing option, Excel turns on *workbook sharing*, meaning that the workbook is set up for multiple users on a network. Workbook sharing is described in greater detail in Hour 21. If you don't have a network, don't worry.

If you select the Highlight Changes on Screen checkbox, a small triangle appears in the upper-left corner of any cells with revised entries. If you have chosen to track changes in your workbook, you can select the Highlight Changes on Screen checkbox at any time to see which entries have been revised; you can also deactivate this option at any time.

Not all changes are recorded. You aren't notified about formatting changes, any hidden (or unhidden) rows and columns, changes to worksheet names, new comments and changes to comments, and certain cell changes related to formula use (as discussed in Chapter 12, "Using Formulas in Excel").

Accepting or Rejecting Changes

If you've chosen to track changes in a worksheet, you can decide either to accept or reject all the changes at any time. If you accept the changes, the revised document becomes the new original version, and the process starts again.

To see all the changes that have been made, select Tools | Track Changes again. Check the List Changes on New Sheet checkbox to see a separate worksheet that identifies the cells in which changes have been made, showing both the old and new entries.

If you reject the changes, you lose the revision history and have only the original document.

Keeping a good revision history is no substitute for keeping backups. It's all too easy for someone to get rid of the revision history inadvertently. To maximize security, it's best to use a locking scheme, as described in Hour 6, "Formatting and Protecting Worksheets."

Summary

Although the methods used to manipulate cells, rows, columns, worksheets, and workbooks within Excel 97 may seem complex, the interface is intuitive and online help is easy to get. If you think there should be an easier way to do a certain task, there probably is. Trying to learn all the formatting techniques before actually beginning a workbook can be counter-productive. Start a workbook, enter some data, and then try various formatting and manipulative techniques on the entries.

5

Workshop

Term Review

copy and paste   To copy the contents of a cell or a group of cells to another location.

cut and paste   To move a cell or group of cells to another location. You can also cut and paste graphic objects and other objects, as discussed in subsequent chapters.

Q&A

Q How can you see more of the spreadsheet at once, or see it in better detail?

A Click the Zoom spin button at the right end of the standard toolbar and adjust the percentages.

Q How can you keep track of changes made to a workbook?

A Choose Tools | Track Changes | Highlight Changes and select the appropriate options in the dialog box.

Q When in doubt about how to carry out a certain task, what should you do?

A Try right-clicking the cell or range to display the popup menu with its numerous options. For general help, press F1 to bring Office Assistant to the rescue.

Exercises

Open up a new workbook in Excel and try the following exercises:

1. Delete Sheet2 and Sheet3.

2. Rename Sheet1 to CapitolsCountries.

3. Enter the following data in the form of a table:

Capitol	Country
Vienna	Austria
Copenhagen	Denmark
Amsterdam	Holland

4. Try cutting and pasting the range to another location in the worksheet. Also try cutting and pasting different rows, columns, and cells.

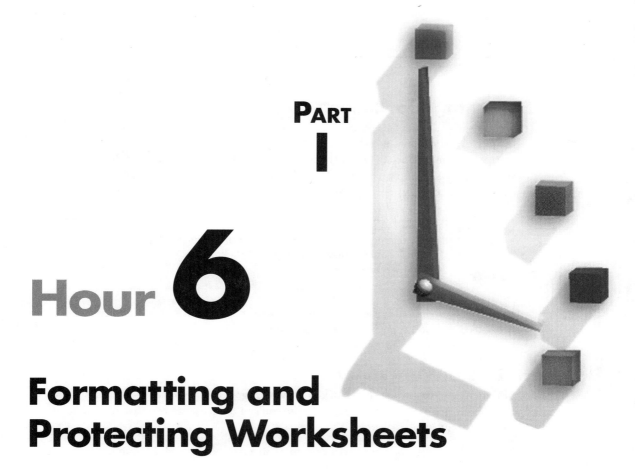

Hour 6

Formatting and Protecting Worksheets

In this hour, you learn how to format worksheets to improve their appearance. A plain black-and-white spreadsheet can convey data, but it can be boring. There are a number of ways to spruce up your Excel files. In this hour, you receive instructions and tips for formatting worksheets and making their contents either accessible or inaccessible to other users and to yourself.

Formatting Worksheets

Select the Format | Sheet submenu from the main menu to see a list of commands you can perform on worksheets. You can rename a worksheet, hide or display a worksheet, and add a background to a worksheet.

Renaming Worksheets

Names such as Sheet1, Sheet2, and Sheet3—the typical names for a worksheet—are not terribly descriptive. Names like July Earnings give a much better idea of what data the worksheet contains. Select Format | Sheet from the main menu and choose Rename from the submenu. Type the new name for the worksheet. The new name can contain spaces, and you can make the name as descriptive as you want within the 31-character limit.

TIME SAVER

As mentioned in Hour 5, "Navigating and Manipulating Excel Documents," you can also rename a worksheet by clicking its tab and then typing a new name.

Although you can't use the Undo command to change a worksheet's name back to its previous name, you can use the Rename command to change the name of a worksheet back to its original name—or to any other name.

Hiding a Worksheet

Hiding worksheets is helpful when you are working with many sheets—especially if they all have lengthy names. By hiding worksheets, you can reduce clutter so that you can focus on the important sheets at hand.

To hide the active worksheet, select Format | Sheet and choose Hide from the submenu.

Note that you cannot hide all the worksheets in a workbook. You must have at least one visible sheet in a workbook at all times.

Displaying a Worksheet

If you've chosen to hide a worksheet, chances are you'll want to see it again sometime. Just choose Format | Sheet from the main menu and then select Unhide.

Setting Backgrounds

You can use backgrounds to add interest to your work while you are preparing the worksheets—even if they don't make it into the final version of the worksheet. Try backgrounds—they're fun!

To put a background into your worksheet, select Format | Sheet and choose Background from the submenu. You can go to any of the graphic files in your directories—whatever their file format—and select the one you want. To see some sample graphic files for your backgrounds, look through this directory:

```
C:\Program Files\Microsoft Office\ClipArt\Backgrounds
```

6

Of course, backgrounds can also add a professional touch to your work, particularly when used in conjunction with other carefully chosen graphics. See Hour 8, "Adding Graphics and Multimedia to Your Excel Documents," for more information about incorporating graphics into your worksheets and for a discussion of how you can create your own graphics for backgrounds and for other uses.

Creating and Applying Styles to Cells

If you've used styles in a word processing program like Microsoft Word, you are familiar with the concept of styles. A *style* is a set of instructions applied to a cell or range that describes the font size, data formatting details, alignment, border, patterns, and protection choices. Every cell has its own formatting style attached to it. The default style is called Normal. To see the different styles available, select Format | Style from the menu. Scroll through the possibilities in the Style dialog box:

Style Name	*Description*
Comma	Accounting format with 2 decimal places
Comma[0]	Accounting format with no decimal places
Currency	Currency format with 2 decimal places (dollars and cents)
Currency[0]	Currency format with no decimal places (just dollars)
Normal	General number format with specific alignment, font, and border options
Percent	Multiplies the contents by 100, adds a percent sign, and uses no decimal places

To apply a style to a cell or group of cells, first highlight the cells. Select Format | Style to display the Style dialog box, select your preferred style, and click OK.

Creating your own styles helps you format your data just the way you want, with a minimum of duplicated effort. Once you create a style, you can apply it to as many cells as you want within your workbook. The following sections describe several ways to create a style.

Creating a Style with the Style Dialog Box

Choose Format | Style from the main menu to display the Style dialog box (see Figure 6.1). As you can see, the default style is called Normal, but you can scroll through the list of style names to see several others.

6

Figure 6.1.

Style name possibilities.

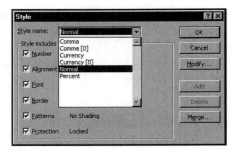

Suppose that you want to create a style called SpecialDate, a style for (surprise!) dates. This style is to display dates in the format dd-mmm-yy with an 18-point Times New Roman font, a blue border in your preferred style, and a red background for the affected cells.

To do this, open the Style dialog box and follow these steps:

1. Select the Style Name box and type **SpecialDate**, replacing the name Normal that was displayed there. Of course, you can enter any name you want for this style.

2. Click Modify to display the Format Cells dialog box shown in Figure 6.2.

3. Make the desired changes in the dialog box. Go through each of the tabs and make selections in each of the categories you want to change.

4. Click OK when you are finished. Depending on your choices, you will see a dialog box similar to the one in Figure 6.3.

5. Click Add. This action adds your newly created style to the list of styles so that you can select it from the Style Name drop-down list box the next time you open the Style dialog box.

TIME SAVER

> If you selected a cell or range before you began to create the style, click OK instead of Add in step 5. Doing so saves the style to use elsewhere in the worksheet and also applies the new format to the highlighted cells.

Now you have a style that you can use repeatedly, for any of your worksheets in any of your workbooks.

To apply the new format, enter the date or dates as usual (if you created a style for other kinds of data, type that kind of data into a cell). Highlight the cells that contain data to which you want to apply the style and choose Format | Style. Scroll through the choices in the Style Name drop-down list box and select SpecialDate (or your preferred style). Click OK.

6

Figure 6.2.
Modifying a style.

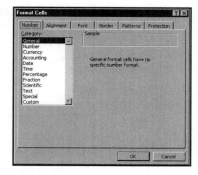

Figure 6.3.
Adding a style.

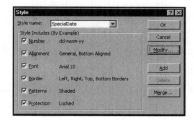

Creating a Style by Example

You can deliberately create a style as described in the preceding section, or you can take a style from a cell you have already formatted.

First you must highlight a cell that is formatted in a way you want to preserve in a style you can apply to other cells. In this example, the selected cell has an orange background and green bold Arial 12-point text. Create a cell like this (or one with your own preferred characteristics) before continuing.

With the formatted cell highlighted, select Format | Style to display the Style dialog box. Position the cursor in the Style Name box and delete the word Normal. You now have a blank space in which you can type the name you want for this style. For this example, type **OrangeGreen**. The formatting you applied to the selected cell is itemized in the dialog box, as you can see in Figure 6.4. Click Add to add this style to your worksheet.

You can now use this style anywhere in your workbooks, just as you can a style created with the instructions in the preceding section.

Figure 6.4.

Creating a style by example.

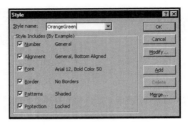

Modifying Built-In Styles

Some of the built-in styles that come with Excel may be *almost* exactly what you want. Rather than create a new style, you may simply want to change a thing or two about one of the built-in styles and continue to use the same style in its modified form. For example, if you want the Normal style for all the cells in your worksheet to be a 12-point Times New Roman font, you can change the Normal style to reflect that. If you do not modify it, the Normal style applies a font of 10-point Arial.

To change a built-in style, open the Style dialog box, select the style you want to modify from the drop-down list, and click the Modify button. The Format Cells dialog box appears as shown earlier in Figure 6.2. Use this dialog box to change the font face, the font size, or other features for the default style.

Deleting a Style

If you've created a style you want to delete, open the Style dialog box, select the style you want to delete from the drop-down list box, and click Delete. You cannot delete a built-in style.

If you have formatted any cells using the style you just deleted, the formatting of those cells changes back to Normal (however that style has been defined for this particular workbook).

Saving a Style for Use with Other Workbooks

The methods described in the preceding sections create styles for use with a particular workbook. If you want to create a style for general use in Excel across several workbooks, you must create a *template*, as discussed in Hour 7, "Using Excel Worksheet Templates."

Copying Formats between Cells and Ranges

There are several ways to copy formats between and among different cells and ranges. Formatting information can be transferred in much the same way data can be. You can also transfer data from cells without transferring the formatting with them.

6

Copying Formats with the Format Painter Tool

The Format Painter tool is likely the easiest way to transfer a formatting style from a cell to another cell or range. The Format Painter tool is in the Standard toolbar; it's the tool that looks like a paintbrush.

To use the Format Painter tool to transfer a formatting style from one cell to another, follow these steps:

1. Select the cell whose format you want to copy.

 2. Click the Format Painter tool on the Standard toolbar.

3. Select the new cell or range and click. The formatting of the cell you selected in step 1 is transported to the new cells.

Copying Formats with the Menu

You can also use the main menu to copy formatting from a cell or a range to another cell or range:

1. Select the cell or range from which you want to copy the formatting.
2. Select Edit | Copy from the main menu. A dashed border appears around the cell or group of cells.
3. Select the cell or range to which you want to copy the formatting.
4. Choose Edit | Paste Special from the main menu.
5. Select the Formats option from the Paste Special dialog box and click OK.

Copying Formats with the Drag-and-Drop Technique

Here's how to copy formats from one cell to another just by using the mouse:

1. Select the cell or range from which you want to copy the formatting.
2. Move the mouse pointer to the bottom of the selected area so that it changes to an arrow.
3. Click the right mouse button and drag the mouse pointer to the location where you want to paste the formatting.
4. Release the mouse button at the new location; a popup menu appears, as shown in Figure 6.5.
5. To copy the formatting only, select Copy Here as Formats Only from the popup menu. Only the formats are transferred to the newly selected range.

Figure 6.5.

Using a popup menu to drag and drop formats.

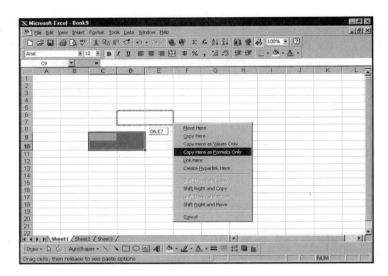

JUST A MINUTE

Note all the other options available from the popup menu. You can also choose to copy or move the data in the selected area without retaining any of the formatting. The right-click drag-and-drop approach is very flexible and can be very valuable.

Changing a Style for Selected Cells

To remove a style from a cell or range, select the area. Display the Format | Style dialog box and choose Normal (or whatever your preference is) from the list of style names.

Note that you can also change any or all characteristics of the formatting of a group of cells without actually changing the style. To do this, select Format | Cells and choose options from the various tabs in the Format Cells dialog box.

Using Cell Styles

If you build up a repertoire of different styles, you can easily format your worksheets in no time. It's a good practice, of course, to use different styles for different types of data. You will likely want a specific style for column headings, one for subtotals, one for worksheet titles, and so forth.

As with desktop publishing, excessive use of different colors and fonts can be distracting and detract from your presentation. So try to curb your flair for wild colors and extraordinary fonts when designing worksheet styles.

6

Adding Comments

Adding comments to your worksheets is another way to help it make sense to others (and yourself). Comments are like having Post-It notes within the file. You can add comments so that your worksheet makes sense to those who are not as familiar with the data as you are. Or you can add comments as reminders to yourself. You can either hide or display your comments.

Here's how to add a comment to a cell:

1. Select the cell to which you want to add a comment and choose Insert | Comment from the main menu.
2. Type your comment in the dialog box that appears.
3. When you finish typing the comment, click outside the box to complete the comment.

You can control the formatting of the comment just as you can anything else that appears in your spreadsheet. Position the insertion point inside the comment box and right-click. The popup menu shown in Figure 6.6 appears. Select Format Comment to make the Format Comment dialog box appear. You can then select the fonts and colors you want for the comment.

You can also display the Format Comment dialog box by positioning the insertion point inside the comment box and choosing Format | Comment from the main menu.

Figure 6.6.

The popup menu that appears in the comment box.

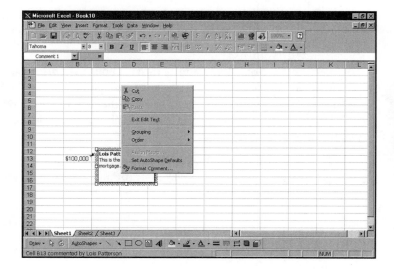

To hide or display the comments in your workbook, choose View | Comments from the menu. Note that you cannot choose which comments to hide or display—it's an all-or-nothing proposition.

If you display all your comments—and particularly if you have a lot of them—your worksheet will tend to look messy and unreadable because the comment boxes obscure the data.

When the comments are hidden, you see a tiny triangle in the corner of each cell that has an attached comment. When you run the cursor over the cell, the comment appears.

You can edit or format a comment by right-clicking the cell that contains the comment; a popup menu appears, from which you can select the desired options.

When you cut or copy and then paste a cell, the comment attached to the cell goes with the cell.

Moving Comments Around

To move a comment to another cell, display it if it is not visible. Then you can click the border of the comment box and drag it to the new cell.

Using the AutoFormat Feature

You can select your own colors and fonts for your worksheet cells, as described in the previous sections, or you can use a number of built-in formats that Microsoft has prepared for different types of tables. Although the AutoFormat option may not be satisfactory if you want a unique look for your worksheets, using it instantly enhances the appearance of your worksheets.

Select the group of cells you want to treat to a built-in set of formats. Select Format | AutoFormat to display the AutoFormat dialog box (see Figure 6.7). Scroll through the list of formats on the left; a sample table appears for each at the right of the dialog box. If you want to use one of the formats, select it and click OK to apply it to your selected cells, whether they are empty or not.

Click the Options button if you want to apply only certain parts of a particular AutoFormat style. The dialog box then displays more options. You can decide whether or not to apply the AutoFormat to each of the following areas:

- ☐ Number
- ☐ Border
- ☐ Font

6

☐ Patterns

☐ Alignment

☐ Width/Height

For example, if you want the Number AutoFormat but not the Width/Height AutoFormat, clear the Width/Height checkbox.

Figure 6.7.

The AutoFormat dialog box, showing a sample format.

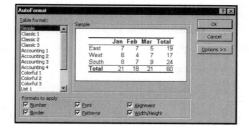

Tables generally share many characteristics. You can start by using AutoFormat and then format particular cells in whatever manner you prefer, referring back to the first part of this hour for suggestions.

Figure 6.8 shows a table formatted in the `Colorful1` format except that the word `Precipitation` was changed to Normal style instead of italicized and its cell was shaded a different color than the months in the column headings.

Figure 6.8.

A table autoformatted with `Colorful1`.

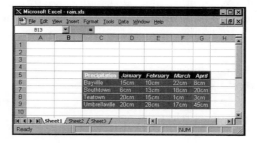

Removing AutoFormat from a Table

To remove an AutoFormat style from a table or a portion of a table, follow these steps:

1. Select the cells of the table that have been autoformatted.

2. Choose Format|AutoFormat from the main menu.

3. Select `None` from the list of choices in the AutoFormat dialog box (this option is at the bottom of the list).

Other Formatting Tips and Tricks

When you work with Excel for a while, you will develop a facility with the different menus and shortcuts to make the formatting process easier for you. The following sections present a few odds and ends that you may find helpful.

Using Color Palettes

When you choose background colors, text colors, or borders for your cells, you have a color palette to work from. You see this palette whenever you are expected to make a choice of colors. There are 56 separate colors from which you can choose at any one time; you can, however, specify which 56 colors you see in the palette.

To change the colors in a color palette, select Tools I Options to display the Options dialog box and click the Color tab. You see the standard palette you use to fill in cells, select text colors, and define borders. If you want a color that is not in the palette, you can replace a color you don't use with the one you want to add. Select the color you want to change, click the Modify button, and choose either the Standard or the Custom tab.

If you clicked the Standard tab, you can click anywhere on the shape shown in Figure 6.9 to get your preferred color.

For finer control over the color palette, click the Custom tab to display the dialog box shown in Figure 6.10. Move the cursor around to choose the desired color and then click to set the color. Alternatively, you can enter numbers in the various boxes to get the precise shade you want. Every color is made up of some proportions of red, green, and blue; you can specify those exact proportions. Another color-specification scheme defines colors by hue, saturation, and luminosity; you can specify those values if you want to define a color in that system.

Figure 6.9.

Choosing a color from the standard palette.

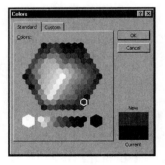

6

Figure 6.10.

Creating a custom color.

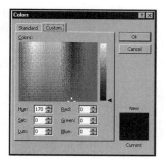

Just a Minute

If you want to go back to the original palette, select Tools | Options from the main menu, click the Color tab, and then click the Reset button.

Doing Double Underlining

To double underline data you are about to enter, press and hold the Shift key and click the Underline tool on the Formatting toolbar. Release the Shift key and enter your data as usual. It will be double-underlined.

To apply double underlines to cells that already contain data, first select the range of cells that contains the data you want double underlined. Then press and hold the Shift key and click the Underline tool.

Note that you can also access the double underline option by selecting Format | Cells and clicking the Fonts tab in the Format Cells dialog box. This tab presents several underlining options.

Centering Data across Several Columns

Here's an easy trick for centering a title across several columns of data. Type the title in a single cell above the columns of data. Select a range that extends across all the relevant columns (see Figure 6.11) and click the Merge and Center tool in the Formatting toolbar.

6

Figure 6.11.

Creating a heading or title across several columns.

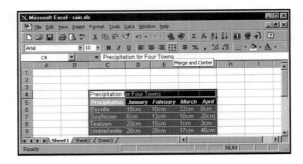

Protecting Worksheets, Workbooks, and Cells

Protecting your files—whether at the level of worksheets, workbooks, or individual cells—makes a great deal of sense, even if you are the only one working on your files.

Opening a Workbook as Read-Only

If you want to make sure that you don't disturb any of the settings or the data in a workbook, you can open it as a read-only file. To open a workbook as read-only, click the Open tool; the Open dialog box appears. Select the file you want to open and click the Commands and Settings icon in the upper-right corner (the icon with the red checkmark). The menu shown in Figure 6.12 appears. Choose Open Read-Only. Now, when the workbook opens, you will not be able to make any changes to the cells, and you will not be able to alter the formatting of the cells.

Opening a workbook in read-only mode helps ensure that you won't mess up the data—but you cannot be sure that anyone else will do the same. You can use the protection schemes discussed in the following sections if you want real protection.

Figure 6.12.

Opening a workbook as read-only.

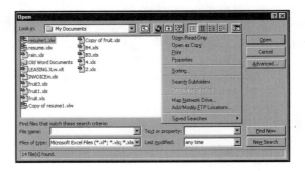

Saving a File as Read-Only

You can save a file with a recommendation that it be read-only, although you cannot enforce this recommendation. Someone can still destroy or alter your data.

To save a workbook with the read-only recommendation, open the workbook file and choose File|Save As from the main menu. Click the Options button, select the Read-Only Recommended checkbox, and click OK.

When you go to open the file, you see a dialog box asking whether you want to open the file as read-only. You can either do so or not. As you can see, the read-only recommendation is no guarantee that someone won't modify the file.

Protecting a Worksheet or a Workbook

Protecting a worksheet or workbook means that you cannot add or change any data or formatting in cells that are *locked*. Because many companies and individuals use Excel for important and sensitive data, being able to protect worksheets and workbooks is a significant help.

To protect a worksheet or workbook, choose Tools|Protection from the main menu. Then choose Protect Sheet or Protect Workbook (depending on whether you want to protect the entire file or only the current worksheet). You can protect any or all of the sheets in a workbook, or you can protect the workbook as a whole. For example, you may want to keep certain worksheets off-limits and make others accessible.

To really protect your files, you have to use passwords, as described in the following section. If you protect your worksheets without using passwords, you can prevent yourself and others from making inadvertent errors, but you cannot stop someone from unprotecting the worksheet and altering or destroying the data in the worksheet. No system of protection is foolproof, of course, and it's possible that an expert could crack the file, or that someone may guess your password.

Using Passwords

The danger of using a password is that you may forget it or lose it. Employees have been fired and much valuable data has been lost because passwords have been forgotten or lost. If you do use a password, keep it somewhere where you can find it. On the other hand, if anyone else finds your password written down, he or she may be able to figure out how to get into your files. Although Excel security is hard to crack, some expert hackers have done so. Don't rely on the password feature to answer all your system security concerns. Also, don't use the same password for your workbook files that you use for other system passwords.

To password protect your worksheet or workbook, first select Tools | Protection and then choose Protect Sheet or Protect Workbook. Then enter your preferred code in the dialog box as shown in Figure 6.13. You will be asked to reenter the password to ensure that you typed what you meant.

Figure 6.13.

Protecting a worksheet
with a password.

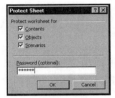

Cell Locking and Unlocking

When you protect a workbook or worksheet, all the cells in the worksheets are *locked* by default. You can *unlock* some or all of the cells if you want, while still maintaining the locked status on the other cells. You can use this feature to make certain parts of a workbook or worksheet inaccessible and other parts accessible. For example, you may want to lock cells that contain column headings, previously entered data, and so forth. You may want to make certain cells available for data entry and lock all of the rest.

You must first unlock the cells you want to be accessible before protecting the rest of the workbook or worksheet. To do this, select the cell or range you want to be accessible. Then select Format | Cells from the main menu and click the Protection tab. Deselect the Locked checkbox and click OK.

After you have unlocked all the cells you want to make accessible, you can protect the workbook or worksheet as described in the preceding section, "Protecting a Worksheet or a Workbook."

Unlocking Locked Cells within a Protected Worksheet

To unlock locked cells within a protected worksheet or workbook, you must first unprotect the worksheet or workbook.

Select Tools | Protection from the main menu and choose Unprotect Worksheet or Unprotect Workbook. If you have password protected the worksheet or workbook, enter the password when you are prompted to do so.

Next, select the cell or range you want to unlock. Select Format | Cells and click the Protection tab in the Format Cells dialog box. Clear the Locked checkbox and click OK.

6

Similarly, follow these steps to lock cells in a protected workbook or worksheet after previously unlocking them:

1. Unprotect the workbook or worksheet.
2. Select the cell or range of cells you want to lock.
3. Select Format|Cells, click the Protection tab of the Format Cells dialog box, select the Locked checkbox, and click OK.

Summary

Excel allows you precise control over how you format and present your worksheets. You can alter the fonts, colors, borders, patterns, backgrounds, and more. Styles are an efficient way to change cell formatting, and you can easily create and delete them. You can also copy formatting from one cell to other cells or ranges. Hour 7, "Using Excel Worksheet Templates," discusses how to use templates, which give you even more formatting options.

Protecting your data and formatting—once you have it in place—is important. You can protect all or part of your worksheets and workbooks. You can also choose to lock or unlock specific cells and ranges.

Workshop

Term Review

comment   A text box that contains descriptive or other information. This text box is attached to a cell. A comment can be displayed or hidden.

lock   You can lock a cell or group of cells to provide some protection from having the data altered or destroyed.

protect   You can protect a worksheet or workbook so that no changes can be made to it.

style   A combination of formatting instructions you can apply to a cell or group of cells as desired.

unlock   You can unlock a cell or group of cells so that you can alter or delete the data in the cell.

unprotect   You can unprotect a worksheet or workbook that has previously been protected so that you can make changes to it.

6

Q&A

Q **What is a style?**

A A style is a particular set of formatting options for a cell that you can save and apply to other cells.

Q **Why use styles?**

A Styles can save you a great deal of work in having to adjust the fonts, format, colors, backgrounds, size, and patterns for cells, especially if you make the same formatting changes to numerous cells.

Q **Why would you use comments?**

A Comments tell the user what the cell or range signifies. Comments are very helpful if more than one person is working on a worksheet.

Q **Why would you want to protect a worksheet or workbook?**

A You may have a large worksheet of which only a small portion should be altered. You can protect the cells that shouldn't be changed and unlock the cells that need to be changed.

6

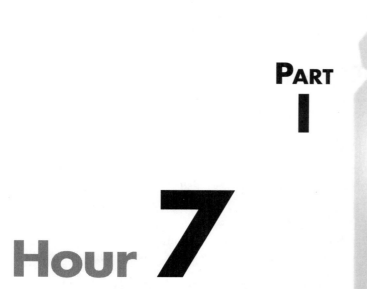

Hour 7

Using Excel Worksheet Templates

Templates allow you to reuse work you or others have done before. You may have noticed that many documents are essentially the same, with only a few differences. A typical business letter, for example, may follow essentially the same format every time—even the content may differ only slightly from letter to letter. Similarly, many companies have prescribed formats for their profit-and-loss statements or other financial and accounting documents. Templates in Microsoft Excel can save you a great deal of work and reduce the possibility of error, as opposed to creating the files from scratch.

In this hour, you learn how to use, create, and modify templates. The Template Wizard with Database Tracking is an add-in you can use to create templates that link to databases and is discussed in Hour 19, "Using Excel with Databases."

Using Templates

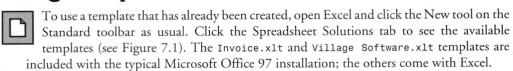

To use a template that has already been created, open Excel and click the New tool on the Standard toolbar as usual. Click the Spreadsheet Solutions tab to see the available templates (see Figure 7.1). The `Invoice.xlt` and `Village Software.xlt` templates are included with the typical Microsoft Office 97 installation; the others come with Excel.

Click once on any template icon to see a preview of the template, if one is available. Double-click the template icon to open up a new file based on that template.

The new file has a standard name such as `Book 1` or `Book 2`, as is normally the case when you open a new document in Excel. You can edit and add data to the new document based on a template just as you can with any other new document without affecting the template itself. Editing a template is discussed later in this hour in the section, "Modifying a Template."

Figure 7.1.

Selecting templates from the Spreadsheet Solutions tab.

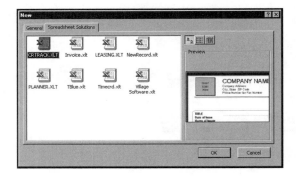

The Templates in Microsoft's Template Library

You can download prepared templates from the Microsoft Excel Web site at `http://www.microsoft.com/excel/work_tpladd.htm`. You can download templates for budget management, financial forecasting, holiday planning, and more. Figure 7.2 shows a template for an employee timecard available from the Microsoft site.

The templates you download are self-executing ZIP files. Save the files to your preferred directories and run the files by entering the path and filename in the Run dialog box (accessed from the Start menu). Most of these files cause a template to be installed in your default template directory. Read the installation instructions on the Web page for more details about individual template files, however.

If you look at the Microsoft site, and elsewhere on the Web, you may find that the templates you need have already been created. Looking at different templates is also a good way to get ideas and to find out what is possible with Microsoft Excel.

7

Figure 7.2.

An employee timecard template available from the Microsoft site.

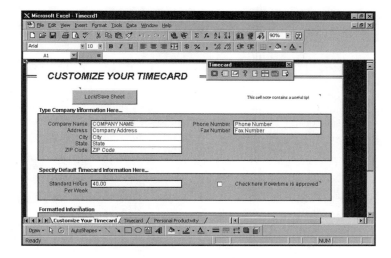

You can also purchase templates for various purposes. For example, if you want a land-value analysis template, you can see a demo template at `http://hollybar.com`; if you like it, you can purchase a full-fledged version. If you want to do financial modeling, you can look at products available for Excel at `http://www.financialcad.com`. Follow the specific installation instructions for these products and any others you may purchase.

In general, if you get Excel templates from another party, copy them into the `C:\Program Files\Microsoft Office\Templates\Spreadsheet Solutions` directory. Template files generally end with the extension `.xlt`.

CAUTION

Macros, which are discussed in greater detail in Part IV of this book, "Using Excel with Other Applications," may contain computer viruses. An Excel *macro* is a program attached to a workbook that performs certain functions. *Viruses* are malicious little programs that become attached to otherwise innocent files and can scramble the contents of not only your Excel files, but other programs and data as well.

Many templates, as well as other Microsoft Office files, contain macros. When you open a file containing macros, you are given the option to disable or enable the macros, or cancel opening the file altogether (see Figure 7.3). If you get the file from a trusted source, the chances of its being infected by a macro virus are likely smaller than if you receive the file from an anonymous source. However, it's always possible that your trusted source has given you files that have been inadvertently infected.

7

Also note that just because you do disable macros, you cannot be certain that your system is safe from viruses. If you don't trust the source of your file, you shouldn't open it.

You can get the latest information about macro viruses and macro virus protection from the Microsoft Excel Web site at `http://www.microsoft.com/excel/productinfo/vbavirus/emvolc.htm`. You can also purchase reasonably priced antiviral software that scans your files for viruses. Many computer users, particularly those with sensitive data, find the security provided by a good antiviral program to be worth the price.

Figure 7.3.

You have the option to disable or enable macros.

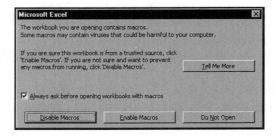

Creating Your Own Templates

You can make any workbook into a template. Create a workbook as you would want it for a template, or open a workbook that you have already created. Modify the workbook as you see fit. You can decide how specific or general you want your template to be.

Figure 7.4 shows a simple worksheet that can be made into a template. This worksheet is used to record company sales of four products. The user can substitute the company name, the particular months for which records are kept, the names of the product, and so forth. You can also create a template with all these fields filled in if you want to do so. The other worksheets in this workbook template have not been altered, but you can do so if you want.

To save the workbook as a template, choose File | Save As from the menu. From the Save As Type list box, select `Template (*.xlt)`. In the File Name box, enter the filename you want to give this workbook as a template. Change the directory to `C:\Program Files\Microsoft Office\Templates\Spreadsheet Solutions`. Click Save.

The next time you click File | New and click the Spreadsheet Solutions tab, your newly created template file is listed there. Click the template file icon to open a new document based on that template.

7

Figure 7.4.

Saving a worksheet as a template.

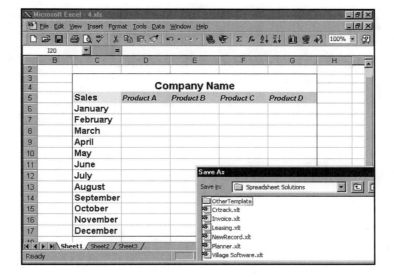

If you have a template file saved in a different directory, you cannot access it as a template unless it has been saved in the C:\Program Files\Microsoft Office\Templates\Spreadsheet Solutions directory (if you installed Excel in the default directory).

COFFEE BREAK

Styles into Templates

If you have created a style, as described in Hour 6, "Formatting and Protecting Worksheets," and you want it to be generally available in Excel, you must save the workbook containing the style in a template.

First, create the style. Then save the workbook as a template. Any new files you open with that template will have that style accessible.

Although it is inconvenient that Excel doesn't allow you to share styles between different workbooks, it generally isn't that much work to re-create the same style in another workbook.

Modifying a Template

To modify a template, open the template file in the same way you open an ordinary file: Choose File | Open from the main menu (or click the Open tool) and then navigate through the directories to get to the templates subdirectory at C:\Program Files\Microsoft Office\Templates\Spreadsheet Solutions. Open the template file you want to modify just as you would any other Excel file. Edit it and save the file again by choosing File | Save As from

7

the main menu. If you want, you can save the file under a different name so that you will have a different template than the original.

Creating a Default Worksheet or Workbook Template

The templates discussed so far have been in respect to an entire workbook. If you want a template that governs all your worksheets on an individual basis, you can create a default worksheet template.

First, create a workbook that has only one worksheet. Format this sheet as desired. Name the file SHEET, and save it in the directory C:\Program Files\Microsoft Office\Office\Xlstart. Make sure that you save the file as a template, as described in the previous section.

When you open Excel the next time, and a new workbook automatically opens, the sheets inside the new workbook will have their ordinary format. If you insert more sheets into the workbook, however, they are based on the template SHEET.

To save a workbook as the default template, create the workbook with the styles and formatting you want for each of the worksheets within it. Save the workbook file as a template under the filename BOOK in the C:\Program Files\Microsoft Office\Office\Xlstart folder. The next time you open Excel and open a new file, the default workbook will be based on the BOOK template.

Inserting Templates for a Worksheet into a Workbook

To insert a worksheet with a particular template into a workbook, right-click one of the sheet tabs to display the popup menu shown in Figure 7.5. Select Insert to see the dialog box that allows you to choose from a variety of different templates for your next worksheet. Select the template whose sheet you want to insert.

If your template has more than one worksheet in it, you add all those worksheets to your workbook at once when you insert the template from the popup menu. If you want to insert templates that contain only a single worksheet, you must create templates that have only one worksheet.

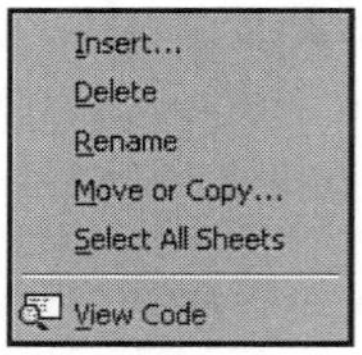

Figure 7.5.

The popup menu that appears when you right-click a worksheet tab.

7

Using Workbook Files as Templates

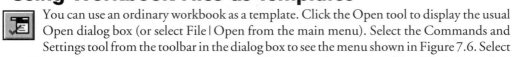

You can use an ordinary workbook as a template. Click the Open tool to display the usual Open dialog box (or select File | Open from the main menu). Select the Commands and Settings tool from the toolbar in the dialog box to see the menu shown in Figure 7.6. Select Open as Copy to open a *copy* of the selected file. Proceed to enter and modify data as usual. When you want to save the file, choose File | Save As from the menu and enter a new name for the file.

Figure 7.6.

You can open a file as a copy and use it as a template.

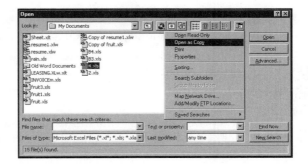

Summary

Templates are an efficient way to save particular formats for worksheets and workbooks so that you can use them repeatedly. You or your company probably has specific requirements for certain documents, so you can readily prepare the basic formats. If you have to modify a template, you can do so easily. You can also purchase templates for various purposes or search the World Wide Web for free or shareware versions of templates.

Part II of this book, "Graphical Manipulation and Display of Data," describes how you can improve the appearance of your workbooks by adding graphics and how you can represent data in meaningful ways with charts, maps, and graphs.

Workshop

Term Review

macro   A program attached to an Excel file that performs particular tasks or functions. Macros may carry a virus.

template   A file that serves as a pattern for a worksheet or workbook. You can reuse a template as many times as necessary.

7

virus A hidden program present in some files, including some Excel files that use macros, which can destroy or modify data. You should use files only from trusted sources to help reduce the possibility of infection by viruses. Installing virus-protection software is also a good idea.

Exercise

The template shown in Figure 7.7 is to be used for the purpose of recording students' grades. In this exercise, you will create this worksheet and save it as a template.

1. Open Excel as usual.

2. Enter the various percentages across the columns in the third row of the worksheet.

 3. Enter the headings in the first two rows of the worksheet and use the Merge and Center tool to adjust them.

 4. Enter the Students label and give it a background with the Fill tool.

5. Enter Lastname, Firstname into the first cell under the Students label. Drag the AutoFill tool down as many additional cells in the column as you want.

6. Choose File | Save As from the menu. Select Template (*.xlt) from the Save As Type drop-down list. Enter the name you want to give this template in the File Name box and click OK.

Figure 7.7.

A template for recording grades.

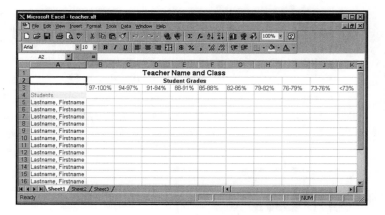

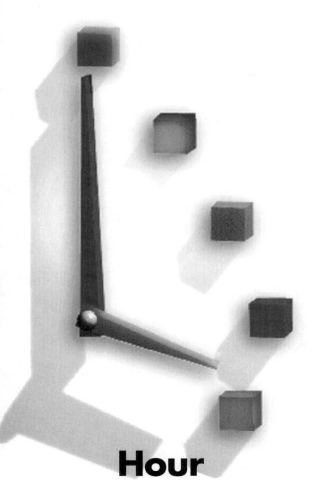

PART

II

Graphical Manipulation and Display of Data

Hour

Hour 8

Adding Graphics and Multimedia to Your Excel Documents

It's the numbers, isn't it? Of course, the actual content of your spreadsheets is what matters ultimately, but you can get your message across more effectively if your work *looks* good. Judicious use of fonts and background colors can go a long way toward improving the appearance of your work. Adding graphics can help even more. You can use graphics to punctuate an important point or just to add visual interest.

You can create your own graphics from scratch, or you can import clipart and modify it as needed. Excel offers many ways in which you can include graphics in your work.

Although graphics are probably the main addition you will want to make to your Excel worksheets, other types of multimedia are also significant. You can include video or animation clips, sound clips, and other objects.

If you are doing an extensive presentation, you may find that a presentation program such as Microsoft PowerPoint 97, used in conjunction with Excel, is best for your purposes. Excel has plenty of features, however, to make great presentations.

This chapter discusses how to use the Drawing toolbar, how to manipulate graphics and multimedia objects, and how to use clipart and external multimedia files.

Using the Drawing Toolbar

The Drawing toolbar is not part of the Excel workspace by default. To display it, select View|Toolbars from the main menu and then select Drawing; a checkmark appears next to the word Drawing to show that it is currently displayed.

To see what all the parts of the toolbar signify, run your pointer along the toolbar. Look at Figure 8.1 to see the various parts of the toolbar.

Figure 8.1.

The Drawing toolbar.

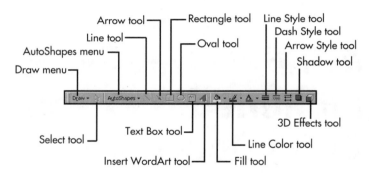

As you can see, the Drawing toolbar is divided into three regions:

- ☐ The region on the left consists of the Draw menu and the Select tool.
- ☐ The region in the middle consists of the AutoShapes menu and the Line, Arrow, Rectangle, Oval, Text Box, and Insert WordArt tools.
- ☐ The region on the right consists of tools you can use to format graphics objects you have already created. For example, there is the Fill tool, the Line Style tool, the Arrow Style tool, the Shadow tool, and the 3D Effects tool, among others.

The following section discusses the middle area first because that is the part used to create *shapes* (also called *drawing objects*).

Creating Shapes with the Drawing Toolbar

You can create shapes with the Drawing toolbar in several ways, as you can see from the tools in the middle. You can use the AutoShapes option, which provides you with many shapes you can adjust for your own use. You can also create lines, arrows, rectangles, ovals, and specially designed word art with the various tools available on the Drawing toolbar.

Using the AutoShapes Feature

The AutoShapes feature provides many premade shapes. Figure 8.2 shows a number of the possibilities, all of which were created with the AutoShapes feature. The AutoShapes feature allows you to include stars, banners, various kinds of polygons, and so on in your Excel documents.

Figure 8.2.

Some of the AutoShapes possibilities you can include in a worksheet.

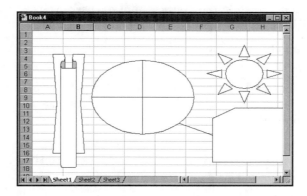

To access the AutoShapes menu, just click the word AutoShapes on the Drawing toolbar. Click the area of the worksheet to which you want to attach the graphic and drag the shape until the graphic is the size you prefer. You can expand and shrink the shape in all directions, as you like.

JUST A MINUTE

When you select a drawing object by clicking it, you see small squares all around the edges of the object. Each of these small squares is called a *handle*. To resize an object or change its configuration, place the cursor on one of the handles and drag until the object looks the way you want it to. The handle you choose to drag affects the way in which the object is distorted.

You can also select an object by clicking the Select tool on the Drawing toolbar and then using the tool to click the object you want to select.

To replace a shape created with the AutoShapes feature, first select the object you want to change. Display the Draw scroll-down menu on the Drawing toolbar (click Draw on the left side of the Drawing toolbar), choose Change AutoShapes, and select the desired shape from the possibilities available.

The following sections describe the various AutoShapes possibilities.

Lines

Choose AutoShapes|Lines from the Drawing toolbar and then select the Freeform or Scribble tool to do freehand drawings.

You can use the Freeform tool to create freehand drawings or polygons. To create polygons, click where you want one of the vertices to be, click at the point of the next vertex, and continue clicking on vertices until you have the shape you want. To close the polygon, click the first vertex again.

To draw freehand, simply drag the Freeform cursor in any shape you want and double-click when you are finished drawing.

You can also draw with the Scribble tool, which works much like a pencil. Select the Scribble tool, click to begin, and drag the pencil to make the shape you want. Double-click when finished.

Any drawing you do with these tools will likely be amateurish in quality compared to what you can do with an actual drawing program. You may be better off creating complex shapes in a drawing program, saving the file, and then importing the object into Excel, as described in the section, "Specially Created Graphics," later in this chapter.

Other tools you can access through the AutoShapes|Lines submenu are a Curve tool, two Arrow tools (one single and the other double-headed), and a Line tool. To use the Arrow and Line tools, first click the tool. Then click where you want one end of the line to go and drag to where you want the other end of the line to go. Release the mouse button when finished. If you clicked the plain Line tool, all you get is a line; if you clicked one of the arrow tools, you get a line with either one or two arrow heads.

To use the Curve tool, select it and then click in the worksheet where you want the starting point of the curve to be. Drag the cursor until you reach the first point at which you want to change the direction of the curve; click there. Continue dragging the cursor until it's time to change direction again and then click again. Continue in this way until you have the curve you want. Double-click when finished.

To change the thickness of any of these borders, select the object and click the Line Style tool on the Drawing toolbar. Choose the line thickness you want from the popup menu.

Connectors

You can use the Connectors tool from the AutoShapes | Connectors menu—as you might expect—to draw connections between objects. Connectors are especially good for flow-charts, particularly when they are used in combination with objects from the AutoShapes | Flowchart menu. Different types of connectors are available: straight and bent lines and arrows.

Choose AutoShapes | Connectors from the Drawing toolbar and select one of the different shapes available. Click the point on the first object at which you want one end of the connector to join; then click the point on the other object to which you want to connect.

Basic Shapes

The shapes you can access from the AutoShapes | Basic Shapes submenu are polygons, a heart, a happy face, and other common symbols. Choose the desired tool from the menu, click in the worksheet at the desired starting point, and then drag the cursor in the appropriate direction to get the shape you want. Click outside the region when finished.

Block Arrows

Like connectors, block arrows are good for diagrams and flow charts. Block arrows differ from connectors in that they do not link *precisely* between the two separate objects.

Select AutoShapes | Block Arrows from the Drawing toolbar, click in the worksheet at the desired starting point, and then drag the cursor in the appropriate direction to get the shape you want. Click outside the region when finished.

Flowchart Shapes

Select AutoShapes | Flowchart from the Drawing toolbar to display the Flowchart submenu, which has 28 different shapes on it. You can choose various shapes from the Flowchart menu to create a flowchart.

The Flowchart shapes are very similar to some of the shapes available on the Basic Shapes menu (or that you can draw with the Line tool). To make the flowchart meaningful, use the Text Box tool to place text inside each of the flowchart shapes.

A typical flowchart needs connectors. If you are describing a process in which some action leads to some other action, you will want to use a connector with an arrow. If you are describing a feedback process, you will want to use a double-pointed arrow connector. You may want connectors that are straight lines or that are bent lines. To choose the connectors you want, select AutoShapes | Connectors from the Drawing toolbar, choose the shape you want, and connect the flowchart objects as described in the previous section, "Connectors."

Formatting AutoShapes Objects

Any AutoShapes object can be formatted. First, select the object you want to modify. You can select the object with the Select tool on the Drawing toolbar, or you can just click the border of the object to select it.

With the object selected, right-click it to display the dialog box shown in Figure 8.3. By using this dialog box, you can adjust the colors and lines, the precise sizes, the protection level, and the properties of your drawing objects.

Figure 8.3.

The Format AutoShape dialog box.

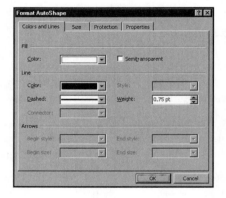

Using the Line, Arrow, Rectangle, and Oval Tools

This section describes the tools you can access from the middle of the Drawing toolbar: the Line, Arrow, Rectangle, and Oval tools.

Select the tool you want, click in the worksheet at the point where you want the object to start, and drag the mouse to get the desired shape and size of the object. Release the mouse button when you have drawn the shape you want.

TIME SAVER

To create perfect circles and squares, press and hold the Shift key while dragging the Oval or Rectangle tool. Release the key when you are finished drawing.

You can create lines that are angled at 15 degrees, 30 degrees, or other multiples of 15 degrees. Press and hold the Shift key while dragging the Line tool at the angle you want. Release the mouse button when the line is as long as you want.

You can format any of these shapes by selecting the object, right-clicking it, and selecting Format AutoShapes from the popup menu that appears. Refer to the preceding section, "Formatting AutoShapes Objects."

Creating Text Boxes

You use the Text Box tool to place text inside drawing objects or other images. Inside a blank space inside the object, the text box can contain text formatted to your specifications.

Here's how to place text inside a drawing object:

1. Click the Text Box tool in the Drawing toolbar. Then click the object in which you want to insert a text box.

2. Drag the cursor until you have a text box the size you want.

3. Type the text you want to appear in the text box. Press Enter when you want to move to the next line in the box. When finished entering text, click outside the box.

4. To change the font and color of the text, right-click within the text box and select Format Text Box from the popup menu. The dialog box shown in Figure 8.4 appears; use it to adjust the fonts as you want.

Figure 8.4.

The Format Text Box dialog box.

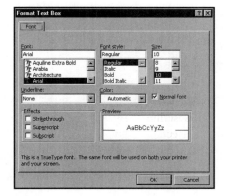

Using WordArt

The WordArt tool turns a word or phrase into an icon of its own by stylizing its appearance. The text is turned into a three-dimensional shape that can look either professional or tacky, depending on how you use it. You can control the color, font size and face, as well as other characteristics of the WordArt object.

To use WordArt, just click the WordArt tool in the Drawing toolbar to display the WordArt Gallery dialog box (see Figure 8.5). You can choose from any of the various WordArt styles in the dialog box. After you select the style you want, the Edit WordArt Text dialog box appears. Enter some text and modify the font as appropriate. Click OK.

At this point, the WordArt toolbar appears. This toolbar offers various tools to manipulate WordArt objects. You can control the color, text, alignment, spacing, and other characteristics of the WordArt object with the tools on the WordArt toolbar.

Figure 8.5.
The WordArt Gallery and toolbar.

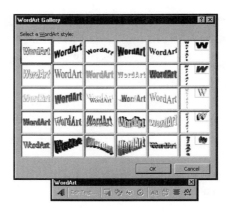

Controlling Object Appearance with the Drawing Toolbar

The right side of the Drawing toolbar is used to manipulate the appearance of objects. You can fill objects with different colors or patterns, change the border color and style, and add shadows and three-dimensional effects.

Filling Objects

To fill an object, first select the object. Then click the Fill tool from either the Standard toolbar or the Drawing toolbar. Choose your preferred color from the palette of colors that appears in the popup menu. You can choose More Fill Colors if you want to create your own custom color. You can choose Fill Effects if you want to fill the object with a particular Fill style, such as one of several gradients, textures, patterns, and even other pictures (see Figure 8.6).

Figure 8.6.
The Fill Effects dialog box.

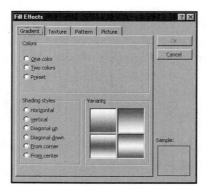

8

8

Changing the Object's Border Color

To change the border color of an object, first select the object you want to modify. Then choose the Line Color tool from the Drawing toolbar. A popup menu appears, showing all the possible colors and the option of choosing patterns. The default line color is black, but you can choose any of the other colors. You can also choose to have no visible border at all by selecting No Line from the popup menu.

Specifying a Line Style, Arrow Style, and Dash Style

You can use the Line Style and the Dash Style tools to change the border around any of your objects.

Select the object whose borders you want to modify. Then select either the Line Style tool (if you want a continuous border) or the Dash Style tool (if you want a dashed border) from the Drawing toolbar. A menu of line style options pops up. Click the style you want, and the border of the selected object changes.

To change the style of an arrow, first draw the arrow with the Arrow tool (in the middle of the Drawing toolbar). Select the arrow by clicking its border. Select the Arrow Style tool and choose the style of arrow you want from the popup menu. You can determine whether the arrow should be single or double-headed as well as other features of its style. You can also use the Line Style or Dash Style tool to change the style of the arrow's line.

Adding Shadows to Objects

Shadows add special effects to your graphics and look ever so impressive. Used excessively, however, they can obscure; used judiciously, they definitely enhance the coolness factor of your worksheets.

To create a shadow around a drawing object, follow these steps:

1. Select the drawing object to which you want to add a shadow.
2. Click the Shadow tool on the Drawing toolbar to display a popup menu.
3. Choose the Shadow option you want to use for your drawing object and click it.

To change the color or position of the shadow, select Shadow Settings from the popup menu. The Shadow Settings toolbar appears (see Figure 8.7). With this toolbar, you can adjust the position of the shadow as well as its color. Notice that the Shadow Color tool has a drop-down menu from which you can select various colors for the shadow you create for your object.

Figure 8.7.

The Shadow Settings toolbar.

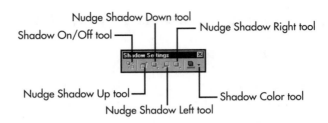

Adding 3D Effects

You can use the 3D Effects tool, at the far right of the Drawing toolbar, to turn ovals into cylinders, spheres, or other shapes and to turn rectangles into prisms or irregularly shaped boxes. Select the object you want to turn into a 3D version and click the 3D Effects tool. The resulting popup menu provides 20 different 3D effects from which you can select to create the shape you want.

If you want to customize a 3D effect, click the 3D Settings option on the popup menu. The 3D Settings toolbar appears. The tools on this toolbar are similar to the tools on the Shadow Settings toolbar: 3D On/Off, Tilt Down, Tilt Up, Tilt Left, Tilt Right, Depth, Direction, Lighting, Surface, and 3D Color (Automatic).

TIME SAVER

> Remember that you can always undo an action by clicking the Undo tool (or pressing Ctrl+Z). Although it's easy to make a change to an object you don't want, you can easily fix it again.

Using the Draw Menu on the Drawing Toolbar

On the left side of the Drawing toolbar is the Draw menu. Click this button to display a menu of options you can use to control the behavior of objects and perform different manipulations on them, either as a group or as individual objects.

Setting AutoShapes Defaults

To set different defaults for AutoShapes, select an object created with AutoShapes that has been modified the way you want it (in terms of fill, borders, shadows, 3D effects, and so forth). From the Drawing toolbar, click Draw and select Set AutoShapes Defaults. The defaults for AutoShapes are now changed to the formats of the selected object. You can change them again by formatting an AutoShapes object to a different specification and repeating the process just outlined.

Suppose that you draw a shape, fill it with a particular color, and then apply a shadow and 3D effect to it. If you select the object and then choose Draw | Set AutoShapes Defaults from the Drawing toolbar, any shapes you draw after that will have the same color, shadow, and 3D effect as the first object. These shapes may be ovals, rectangles, AutoShapes, or others.

Editing Freeform Drawings

You can use the Edit Points tool to edit freeform drawings. Select the object drawn with the Freeform tool that you want to modify. From the Drawing toolbar, select Draw; from the drop-down menu that appears, choose Edit Points. Now click a point in the freeform object (see Figure 8.8) and drag it in various directions, depending on how you want to edit the figure.

Figure 8.8.
Using the Edit Points tool to modify a freeform object.

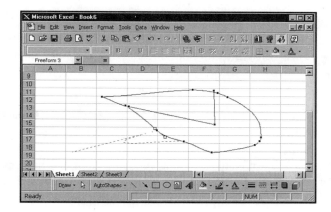

Rerouting Connectors

To change the location or route of a connector, first select it. From the Drawing toolbar, select Draw; from the drop-down menu that appears, choose Reroute Connectors. Now you can move the connector anywhere you see fit.

Changing the Order of Drawing Objects

Frequently, you may want to place objects in front of or behind other objects. You may want one object to overlap others. Of course, you can draw objects in the order you want them in, in the first place. However, if you want to rearrange the objects after they have been drawn, you can do so by following these steps:

1. Make sure that the objects are positioned together, with some overlap between them.
2. Select the object you want to reposition relative to the other objects.

3. From the Drawing toolbar, select Draw; from the drop-down menu that appears, choose Order. The Order submenu provides several options:

Option	Description
Bring to Front	This option moves the object to the very front of all the objects.
Send to Back	This option sends the object to the very back of all the objects.
Bring Forward	This option moves the object forward one place, in front of the next object (rather than moving it to the very front).
Send Backward	This option moves the object backward one place, behind the object just behind it (rather than moving it to the very back).

Select the move option you want from the Order submenu.

4. Continue selecting and rearranging objects. Depending on the size of the various objects, some objects may completely cover other objects.

Grouping, Ungrouping, and Regrouping Drawing Objects

You can manipulate several objects together as a group. You *group* objects together so that you can manipulate them together. When you scale the grouped objects up or down, move them in different directions, rotate them, or otherwise make changes to the objects, all the objects in the group change in the same way. Grouping objects together helps you synchronize the appearance of a group of drawing objects.

After you group objects together, you can also *ungroup* them so that you can deal with the objects individually. If you then want to deal with the objects as a group again to do further manipulations, you can *regroup* them.

Here's how to group objects:

1. Select the various objects you want to group together: Press and hold the Shift key and select the first object. Continue to hold the Shift key as you select the other objects you want in the group. Release the Shift key.

2. From the Drawing toolbar, select Draw; from the drop-down menu that appears, choose Group.

   The selected objects now have a new set of handles that works for all the objects together. You can drag this collection of objects to resize them or move them together. These objects remain a group until you ungroup them again.

3. To ungroup a set of grouped objects, first select the group. From the Drawing toolbar, select Draw; from the drop-down menu that appears, choose Ungroup.

8

4. To regroup the objects after ungrouping them, select one of the objects in the original group. From the Drawing toolbar, select Draw; from the drop-down menu that appears, choose Regroup. It doesn't matter if you have altered the same or other objects after previously ungrouping the objects.

Rotating and Flipping Objects

You can rotate or flip any graphic object. To do so, select the object and click a handle. Select Draw from the Drawing toolbar; from the drop-down menu that appears, choose Rotate or Flip to display yet another submenu.

Choose one of the directional options. If you select Free Rotate, green handles appear around the selected object. Click one of the green handles and drag the object through a rotation until it is tilted the way you want it. If you choose one of the other directional options from the submenu (such as Rotate Left, Rotate Right, Flip Horizontal, or Flip Vertical), the rotation happens automatically.

Using the Snap Feature

You can "snap" an object to either the gridlines or to another object by choosing Draw from the Drawing toolbar and then choosing Snap from the drop-down menu that appears. A submenu appears. To automatically align objects with the vertical and horizontal edges of other shapes when you move or draw them, click To Shape from this submenu. To automatically align an object with the gridlines of the worksheet, click To Grid from the Snap submenu.

TIME SAVER

You can also make objects snap to the gridlines by pressing the Alt key while dragging the objects.

When creating objects, you can activate either the Snap | To Grid option or the Snap | To Shape option. All objects created after you make that selection will snap either to the grid or to shapes they overlay.

Using the Nudge Feature

You can use the Nudge feature with both shadows and objects to make slight changes to their positions.

Select the object you want to nudge. From the Drawing toolbar, select Draw; from the drop-down menu that appears, choose Nudge; a submenu appears. The options on the Nudge submenu are up, down, left, and right.

Click the direction in which you want to nudge the object; the object moves slightly. If you don't move the object as far as you want with the first nudge, repeat the process.

Manipulating Objects

When you work with graphics and multimedia objects in Excel, you must be able to select them, move them around, and copy, delete, and paste them. The principles involved are easy and intuitive, particularly if you understand how to manipulate cells and ranges. The rules for manipulating objects are very similar to those for manipulating cells.

TIME SAVER

A general rule for manipulating objects in Excel is to select the object and then right-click to display a popup menu of the options available for that object.

Deleting Objects

To delete an object, select it and press the Del key (or select Edit | Clear | All from the main menu).

Cutting Objects and Cells Together

By default, objects and cells are not cut or copied as a unit when an area is selected. You can change the options so that objects and cells are processed together, however.

Select Tools | Options from the main menu to display the Options dialog box. Click the Edit tab and either check or uncheck the Cut, Copy and Sort Objects with Cells checkbox.

Copying Objects

There are several ways to copy objects. Here is the simplest way:

1. Select the object.
2. Right-click the object; from the resulting popup menu, click Copy.
3. Move the cursor to the desired new location.
4. Right-click the new location; from the resulting popup menu, click Paste.

Using the drag-and-drop method to copy objects is very similar to the method for copying a range of cells:

1. Select the object.
2. Press and hold the Ctrl key as you drag the object to its new location.
3. Release the Ctrl key and the mouse button when you are finished.

Of course, you can always use the main menu to copy an object:

1. Select the object.
2. Choose Edit I Copy from the menu. Alternatively, press Ctrl+C.
3. Move the cursor to the desired new location in which you want to copy the object.
4. Select Edit I Paste from the menu. Alternatively, press Ctrl+V.

Moving an Object

The easiest way to move an object is simply to select the object and drag it to its new location.

You can also select the object, choose Edit I Copy from the main menu (or press Ctrl+X), move the cursor to the new location, and select Edit I Paste (or press Ctrl+V).

JUST A MINUTE

> You can lock and unlock objects, just as you do cells. First, protect the worksheet or workbook, as described in Hour 6, "Formatting and Protecting Worksheets." Select Format I Object from the menu to display the Format Objects dialog box. Select the Protection tab and then check or uncheck the Locked checkbox.

Resizing Objects

To resize an object, first select it with the mouse. Move the mouse pointer over one of the handles and drag the handle to resize the object. You can move the handle in or out to adjust the size and shape of the figure.

Using the Format Painter Tool to Format Objects

You can transfer formatting from one object to another in a manner similar to the way you transfer formatting between cells: You use the Format Painter tool to copy the formatting for one object to another.

1. Select the object whose formatting you want to copy.

2. Click the Format Painter tool from the Standard toolbar.

3. Click the object to which you want to copy the format.

Controlling Object Display

When working with a spreadsheet, you may prefer not to see all the drawing objects because they may distract you from the main purpose of the worksheet (manipulating data). To hide the drawing objects, choose Tools I Options from the main menu to display the Options dialog box. Click the View tab to see the three options for viewing objects:

□ **Show All:** All the objects are displayed.

□ **Show Placeholders:** A small icon appears at each spot where there is an object. You can click the icon to see the object.

□ **Hide All:** All the objects are hidden.

Select the option you want and click OK to close the Options dialog box.

Using Clipart and External Files

Clipart is a good way to include professional-quality graphics in your work. (You can obtain clipart files from Microsoft or from other sources.) You can also include graphics files you or others have created using various image-creation and image-editing programs.

Microsoft Clipart

The Microsoft Office 97 CD-ROM offers a goodly sized collection of clipart that you can easily place in your Excel documents. Select Insert | Picture and choose Clipart from the submenu. Some of the clipart is shown in Figure 8.9. If you have not done a full installation, you won't be able to access much of the clipart without inserting the CD-ROM.

Figure 8.9.

Some of the clipart available from Microsoft Office 97.

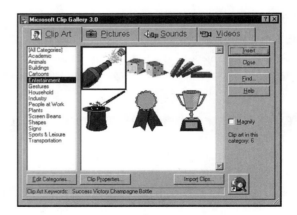

Specially Created Graphics

You can create your own graphics with any graphics program, such as Adobe Illustrator, CorelDRAW!, Macromedia Freehand, Paint Shop Pro, or one of many others. You can then insert the graphics in your Excel worksheets.

To insert in an Excel worksheet a graphic file you have created, start Excel and open the worksheet you want to receive the graphics file. Position the cursor at the location in the worksheet where you want the graphic to appear. Choose Insert | Picture from the main menu

8

8

and choose From File to display the dialog box shown in Figure 8.10. Search the directories until you find the graphics file you want to insert. When you highlight the filename, you can see a preview of the graphic as you search through the directories. When you find the graphics file you want, click Insert; the graphic appears at the selected location in the worksheet.

Figure 8.10.

Inserting a graphic from a file.

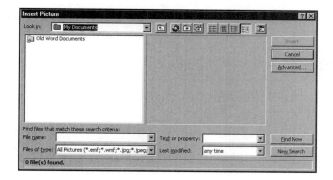

JUST A MINUTE

If you choose Insert|Object and then select Bitmap Image from the scroll-down menu, the Microsoft Paint application opens up within Excel (see Figure 8.11). You can use Paint to create an image on the spot. When finished, click outside the Paint program box to return to Excel and the Excel menu bars.

Figure 8.11.

Creating a bitmap image within Excel.

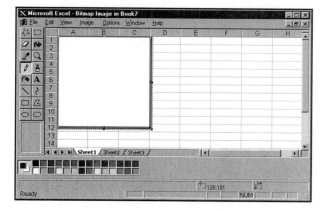

External Clipart

Many companies, such as Corel, offer clipart packages that contain premade art you can use in your Excel worksheets. Put the CD-ROM that contains the third-party clipart into your CD-ROM drive, start Excel, and open the workbook you want to receive the clipart. Select Insert|Picture from the Excel main menu, select From File from the submenu, and then navigate through the files on the CD-ROM. Excel can import the file types shown in Table 8.1. The clipart package may have its own specific instructions as well.

Table 8.1. The types of files Excel can import as graphics.

File Extension	File Type Description
.BMP, .DIB, .RLE	Windows Bitmap
.CDR	CorelDRAW!
.CGM	Computer Graphics MetaFile
.DRW	Micrographix Designer/Draw
.EMF	Enhanced MetaFile
.EPS	Encapsulated PostScript
.GIF	Graphic Image Format
.HPGL	Hewlett-Packard Graphics Language
.JPEG or .JPG	Joint Photographers' Expert Group
.PIC	Lotus 1-2-3 Graphics
.PCT	Macintosh PICT Filter
.PNG	Portable Network Graphic
.PCX	PC Paintbrush
.TIFF or .TIF	Tagged Image Format
.WPG	WordPerfect Graphics
.WMF	Windows MetaFile

The Picture Toolbar

When you insert a graphic, whether it is a piece of clipart or a graphic created with another drawing package, the Picture toolbar appears in your Excel worksheet (see Figure 8.12). To use a tool in the Picture toolbar, first select the graphic and then click the tool. You see a menu of options from which you can choose.

8

Figure 8.12.

The Picture toolbar.

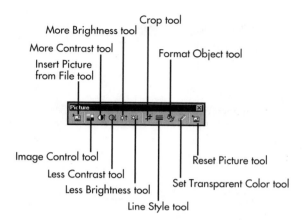

To use the tools on the Picture toolbar, click the border of the picture object to display the handles of the object. The Picture toolbar has the following tools:

Tool	Description
Insert Picture from File	Click this tool and you can insert a picture file located on your computer.
Image Control	Click this tool and you can choose any of the following options: Automatic (the default), Grayscale, Black & White, and Watermark (turns the image very pale).
More Contrast	Click this tool to increase the contrast of the image.
Less Contrast	Click this tool to decrease the contrast of the image.
More Brightness	Click this tool to increase the brightness of the image.
Less Brightness	Click this tool to decrease the brightness of the image.
Crop	Click the tool and drag the resulting pointer over a handle of the image to crop the picture.
Line Style	Click this tool and choose the desired line thickness to place a border around the picture.
Format Object	Click this tool and the Format Picture dialog box appears. You can then adjust various features with the following tabs: Colors and Lines, Size, Picture, Protection, and Properties.
Set Transparent Color	If you have a bitmap image, you can click the color that you want to be transparent (meaning that objects located under that color can also be seen).

Tool	Description
Reset Picture	Changes the picture back to what it was when the image was initially inserted into the worksheet.

The Picture toolbar has enough tools to be like a small image-editing program. If you want to do a comprehensive job of editing the images, however, consider using an image-editing program such as Adobe PhotoShop and then import the images—precisely the way you want them—into Excel. If you lack an image-editing program, however, the Picture toolbar is a relatively powerful substitute.

Adding Video, Sound, and Other Multimedia

You are not limited to adding simple drawing objects to your worksheets. You can add animations, video, and sound clips, as well as other media.

To insert other types of multimedia objects in your Excel worksheets, select Insert|Object from the main menu. There is a variety of different objects you can add to your Excel worksheet, as you can see from the resulting dialog box. To view these objects, however, you must have an appropriate program to view them with. For example, if you insert a video clip into your document, you must have a viewer program to see the video clip.

Once multimedia objects are inserted in your Excel worksheet, you can manipulate them in much the same way you manipulate graphic objects. To see how you can manipulate a particular multimedia object, select the object and right-click it. A popup menu containing the various options currently available for that object appears. You can also manipulate various features of how the object looks within the Excel worksheet by using the Picture toolbar.

If you have recording equipment, you can even add your own voice annotations to different cells. Create a sound clip with whatever information you want and save it in the appropriate format. Import the sound clip as you would any other object.

Summary

Including graphics and other multimedia objects in your worksheets can greatly enhance the appearance and usability of your Excel documents. Excel makes the process easy because it includes so many ready-made drawing objects and clipart, which you can customize to meet your specific needs. Excel also allows you to include sound, video, animation, and other multimedia objects, which means that you can create a top-quality presentation with pizzazz. Hour 9, "Creating Excel Charts," discusses charts, another way to emphasize your data and enhance your presentation.

Workshop

Term Review

AutoShapes   A variety of shapes, available from the Drawing toolbar, you can use in your Excel worksheets. These shapes include banners, ribbons, stars, connectors, and others.

clipart   Ready-made art in the form of various graphics files. Some clipart images come with the Office 97 CD-ROM. You can also buy clipart from other vendors such as Corel.

drawing objects   Graphics objects you draw with the tools on the Drawing toolbar, such as AutoShapes, circles, ovals, lines, and so on. These objects are also called *shapes*.

group   You can group a selection of graphics objects together so that they all can be manipulated together.

handle   When you activate a graphics object by clicking its border, small squares called handles appear at the edges of the object. Place the mouse pointer on one of these handles and drag it to resize or reshape the object.

regroup   To activate a previously used grouping of objects.

ungroup   To remove the grouping from a selection of graphics objects that have been grouped together.

Q&A

Q What do you use to create and modify graphics?

A The Drawing toolbar has most of the tools you need. You can also create graphics in other programs and import them into your Excel worksheet.

Q What's a good tool for creating fancy text?

A You can use the WordArt tool to create colorful, three-dimensional text.

Q How can you use graphics from other programs?

A Choose Insert|Picture from the main menu, choose Clipart or From File from the submenu, and use the dialog box to locate the file.

Q Can you include sound and video in your worksheets?

A Yes. Graphics, video clips, sound clips, and other multimedia files are all objects you can insert in your worksheets. Once they are inserted in the worksheet, you can cut, copy, paste, and otherwise manipulate them.

Exercise

Try creating the shapes shown in Figure 8.13. Start by displaying the Drawing toolbar.

☐ Here's how to create the oval:

1. Select the Oval tool. Click the worksheet and drag the shape to the size you want.

2. Select the oval. Click the Line Style tool and choose the style you want from the popup menu to change the border.

3. Select the oval. Click the Line Color tool and choose the color you want from the popup menu to change the color of the border.

4. Select the oval and use the Fill tool to fill the object with the color white (or whatever color you prefer). By filling the oval, you obscure the gridlines.

☐ Here's how to create the WordArt object:

1. Place the cursor in the location where you want the WordArt object to appear. Select the WordArt tool. Choose the style you want from the resulting dialog box and click OK.

2. The Edit WordArt dialog box appears. Change the font and size as desired. Type the text you want and click OK.

3. You can further adjust and rotate the WordArt with the tools on the WordArt toolbar.

☐ Here's how to create the 3D shape:

1. Select the Rectangle tool from the Drawing toolbar. Click the worksheet and drag the shape until it has the dimensions you want.

2. Select the 3D tool from the Drawing toolbar; from the submenu that appears, choose the shape you want the rectangle to transform into.

Figure 8.13.

What the Drawing tools can do.

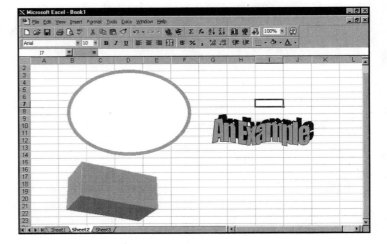

8

Hour 9

Creating Excel Charts

Charts are an excellent way to present data in a powerful way. If you want to make sure that your data is understood, you should present it in more than one way. Some people find a basic table easiest to understand; others prefer the stark graphic evidence of a chart. Quarterly earning reports, scientific data, population data, changes in house prices, and innumerable other types of data look good when converted into charts.

With Excel, you can link the charts to the data, so that if the data changes, the chart does as well.

Many different types of charts are possible, and there are many different things you can do with them. This hour provides only a basic introduction to charts because Excel provides so many options and possibilities.

Creating Charts

To create charts, you first need the data. A typical worksheet that represents various relationships can generally be changed into a chart quite easily. If you have the data arranged in a tabular format, you can readily change it into a chart. It's even easier if you label the rows and columns containing the data.

Excel is quite good at figuring out a suitable chart automatically. The data in Figure 9.1 represents the normal minimum and maximum January temperatures for five U.S. cities, taken in degrees Fahrenheit. To create the table shown in Figure 9.2, simply select one of the cells within the table you want to turn into a chart. Then press the F11 key, and Excel automatically creates a new chart sheet. That's the easy way, but you can manufacture charts in other ways as well, as described in the rest of this hour.

Figure 9.1.

A simple table in an Excel worksheet.

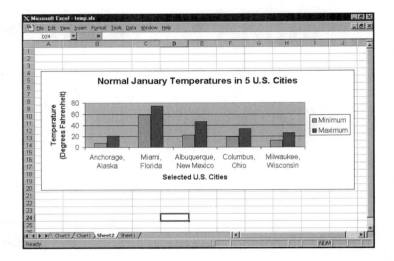

Figure 9.2.

The table turned into a chart.

JUST A MINUTE

A *data point* consists of the data in one cell. A *data series* is the collection of data that corresponds to a single label. In the chart in Figure 9.2, 21 is one of the data points; all the Minimum values form a data series.

9

Using the Chart Wizard

To create a chart from the data shown in Figure 9.1 using the Chart Wizard, begin by selecting a cell within the table.

Step 1 of the Chart Wizard

Click the Chart tool on the Standard toolbar or choose Insert | Chart from the main menu. The first dialog box of the Chart Wizard appears (see Figure 9.3). A *wizard* is just a tool that facilitates a particular process by walking you through the various steps. When you invoke a wizard, it displays a dialog box that asks for information. You enter the information, or accept the defaults, and continue through all the wizard's dialog boxes that ask for information. If you just follow the requests for information in the Chart Wizard dialog boxes, the process is easy.

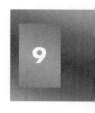

JUST A MINUTE

Note that when you select a chart, the main menu changes: The Data menu option is replaced with the Chart menu option. You can choose various options from the Chart pull-down menu, including options that allow you to change the type of chart, the source data, the chart options, and where the chart is placed.

From the first screen of the Chart Wizard, click the Standard Types tab if it is not already displayed. From the Chart Type list, choose your preferred style of chart. The type of data in the table shown in Figure 9.1 is best suited to a column or bar presentation. For this example, select Column from the Chart Type list and select Clustered Column (the top-left image) from the Chart Sub-type list, as shown in Figure 9.3.

Figure 9.3.

Step 1 of the Chart Wizard dialog box.

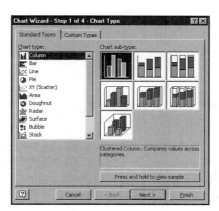

To see how your data will look as presented in different kinds of charts, choose a chart type and then click the Press and Hold to View Sample button. Continue selecting chart types and viewing samples until you are pleased with the selected chart type.

The Kinds of Charts Available

The Step 1 dialog box shows the various types of charts you can create. Scroll through the possibilities to see what is available. Each of the different standard types has a variety of subtypes.

Certain types of charts are good for particular types of data. For example, Figure 9.4 shows a pie chart graphing the educational attainment of the employees in a fictitious corporation. Because the chart is supposed to represent all the employees, a pie chart makes sense. Bar charts and column charts are good for representing specific quantities, such as temperatures, sale amounts, precipitation, and so forth. Line charts are good when you want to interpolate between the data points, as you need to do with many scientific experiments. Three-dimensional charts are good for complicated data that you want to view from different perspectives.

Figure 9.4.

An example of a pie chart.

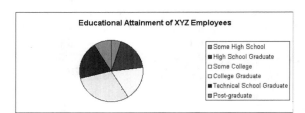

Step 2 of the Chart Wizard

Click the Next button at the bottom of the Chart Wizard dialog box to display the next screen, Step 2 of 4 (see Figure 9.5). The selection you make for Series In, whether Rows or Columns, determines how the data is oriented (that is, which data label goes on the bottom axis of the chart).

The sample data table has the labels Cities, Minimum, and Maximum in a row at the top of the table. The names of the cities are in a column along the left edge. If you choose a column chart, the default presentation of this data is to have the names of the cities along the bottom axis and the temperatures along the left axis. The temperatures are displayed in vertical bars for each city.

9

Figure 9.5.

Step 2 of 4 of the Chart Wizard dialog box.

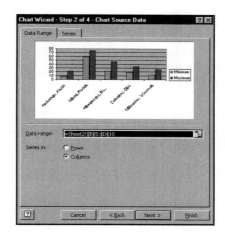

If you want to change the orientation of the way the data is presented, click the Rows button in the Step 2 dialog box to place the labels Minimum and Maximum on the bottom axis and the city names in a legend box alongside the chart.

 You can change the data range included in the chart. Click the Collapse Dialog icon (at the end of the Data Range text box) so that the Chart Wizard dialog box moves out of the way. When the dialog box is collapsed, it looks like Figure 9.6.

Figure 9.6.

A collapsed dialog box.

You can then view your worksheet again. The data in the worksheet that Excel has selected for use in the chart is surrounded by dashed lines. If you want the chart to use a different set of data, you can select the area of the worksheet you want. Click the Expand Dialog icon (located at the right edge of the collapsed dialog box) to get back to the dialog box.

You can also change the area of the worksheet that is used by the chart by editing the Data Range string within the dialog box. In this case, the range Excel selected is =Sheet1!$C$8:$E$13 because the data is located in Sheet1, with the upper-left corner of the range at C8 and the bottom-right corner at E13.

The addressing system used in the Data Range string uses an ! symbol after the worksheet name and $ symbols after each of the column and row references. Using the $ makes the reference an *absolute reference*, meaning that the cell reference does not change if the cells are moved around. $C$8 is another way of writing the cell reference C8. You can change any part of the string so that you have a different worksheet, a different upper-left corner, or a different bottom-right corner. For example, if you want the chart to use the data in Sheet1 in the range D8:E12, you would change the Data Range string to =Sheet1!$D$8:$E$12.

Step 3 of the Chart Wizard

When you have the chart's orientation the way you want and have selected the data you want to chart, click Next to display the next Chart Wizard dialog box (see Figure 9.7). You use the tabs in this dialog box to format the chart according to your preferences.

Figure 9.7.

Step 3 of 4 of the Chart Wizard dialog box.

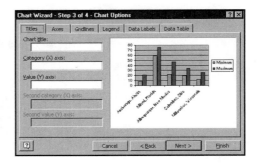

You use the Titles tab to label the chart and its axes. For this chart, a good title is Normal January Temperatures in 5 U.S. Cities. Type the title for the x axis in the Category (X) Axis text box; a good title for this example is Selected U.S. Cities. Type the title for the y axis in the Value (Y) Axis text box; because these values are the temperatures in degrees Fahrenheit, a good title for the y axis is Temperature (Degrees Fahrenheit).

You use each of the other tabs in this dialog box to control different aspects of the chart. On the Axes tab, you can control whether the labels for the values on the axes will show up—in addition to other features. On the Gridlines tab, you can get rid of gridlines entirely, make the grid finer, or display gridlines for only one direction. On the Legend tab, you can control whether or not the *legend box* (in this example, the box that describes which column shading shows the minimum values and which column shading shows the maximum values) is displayed and where it is placed. You can use the Data Labels tab to control whether the actual data numbers (in this case, the degrees Fahrenheit) are displayed within the chart and whether the corresponding data labels (in this case, the city names) are displayed. You can use the Data Table tab to specify whether or not a formatted table of the data is included along with the actual chart.

Step 4 of the Chart Wizard

When you have made all your choices, click Next to display the final wizard screen, shown in Figure 9.8.

On this, the last screen of the Chart Wizard, you can choose to embed the chart as an object in one of the worksheets or to place the chart in a separate worksheet.

9

Figure 9.8.

Step 4 of 4 of the Chart Wizard dialog box.

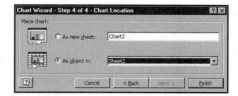

Here is the difference between these two types of charts:

☐ **Embedded charts** are linked to the data from which they are created, and they change if the data changes.

☐ **Chart sheets** are charts placed on separate worksheets. Like embedded charts, the data in the chart sheets is also linked to the underlying data. If you choose this option, the chart is centered in the middle of a new worksheet, but you cannot control its placement any more than that.

Click the Finish button when you are done.

TIME SAVER

> In any of the Chart Wizard dialog boxes, you can click the Finish button to end the wizard and create a chart that uses the default selections for any of the options you have not specified.

Creating Custom Charts

To create your own custom chart, first select the data in the worksheet that you want to chart. Start the Chart Wizard by clicking the Chart tool or choosing Insert | Chart from the main menu and then click the Custom Types tab.

From the Chart Type list, you can select different possibilities; a sample on the right side of the dialog box shows what your selected data will look like when presented in that kind of a chart. Again using the data in Figure 9.1 for this example, select the B&W Column option from the Chart Type list to see your data presented in a good-looking and meaningful way (see Figure 9.9).

Creating a User-Defined Custom Chart

You can add your own user-defined chart to the list of Custom Types. To do so, you first create the type of chart you want to reuse and then add it to the list, as described in these steps:

1. Create a chart of the type you want, using the Chart Wizard as described in the previous section. You can alter the axes, size, and any other features of the chart as you want.

Figure 9.9.

A B&W column chart shown in the Custom Types tab of the Chart Wizard dialog box.

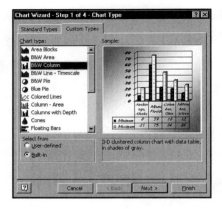

2. Select that chart and right-click it to display the Chart Type dialog box.
3. Click the Custom Types tab to display the dialog box shown in Figure 9.10.
4. Click the Add button; you are prompted for a title and description.
5. Click OK when finished.

Figure 9.10.

The Custom Types tab on the Chart Wizard dialog box.

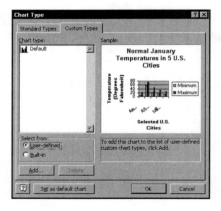

 When you want to use the chart type you just created, display the Chart Wizard by clicking the Chart tool or choosing Insert | Chart from the main menu. In the Step 1 dialog box, click the Custom Types tab. Select the User-Defined radio button to display the chart type you created. Select it and click Next to go to the Step 2 dialog box and continue as usual.

Changing the Default Chart Type

The *default chart type* is the type of chart you get if you accept the defaults when creating a chart with the Chart Wizard. The default chart type is Clustered Column—a good choice for a standard chart, but you may prefer another type of chart to be your default.

TIME SAVER

To create a chart on a separate chart sheet with the usual defaults, just select a cell of the data and press the F11 function key to make an instant chart.

Here's how to change the default chart type:

1. Create the chart you want to set as a default by using the Chart Wizard as usual and embedding the chart within a worksheet. Then select the chart by clicking its border.

2. Right-click the chart to display the popup menu; select Chart Type to display the Chart Type dialog box.

3. Click the Custom Types tab (refer back to Figure 9.10).

4. Click Set as Default Chart. You are asked whether you really want to set the new default. Click Yes if you do.

Creating Charts from Data in Noncontiguous Cells

You can create charts using data in cells that are not contiguous. Select the first group of cells you want to include in the chart; press and hold the Ctrl key while selecting the other groups of cells you want to include in the chart. If you wanted to include in your chart only the cities west of Chicago, you would select the cities and labels shown in Figure 9.11.

Figure 9.11.

Selecting noncontiguous cells to make a chart.

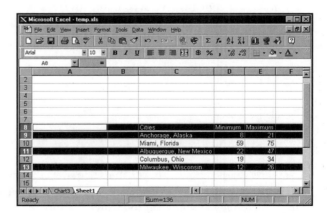

Choose Insert | Chart to start the Chart Wizard and continue as usual; alternatively, press the F11 key to make a default chart sheet.

Adding Data to a Chart

To add data to a chart, follow these steps:

1. Select the range of cells in the worksheet that represents the data you want to add. The data range you select does not have to be contiguous with the rest of the table that defines the chart.

2. Choose Edit | Copy from the main menu to copy the selected data to the Clipboard.

3. Click the chart's *plot area* (the area in which the graphic part of the chart appears).

4. Choose Edit | Paste from the main menu. The data you copied in step 2 is added to the chart in accordance with its position on the worksheet. Thus, if the new data is below the other data in the data table, it appears at the furthest right (if a column chart is used) or at the bottom (if a bar chart is used). If the new data is above the other data in the table, it appears at the furthest left or at the top of the chart.

Changing Data by Changing the Chart

You can also change data by changing the chart. Select a data point in the chart and then drag the handles to resize it. Resizing the data point—whether it is a column, a bar, a line, or other representation—increases or decreases the quantity in the worksheet. For example, if you select the column in the chart that plots Anchorage's maximum January temperature at 21 degrees Fahrenheit and drag it up to the 60-degree line, the data in cell E9 in the worksheet also changes to 60 so that the chart and the worksheet are always in accord.

Modifying Chart Components and Chart Types

A typical chart contains several components (see Figure 9.12):

- ☐ Chart title
- ☐ Chart area (this is the chart as a whole)
- ☐ Legend
- ☐ Value axis and value axis title
- ☐ Category axis and category axis title
- ☐ Plot area and plot area gridlines
- ☐ Data series and data points

To modify chart components, you must first select the chart. Then right-click the component you want to modify in the chart. A popup menu appears. Select Clear if you want to erase the selected item. If you want to change the formatting of the component, select Format

9

Chart Component to display the appropriate dialog box that allows you to change that component.

Figure 9.12.

The components of a chart.

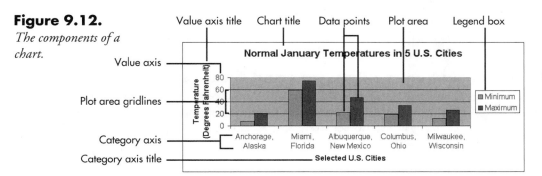

You can also select the component you want to modify in the chart and press Ctrl+1 to display the appropriate tab of the Chart Options dialog box.

TIME SAVER

You can also bring up the Chart Options dialog box to make modifications to the chart. Right-click anywhere on the chart area to display the popup menu and select Chart Options to display the Chart Options dialog box (see Figure 9.13). You can modify a number of features with this dialog box.

Figure 9.13.

The Chart Options dialog box.

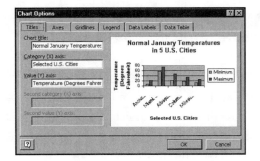

Formatting Titles

When you right-click one of the axis titles or the chart title and then select Format *Chart Component* from the popup menu, the dialog box that appears has three tabs: Patterns, Font, and Alignment. Click the tab that identifies the category of formatting changes you want to make to the selected title and make selections as appropriate. The dialog box is very similar to the one used for formatting cells.

Formatting Axes

When you right-click either the category axis or the value axis and then select Format *Chart Component* from the popup menu, the dialog box that appears has five tabs: Patterns, Scale, Font, Number, and Alignment. All of these formatting categories except for Scale will be familiar to you from working with cells. The Scale tab applies to axes that control numerical values. You can change the scale and other values as you see fit.

Formatting the Plot Area and Gridlines

You can format the plot area by choosing different colors and patterns. Right-click the plot area and select Format Plot Area from the popup menu to display the Format Plot Area dialog box. This dialog box allows you to choose the colors and patterns used in the plot area. Make your selections and click OK.

You can also change the gridlines used in your chart. Right-click one of the gridlines and choose Format Gridlines from the popup menu to display the Format Gridlines dialog box. The Patterns tab has features that allow you to change the look of the gridlines; the Scale tab allows you to change the scale of the gridlines.

Formatting the Chart Area

To change the fonts and patterns in a chart, select the chart and right-click it to display the popup menu. Select Format Chart Area to display a dialog box. Depending on what you want to change, click either the Patterns tab or the Fonts tab. Each tab offers a number of different choices, which are similar to those you see when you want to modify cells.

If you protect the workbook as a whole, the chart is also protected by default. Of course, you can unlock it. To unlock or protect a chart, first select the chart. Choose Format | Selected Chart Area from the main menu (or press Ctrl+1) to display a dialog box. Click the Properties tab and either check or uncheck the Locked checkbox.

Formatting Data Series

To format a data series in a chart, right-click one of the data points to display the popup menu. Select Format Data Series to display a dialog box with six tabs:

- [ ] Use the Patterns tab to manipulate the appearance and color of the data series.
- [ ] Use the Axis tab to include a secondary axis to plot data if you need one.
- [ ] Use the Y Error Bars tab for experimental data for which you want to display error ranges. This option puts error bars on your data points, with the error range that you specify.
- [ ] Use the Data Label tab to add more labels to the data.
- [ ] Use the Series Order tab to change the order in which the data series is displayed. For example, with the sample chart shown in Figure 9.12, you can reverse the order of the minimum and maximum bars.

9

☐ Use the Options tab to control whether data series will overlap and how much space there will be between them.

To format a single data point, select it with a single left click. After selecting it, right-click it to display the Format Data Point dialog box. This box has three tabs: Patterns, Data Label, and Options. Each of these tabs works in the same way its counterpart does in the Data Series dialog box, as just described.

Using the Chart Toolbar to Modify a Chart

You can use the Chart toolbar, shown in Figure 9.14, to alter any component of the chart or to make other modifications.

Figure 9.14.

The Chart toolbar.

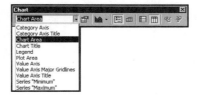

Use the Chart Objects drop-down menu to select which component of the chart you want to modify. The other tools on the toolbar are described in Table 9.1.

Table 9.1. The tools in the Chart toolbar.

Icon	Name	Description
	Chart Objects	Displays a drop-down menu that allows you to choose a particular chart component to modify.
	Format *Selected Object*	Displays the appropriate dialog box, depending on the chart object you selected from the Chart Objects drop-down menu.
	Chart Type	Displays a drop-down list of chart types from which you can select to change the type of chart you are using.

continues

Table 9.1. continued

Icon	Name	Description
	Legend	Hides or displays the legend.
	Data Table	Hides or displays the corresponding data table.
	By Rows	Changes the orientation of the data.
	By Column	Changes the orientation of the data.
	Angle Text Up	Alters the position of the text in the chart.
	Angle Text Down	Alters the position of the text in the chart.

Manipulating Chart Objects

You can manipulate charts in much the same way you can manipulate graphic objects, cells, and ranges. Follow these steps:

1. Select the chart object by clicking its border. Drag the chart to move it.

2. To see the manipulation options available to you, select the chart object and then right-click it to display the popup menu shown in Figure 9.15.

To resize a chart, select the chart and then drag one of the handles in the direction you want to stretch or contract the chart.

To delete a chart, select the chart and then press the Delete key.

To cut and paste a chart to a new location, follow these steps:

1. Select the chart.

2. Select Edit | Cut from the main menu (or press Ctrl+X). The chart is cut from its original location.

3. Move the cursor to the new location in which you want the upper-left corner of the chart. Select Edit | Paste from the main menu (or press Ctrl+V). The chart appears in its new location.

Figure 9.15.

The popup menu for manipulating chart objects.

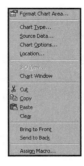

To copy and paste a chart to a new location, follow these steps:

1. Select the chart.

2. Select Edit | Copy from the main menu (or press Ctrl+C). A copy of the chart is made.

3. Move the cursor to the location in which you want the upper-left corner of the chart. Select Edit | Paste from the main menu (or press Ctrl+V). A copy of the original chart appears in its new location.

To change the chart type, follow these steps:

1. Select the chart.

2. Right-click the chart to display the popup menu and select Chart Type. Alternatively, choose Chart | Chart Type from the main menu. The Chart Type dialog box appears.

3. Change the chart and its data to any of the many formats offered on the Standard Types or Custom Types tab of the Chart Type dialog box.

You can control some aspects of the behavior of your chart objects by choosing Tools | Options from the main menu and clicking the Chart tab of the Options dialog box. You can decide whether empty cells in the chart's data range should be ignored or whether they should be plotted as zeros. You can also decide whether or not only visible cells in the data range should be plotted. You can decide whether or not the names and values should be displayed on the chart tips. If enabled, a *chart tip* appears when you move your mouse over a data point and displays the name and value of that data point. Check or uncheck the boxes as needed.

Looking at Other Chart Types

This hour has focused largely on simple charts created by the Chart Wizard. You have other options as well. Organizational charts are good for working out and representing flowcharts and hierarchical organization. Picture charts are yet another way to represent data in a way that makes sense to your intended audience.

Organizational Charts

To insert an organizational chart into your worksheet, choose Insert | Picture from the menu and select Organization Chart from the submenu.

A separate program opens within Excel (see Figure 9.16). Use this program to create and modify an organizational chart. Don't worry about altering the size of the chart itself—you can do that when you return to Excel. Use the buttons on the menu (underneath Excel's main menu) to change various features of how the chart looks. You can reorganize boxes, type names and information in the boxes, change the colors and line styles, and so forth. When you are finished creating your organizational chart, choose File | Close and Return to *filename.xls* from the main menu. Click Yes if you want the chart to be included in your Excel workbook file.

Figure 9.16.

Creating an organiza-tional chart in Excel.

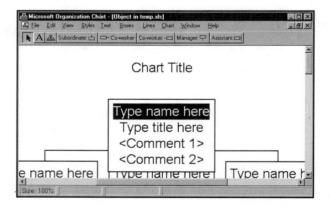

Once you return to your Excel worksheet, you can modify the chart by dragging its handles and cutting and pasting it to a new location. You can also change the appearance of a chart with the tools in the Picture toolbar. To display the Picture toolbar, choose View | Toolbars | Drawing from the main menu.

You can display the chart as an icon in the worksheet rather than at full size. To do this, right-click the organizational chart and choose MS Org Object | Convert from the popup menu; then select the Display As Icon checkbox. To view the chart again, double-click the icon.

9

TIME SAVER

You can place a comment box next to the icon to inform the user that he or she can view the chart by double-clicking the icon.

Creating a Picture Chart

Using picture charts is another way to add visual appeal to your worksheets. Suppose that you have a worksheet that shows the records of the Christmas tree sales for your company for the last five years. This data looks rather plain as an ordinary chart. You can replace the bars with something that makes pictorial sense—such as a Christmas tree—as shown in Figure 9.17.

Figure 9.17.

Creating a picture chart.

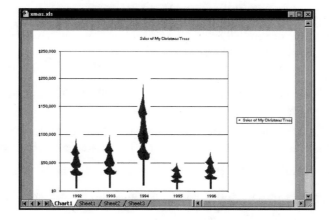

To make a pictorial chart from a chart that already exists, follow these steps:

1. Create a standard Excel chart for the data you want to display pictorially. Column or bar charts work the best.

2. Find or create the graphic you want to use to replace the data series bars in the chart. You can create or insert this graphic object within Excel, or you can open another application that contains the object.

3. In the other application (or within Excel, if that's where you created the object), select the graphic object by clicking its border. Choose Edit | Copy from the main menu of the application to copy the object to the Clipboard.

4. Select the data series or data point in the chart that you want to replace with the graphic picture.

5. Choose Edit | Paste from the main menu. The graphic replaces the standard bar in the Excel chart.

Summary

Charts are an effective way to add visual "oomph" to your data and to translate dull-looking columns and rows into a meaningful and immediately understandable representation. Excel offers a number of different chart varieties and almost completely automates the process of creating charts. You can customize charts and chart components to fit your specific requirements, and you can easily update charts with new information. Maps, discussed in the following hour, are another way to represent data in a visual way.

Workshop

Term Review

chart component   One of the following parts of a chart: chart title, chart area (the chart as a whole), legend, value axis, value axis title, category axis, category axis title, plot area, plot area gridlines, data series, and data points.

chart object   A term that refers to an entire chart as a graphic object that you can manipulate as you can any other graphic object.

chart   A graphical representation of data values stored in a table. A chart can take the form of a bar chart, a column chart, a line chart, or one of many other forms.

data point   A single unit of data—the data in a single cell.

data series   A group of data points corresponding to a single label.

gridlines   Vertical and horizontal lines that extend through the plot area of a chart.

legend box   An accompanying box in a chart that indicates what various graphical symbols represent.

plot area   The area of a chart that displays the actual data points.

Q&A

Q What are charts good for?

A Charts present data so that you can interpret what it means at a single glance.

Q What kinds of charts can you make?

A The most common kinds of charts are column, bar, and pie charts. You can make a number of other types of charts, however, such as line, scatter, bubble, and many others. Your charts can also be three dimensional.

Q Can you convert charts from one type to another?

A Yes. However, the chart type you choose should make sense in relation to the data it is presenting.

9

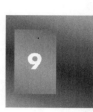

Exercise

Make a pie chart with the information shown in Figure 9.18.

1. Create the tabular data.

2. Select any data cell in the chart.

3. Choose Insert | Chart from the main menu.

4. Choose Pie as the chart type and choose your preferred chart subtype from the menu from the first dialog box in the Chart Wizard. Click Next.

5. Continue through the remaining dialog boxes in the Chart Wizard. Although you can accept the defaults for the other dialog boxes, in the third dialog box, type the title of the chart. Click Finish when you are done.

6. If you don't like where the chart is situated, move it in the same way as you do any other graphic object.

Figure 9.18.

Some data and its accompanying pie chart.

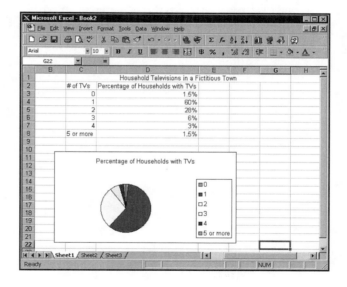

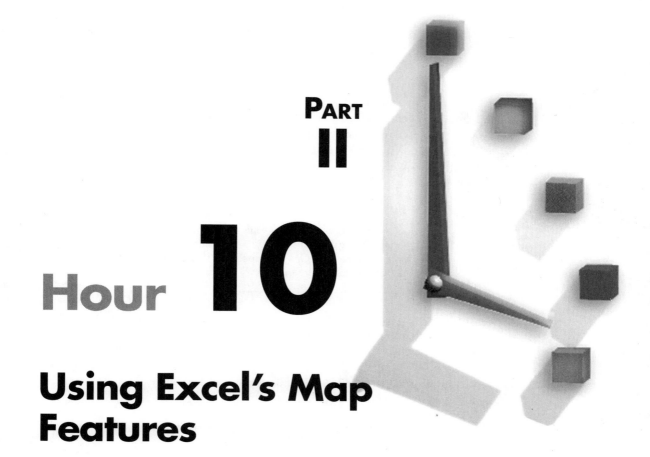

Hour 10

Using Excel's Map Features

Maps are a good way to represent data that has a geographical basis. A Microsoft map is a special kind of chart. The Microsoft Map module is included in Excel 97 and includes maps for the following regions:

- [ ] Australia
- [ ] Canada
- [ ] Europe
- [ ] Mexico
- [ ] North America
- [ ] Southern Africa
- [ ] UK and ROI (Republic of Ireland) countries
- [ ] United States (Alaska and Hawaii inserts)
- [ ] World Countries

As you can see, many countries and some continents have been left out of the basic Map module. You can purchase more maps, however, and install them as part of the Microsoft Map module. For more information, check the MapInfo Corporation Web site at http://www.mapinfo.com. You can even buy a product from MapInfo so that you can make your own map. The MapInfo Web site also has information about how to do demographic data analysis.

JUST A MINUTE

> A typical installation of Microsoft Office does not include the Microsoft Map module. To add this module, you must add this component by custom installing it from the CD-ROM (or floppy disks). To find how to install an individual component, refer to Hour 2, "Installing Excel 97."

In addition to using Microsoft Map to represent data, you can also add a map to your worksheet without linking the map to any data. Figure 10.1 is a map that shows where all the Canadian airports are located. You can then use the Map Label button, described later in this hour, to tell you the names of all the airports. The Map module also has maps showing highways in North America, the UK, and Europe, as well as other features. The maps are worth a look just for general interest and information.

Figure 10.1.

A map of Canadian airports.

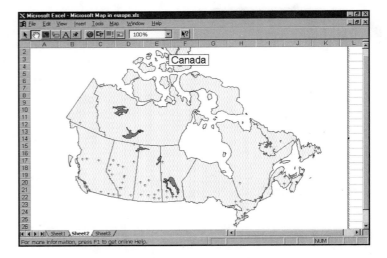

10

How to Create a Map

To create a map, you first need a tabular set of data with a geographical basis. A typical example is product sales broken down by country or state, or a list of your organization's membership in various states or countries.

One column in this tabular set of data must contain geographical information. Use standard names for the countries, states, provinces (for Canada), or counties (for the UK and ROI). The Microsoft Map module does not recognize cities (or most other geographical units) for the entries in this column. The "standard names" are listed in the `mapstats.xls` file, which is installed with your Microsoft Map module. Here is its default location:

```
C:\Program Files\Common Files\ Microsoft Shared\Datamap\Data\mapstats.xls
```

Set up your data as you would for any other table. Typically, you have data such as sales figures, population, precipitation, or other quantities that correspond to a geographical region.

Once the table is set up, select a cell in the table. Next, choose Insert | Map from the main menu or click the Map tool in the Standard toolbar. Excel should recognize your data and either choose or give you an option of the appropriate maps. If you have misspelled a geographical name or used a nonstandard spelling, Excel cannot recognize it and presents you with a list of options for various maps.

Drag the mouse cursor across the worksheet to create a box the size you want the map to be, or double-click the worksheet to get the default size. A map that looks something like the one in Figure 10.2 appears (in this figure, you can see the tabular data as well).

Figure 10.2.

A typical map and associated tabular data.

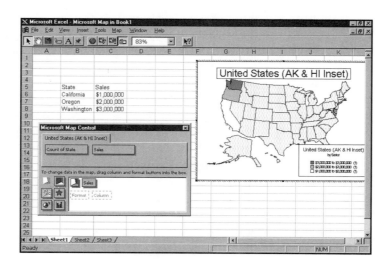

JUST A MINUTE

When you are working with Microsoft Map, you see a different set of toolbars than when you are working with Microsoft Excel, as you can see from Figure 10.2. To get back to the Excel toolbars, just click the worksheet outside the map.

COFFEE BREAK

Microsoft Map Tips

For more information about using Microsoft Map, select Help from the main menu and choose Microsoft Map Help Topics.

It's often a good idea to place your maps in a separate worksheet than the one that contains the actual tabular data. Because the map generally has to be fairly large for the user to make out any details on it, it can often obscure the tabular data. It's easier to work with maps if they are located in a location separate from the data.

Microsoft Map does not have an Undo feature like the Excel program itself does. However, to cancel the last change you have made, select View | Previous from the Map module's main menu (or press Ctrl+Y).

The Microsoft Map Toolbar

The Microsoft Map toolbar, shown in Figure 10.3, allows you to manipulate the map object in various ways. The following sections describe the tools in the Map toolbar.

Figure 10.3.

The Microsoft Map toolbar.

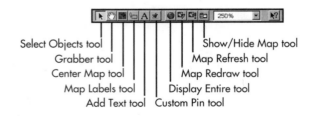

The Select Objects Tool

The Select Objects button is used to select a map object for further manipulation. You can achieve the same effect by clicking the border of the map object.

The Grabber Tool

When you create a map, you draw a rectangular box in which the map is placed. With a name like a character in a bad horror movie, the Grabber tool is used for picking up the map and moving it within this rectangular box.

Note that you can use the Grabber to hide certain parts of a map. Suppose that you want to show only the Western United States in the map boundary. Simply use the Grabber tool to push the Eastern states out of the map boundary, as shown in Figure 10.4.

Figure 10.4.

Using the Grabber tool to "crop" a map within the map border.

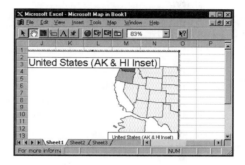

The Center Map Tool

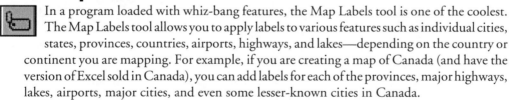

Click the Center Map tool to fix the center of the map. The mouse pointer changes to a special cursor. Use this cursor to click the map where you want the center of the map to be. Suppose that you want a map of the United States to be centered around Wyoming rather than Nebraska or Kansas (the default center). To do so, click the Center Map tool and then click the state of Wyoming in the map. The map moves within the boundary box so that Wyoming is in the center of the box.

The Map Labels Tool

In a program loaded with whiz-bang features, the Map Labels tool is one of the coolest. The Map Labels tool allows you to apply labels to various features such as individual cities, states, provinces, countries, airports, highways, and lakes—depending on the country or continent you are mapping. For example, if you are creating a map of Canada (and have the version of Excel sold in Canada), you can add labels for each of the provinces, major highways, lakes, airports, major cities, and even some lesser-known cities in Canada.

First, create the map of the area. To add labels to the map, click the Map Labels tool or choose Tools | Labeler from the main menu to display the Map Labels dialog box. From the drop-down menu in this dialog box, choose the features you want to label and click OK.

The mouse pointer changes to a cross hair. Run the cross-hair pointer over the map to see the corresponding labels. Click the map when you see a label you want to include. If you have a map of Europe, for example, you have the option of labeling European countries from the Map Labels dialog box. If you run the special cursor over each country, the name of the country appears.

The Add Text Tool

To add text to a map, click the Add Text tool. Move the cursor to the spot in the map where you want to add text, click, and start typing. If you want to change the font of the text you are adding, right-click the text to display the Format Font dialog box; make your selections and click OK.

The Custom Pin Tool

The Custom Pin tool lets you customize your maps to a greater degree than the Add Text and Map Labels tool. Suppose that you have a map of the United States on the wall in your office and wanted to mark each of the states in which you managed to sell one million dollars' worth of product last year. You could stick straight pins in the relevant states to accomplish your goal.

Similarly, you can place a pin-like marker in any geographical location on one of your maps. If you have a good eye for detail, you can place these pins in the vicinities of certain cities.

Here's how to add custom pins to an existing map:

1. Make sure that you can see the Excel toolbars and not the Map program toolbars. Select the map and right-click to display the popup menu. Choose Microsoft Map Object and then choose Edit from the popup menu to change to the Map program and see the Microsoft Map toolbars. Once you have the Map toolbars, click the Custom Pin tool.

2. Excel prompts you for a name for your custom pin map. Type the name you want and click OK. Obviously, it makes sense to choose a name that reflects what the map is about, such as EuropeSales.

3. Use the stick-pin cursor and click wherever you want to stick a pin on the map. Stick pins wherever you see fit on your map.

4. If you want to either clear or format a stick-pin, right-click the stick-pin to display the popup menu. Choose Clear to erase the pin; click Format to display the Symbol dialog box. You do not have to use pin-shaped graphics; you can choose one of a variety of different symbols from the Symbol dialog box and then click OK.

To remove a Custom Pin map you have created, choose Map | Delete Custom Pin Map from the main menu to display the Delete Custom Pin dialog box. You can then choose the Custom Pin map you want to delete from the pull-down menu on this dialog box. The map returns to its original state (the state it was in before you put the pins in it).

You can choose to close a Custom Pin map by choosing Map | Close Custom Pin Map. Closing the Custom Pin map returns you to the same map, but without the pins in place. After closing a Custom Pin map, you can elect to see it again by choosing Map | Open Custom Pin Map from the main menu; the Custom Pin Map dialog box appears. Select the Custom Pin map you want to reopen by selecting the name of the Custom Pin map from the drop-down menu.

The Display Entire Tool

You can click the Display Entire tool or press Ctrl+Spacebar to display the entire map within one screen. If the map covers more than one screen, the scale of the map is reduced. If you have moved part of the map out of view with the Grabber tool, clicking the Display Entire tool brings the entire map back in the boundary box.

The Map Redraw Tool

The Map Redraw tool is useful when you have changed the position of a map by using the Grabber tool. When you have a map on a flat surface, certain areas are "stretched." If you use the Map Redraw tool after using the Grabber tool, you can minimize the stretching.

The Map Refresh Tool

Use the Map Refresh tool when you change the tabular data represented in the map. Unlike the Chart tool (which updates a chart automatically if you change the tabular data used to create the chart), the Map feature does not automatically update the map image when you change data in the table. To update the map image after you make changes to the map's tabular data, click the Map Refresh tool or choose Map | Refresh from the main menu.

The Zoom Box

You can increase or decrease the magnification of your map by clicking the drop-down Zoom menu at the right end of the Map toolbar. Select the percentage you want or type a custom percentage and press Enter.

JUST A MINUTE

The size of the rectangular box remains the same when you change the Zoom factor. What the Zoom factor essentially allows you to do is to display one part of the map at a larger or smaller scale. The rest of the worksheet is unaffected by the scale you choose for the map.

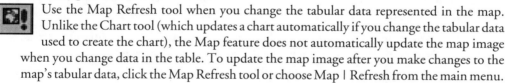

You should decide on the zoom factor you want your map to have *before* applying any labels. If you add labels to the map, change the zoom factor, and then add more labels, the last labels you added will not match the earlier labels.

More Map Manipulation

You can manipulate maps just as you can any other graphic object. You can cut, copy, and paste maps in the same way you do for clipart or drawing objects. First select the map object by clicking the border of the map or by clicking the Select Objects tool.

If you want to move the object, simply drag it to its new location by holding the cursor at the serrated edge of the rectangular box that contains the map.

If you want to copy and paste the object, select the map and choose Edit | Copy from the main menu (or press Ctrl+C). Move the cursor to the new location and choose Edit | Paste from the main menu (or press Ctrl+V). A second copy of the map appears at the new location.

To return to the Excel worksheet menu from the Microsoft Map menu, simply click outside the map object, anywhere in the worksheet. Once you are back within Excel, you can click the map once to display the graphics handles (just as you can for any graphic object). You can drag these handles to increase or decrease the size of the map object.

To return to Microsoft Map from the Excel worksheet, right-click the map to display the popup menu. Select Microsoft Map Object and then select Edit to open up the Map program within Excel and have the Map program take over the toolbars.

You can also open up the Microsoft Map program separately, in addition to Excel, so that each program has its own window. To do this, follow these steps:

1. Right-click the map to display a popup menu.
2. Select Microsoft Map Object from the popup menu and then select Open. The Map program opens in a window separate from Excel. Each program has its buttons on the Windows 95 toolbar, and you can move back and forth between the windows with ease.

Modifying Legends

If your map represents data from a table, a *legend box*, which explains the data representation, is included with your map. In Figure 10.2, earlier in this chapter, the legend box is on the bottom right of the map; it explains the various shadings based on product sales.

10

To change how a legend is displayed, right-click the legend box to display a popup menu of options. You can choose Hide, Edit, or Compact. The Hide option, as you might expect, hides the legend box. The Compact option changes the legend box so that it displays only a single brief title. If you select Edit, the Format Properties dialog box appears, and you can change the contents and appearance of the legend box.

Here are some other ways you can modify the legend box:

☐ To resize the legend box, move the mouse pointer to the corner of the legend box until the pointer becomes a double-headed arrow. Click and drag the box to the size you want.

☐ To show the legend after hiding it, choose View | All Legends from the main menu.

☐ To make compact legends the default, choose Tools | Options from the main menu and select the Compact Legends by Default checkbox.

☐ To format the legend, choose Edit to display the Format Properties dialog box shown in Figure 10.5. Use this dialog box to change the font as well as other features of the legend box. If you click the Value Shading Options tab, you can control the value ranges for which different shading options apply. The Map program chooses reasonable ranges for the different shading options, but you can tweak these ranges as you see fit. You can also control the colors used to shade various parts of the map. If you click the Legend Options tab, you can change the title, subtitle, fonts, format, and legend entries.

Figure 10.5.

The Format Properties dialog box for a map legend.

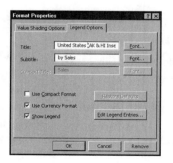

Modifying the Map Object as a Whole

You can change the colors, size, protection, and properties of the map object as a whole with the Format Object dialog box, just as you can change these properties for any graphic object.

To display the Format Object dialog box, you must be within the Excel worksheet. Right-click the map to display the popup menu. Choose Format Object from the popup menu, and the Format Object dialog box appears. You can use the Size tab of the dialog box to change the size of the map. You can use the Picture tab to crop the picture and change other properties. You can use the Protection tab to lock or unlock the map object to protect it from inadvertent modification. You can use the Properties tab to control how the map object is positioned in relation to the cells.

Changing Map Options

You can change various options for your map by choosing Tools | Options from the Microsoft Map main menu. The Microsoft Map Options dialog box appears (see Figure 10.6). You can make the map change automatically when new data is added by selecting Automatic from the Data Refresh area and clicking OK. The Map Matching choices let you control how much time Excel should take to match the data to a map. Most of the time, this choice is not significant—unless you have an enormous data table. You can determine the sizing units used, which may be significant if you are preparing figures to a precise standard. You can also compact the legends if necessary.

Figure 10.6.

The Microsoft Map Options dialog box.

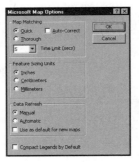

Adding, Changing, and Deleting Map Data

To add data to your map, add another entry to your worksheet as usual. Make sure that the data you enter has both the geographic value and the numeric value. Right-click the map to display the popup menu, select Microsoft Map and then select Refresh Data. Similarly, if you change or delete data from the worksheet table that will affect the map, bring up the popup menu, select Microsoft Map, and then select Refresh Data.

Adding and Removing Features

To add or remove features from your map, right-click within the map object to display the popup menu and then select Features or Add Features. Alternatively, you can choose Map | Features or Map | Add Features from the main menu. If you are using the United States (with AK and HI Inset) map, you will see the dialog box shown in Figure 10.7.

10

Figure 10.7.

Adding or removing map features.

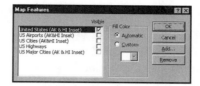

Each geographical map has a number of features you can add or remove from the map. Select the boxes for the features you want visible and click OK. Not all the maps have all the features, but you can pick and choose from what is available for each individual map.

The Show/Hide Microsoft Map Control Dialog Box

If you generated a map from data in a table, the Microsoft Map Control dialog box appears (see Figure 10.8). If you insert a map with no relationship to any data, the Microsoft Map Control dialog box does not appear. You can hide or display the Microsoft Map Control dialog box by choosing View | Microsoft Map Control from the main menu or clicking the Show/Hide Microsoft Map tool. The Microsoft Map Control lets you control the shading of the regions in the map. In a map that represents data, geographical regions are shaded in different ways corresponding to the numerical value of the data. You can shade the map by assigning different colors to the regions based on the corresponding value of the region, by filling in the regions with different dot densities depending on the value of the region, or in some other way.

Figure 10.8.

The Microsoft Map Control dialog box.

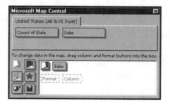

Changing the Shading of Different Regions

You can change the way different regions representing different data values are shaded for your map using the buttons in the Microsoft Map Control dialog box. These buttons are located on the left side of the dialog box. With each of these options, a legend box appears alongside the map, explaining which color or shade belongs to which data value. In addition to the Pie and Column Chart buttons described in the next section, you have four options:

- [ ] **Value Shading (the default).** This button displays the various regions of the map that have corresponding data values in various shades of black, gray, and white. The largest values have the darkest shades; the smallest values have the lightest shades.

- [ ] **Category Shading.** This button produces a more colorful map. The areas of the map are displayed with different colors. You have to look at the legend to determine what each color means.

- [ ] **Dot Density.** This button displays the areas of the map by shading them with dots; the density of the dots in the area is in proportion to the quantity measured for that area. The legend explains the number each dot stands for (for example, 1 dot = 40 units).

- [ ] **Graduated Symbol.** This button places symbols on the map in the locations specified by the tabular data. The size of the symbols is in proportion to the quantity measured for that area. For example, if you have several states with sales data on your map, and Nevada has the most sales, the graduated symbol for Nevada is the largest of all the symbols on the map. To change the graduated symbol used, right-click in the legend box and choose Edit from the popup menu. A Format Properties dialog box appears; click the Graduated Symbol Options tab and make your choice.

If you want to change the default style of your map, click the button you want (for example, click the Graduated Symbol button—the star button) and drag it to the white work area, on top of the dashed Format button, as shown in Figure 10.9. From the top of the dialog box, drag the button that represents the category values you want to format (in this case, the Sales button) into the white work area on top of the dashed Column button.

To remove this formatting, drag the Graduated Symbol button from the white area on the Microsoft Map Control dialog box back to its original position. Your map will once again use the default Value Shading option.

Adding a Column or Pie Chart to a Map

You can add a column or pie chart to a map for extra emphasis on what the data means. Suppose that you have tabular data that represents the sales of a hypothetical product in California, Oregon, and Washington. To add a column chart to the map, drag the Column Chart icon from the left side of the Microsoft Map Control dialog box to the white area on the right side of the dialog box. Drag one of the buttons from the top of the dialog box—in this case, the Sales button—to the Column Chart icon. These actions produce the column chart shown in Figure 10.10. To add a pie chart to the map, drag the Pie Chart icon instead of the Column Chart icon and continue as outlined here.

10

Figure 10.9.

Using the Graduated Symbol button to format the map data.

Graduated symbols

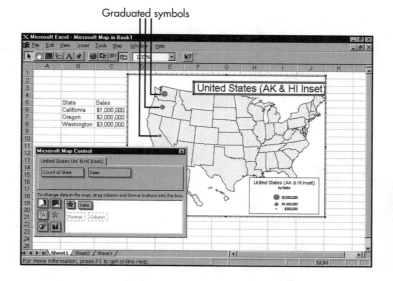

Figure 10.10.

Adding a column chart to a map.

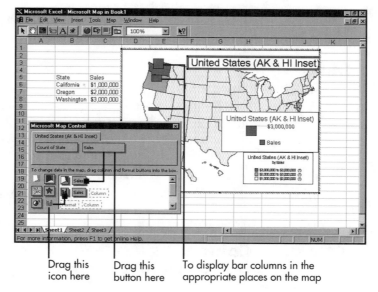

Drag this icon here   Drag this button here   To display bar columns in the appropriate places on the map

10

Summary

Maps are another useful way to add interest, pizzazz, and meaning to your Excel worksheets. Use graphics, charts, and maps to make your data come alive. If your data has a geographical basis, and you have a corresponding map for the regions, you can create a map that displays your data in a meaningful way. You can link maps to your data and change the map with each new addition to your worksheet. Maps, however, take up a lot of disk space and can slow down your work considerably—particularly if you are short on memory or processing power.

Workshop

Term Review

legend   A box, automatically generated when you create a map from data, that explains the shading of different regions in relation to the corresponding numerical values.

map   In Excel, a graphical representation of a geographical region that can be linked to data in a worksheet.

stick-pin   If you want to highlight a particular region of a map, Excel lets you place a graphic that resembles a stick-pin on that location.

Q&A

Q Why are maps useful?

A You can represent data that has a geographical basis in a graphical format. Maps can be shaded to represent different data values for different regions. You can also create maps that serve solely as visual aids, rather than as graphical representations of data.

Q What types of maps can you create?

A Excel includes maps for every continent, as well as maps that display the entire world.

Q Can you label parts of a map?

A Yes. Excel allows you to add labels for some or all of the following features: countries, states, provinces, airports, highways, cities, and lakes.

10

Exercise

Create a map showing all the major highways of Australia. For this exercise, you don't need any data.

1. Select Insert | Map from the main menu.

2. Click anywhere in a blank worksheet. The toolbars switch to indicate that you are now in the Microsoft Map module.

3. Select Australia from the dialog box that comes up and click OK. A map of Australia appears in a window.

4. Right-click the map and choose Features from the popup menu.

5. Select the Australia Highways checkbox and click OK.

6. Resize the map as desired. When finished, click outside the map box to return to your Excel worksheet. You can move and manipulate the map as you can any other object.

10

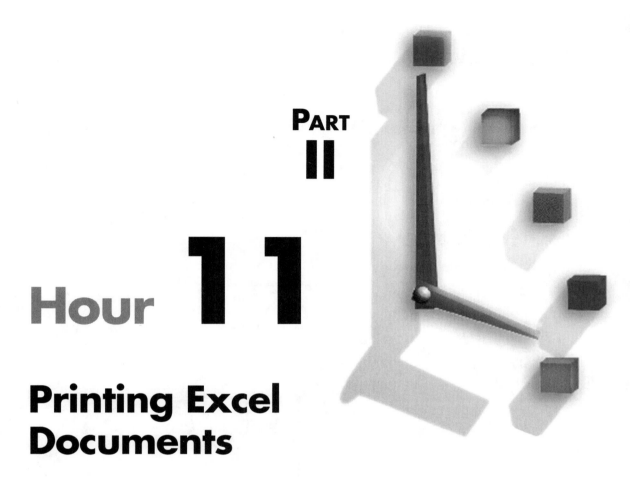

Hour 11

Printing Excel Documents

Your Excel spreadsheets likely seem at their best and most interactive when you work with them on-screen. However, there are plenty of reasons why you might have to print them.

For many documents, of course, you do not print the worksheets directly; you print them as part of a larger document, such as one created in Microsoft Word. Using Excel with other applications is discussed in Hour 18, "Using Excel Data in Other Office 97 Applications."

JUST A MINUTE

> The discussions in this hour assume that you have set up your printer so that it works with your operating system; this chapter does not discuss the use of specific printers.

The quick-and-easy way to print your Excel worksheet is simply to click the Print tool in the Standard toolbar. However, this approach to printing may result in extra blank pages being printed; you also lack control over the output—*everything* is printed!

There are several ways to control your printed output and a number of related dialog boxes. Selecting File | Page Setup, File | Print Preview, and File | Print from the main menu gives you access to most of the printing options, as discussed throughout this hour.

Print Preview

 Click the Print Preview tool, located in the Standard toolbar, or choose File | Print Preview from the main menu to see how your document will look when printed. Your worksheet will look something like the one shown in Figure 11.1.

Figure 11.1.

Viewing a document in the Print Preview window.

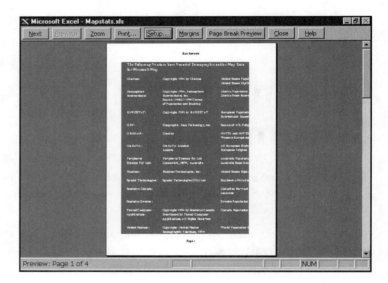

The buttons across the top of the Print Preview window allow you to navigate your worksheet, make changes to it, or print it.

Excel worksheets can have both horizontal and vertical page breaks. Excel numbers the pages from top to bottom first and then goes from left to right. Here is how a typical document is numbered, if the document has one vertical page break and two horizontal page breaks:

```
1        4
2        5
3        6
```

11

In the Print Preview window shown in Figure 11.1, only one page appears at a time. You can see other pages of your worksheet by using the Next and Previous buttons, located across the top of the window; the other buttons also provide helpful features:

- [ ] Click the Next button to go to the next page in your document; click the Previous button to go back one page.

- [ ] Click the Zoom button to increase or decrease the portion of the worksheet you can see at one time.

- [ ] Click the Print button to display the Print dialog box, discussed later in this hour.

- [ ] Click the Setup button to display the Page Setup dialog box, discussed later in this hour.

- [ ] Click the Margins button to display a screen similar to the one in Figure 11.2. You can move the margins in and out, and make more or less space available for the worksheet data on the page. To move the margins, click the dashed bars and drag them in the direction you want to move the margins.

Figure 11.2.

Changing the margins in Print Preview.

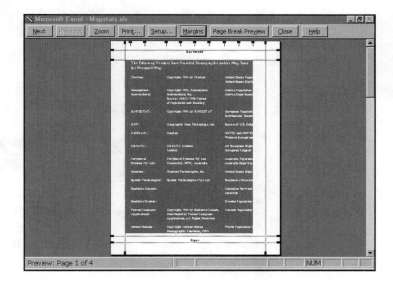

- [ ] Click the Page Break Preview button to see where the page breaks are located. You learn how to change the page breaks in the following section.

- [ ] Click the Close button to return to the standard worksheet view.

- [ ] Click the Help button to display the Microsoft Excel Help Topics screen.

Changing Page Breaks

Excel automatically breaks pages as needed. You may prefer to manually specify where you want the pages to break, however, so that certain portions of data are kept together.

To see where your pages are going to break, use the Page Break Preview feature of Excel: Select File | Print Preview from the main menu (or click the Print Preview tool) to display the Page Preview view of the worksheet. Then click the Page Break Preview button at the top of the screen. You see a preview screen like the one in Figure 11.3. Just as the dialog box instructs you to do, click and drag the dashed lines to change the location at which the page is broken.

Figure 11.3.

Changing page breaks.

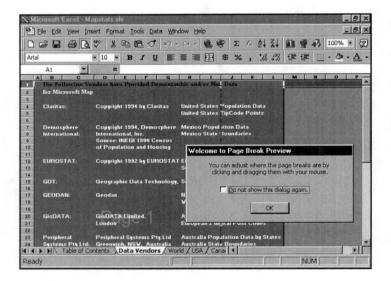

In Figure 11.3, the worksheet is broken into pages both horizontally and vertically. The vertical blue dashed line at the start of column J near the right edge represents the vertical page break. The horizontal page break is not visible in Figure 11.3, but it is represented by a horizontal blue dashed line. Excel cannot print the entire width of the worksheet without reducing the size of the text. If you move the vertical dashed line all the way to the right, in the example in Figure 11.3, past column L, to force the entire width of the worksheet on one page, the text must be printed smaller than it otherwise would. Excel adapts the scale of the page so that all the information fits as you require. Of course, you may find the print too small if you try to fit too much on a page.

You can also display the page breaks on the worksheet itself. Select Tools | Options from the main menu, click the View tab in the Options dialog box, select the Page Breaks option (deselect it if you want to remove the page breaks from the worksheet), and click OK.

11

To adjust page breaks, click the Page Break Preview button. Then right-click a cell to display a popup menu that allows you to Insert Page Breaks or Reset All Page Breaks. You can do either one. To remove a specific page break, right-click the break itself to display a popup menu from which you can select the Remove Page Break option.

Using the Page Setup Dialog Box

When you want to print your workbook, you may want to make specific changes or additions to improve the clarity of the final printed product. Set up your workbook for printing by choosing File | Page Setup. The Page Setup dialog box appears. There are four tabs on the Page Setup dialog box: Page, Margins, Header/Footer, and Sheet.

Each of these tabs has a Print, a Print Preview, and an Options button. The Print button displays the Print dialog box (described later in this hour in the section "Using the Print Dialog Box"). The Print Preview button changes your view of the worksheet to the Print Preview screen, described earlier in this hour. The Options button displays a dialog box you can use to alter the settings of your particular printer. Make changes to the various tabs in the Page Setup dialog box, as described in the following sections, and click OK when you have made your changes.

The Page Tab

The Page tab of the Page Setup dialog box is shown in Figure 11.4. You can use this tab to change a number of characteristics controlling how your page prints:

☐ **Orientation.** By default, a page prints in Portrait mode. You can change the orientation to Landscape so that a worksheet prints "sideways."

☐ **Scaling.** You can scale the worksheet so that it prints at some fraction of its actual size. You can also scale the worksheet so that it prints on a specific number of pages in both width and height.

☐ **Paper Size.** Most worksheets are printed on letter-size paper. However, you can change the paper size to whatever suits your current purposes.

☐ **Print Quality.** You can control the quality of print with this option's drop-down list. For my printer, I have the option of choosing between 360 dpi and 180 dpi. Depending on your printer, you may have several print-quality options from which you can choose. The higher the number of dots per inch, the greater the print resolution, and the better your final product appears. Of course, printing with more dots per inch is more expensive and may take somewhat longer, depending on your printer.

11

☐ **First Page Number.** You can specify the first printed page number if you do not want the default choice of page number 1. When you specify a new first page number, you must use either an integer or a decimal value, such as 2 or 3.4. You may want to change the default page number for a number of reasons. Suppose that your document is going to be pages 8 and 9 of another, larger, document. In that case, enter **8** in the First Page Number field.

Figure 11.4.

The Page tab of the Page Setup dialog box.

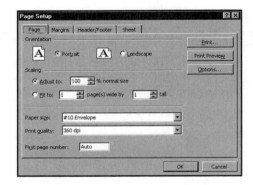

The Margins Tab

The Margins tab of the Page Setup dialog box is shown in Figure 11.5. Use this tab to change the various margins for the page: top, bottom, left, right, header, and footer. The header margin specifies how far down the page the header begins; the footer margin specifies how far up from the bottom of the page the footer begins. The top margin specifies how far down from the top of the page the actual content of the worksheet begins; the bottom margin specifies how far up from the bottom of the page the content ends. The left and right margins determine the placement of the content within those parameters.

Figure 11.5.

The Margins tab of the Page Setup dialog box.

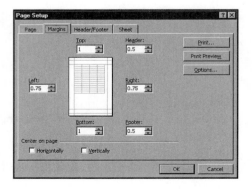

11

It's often easier to change the margins from the Print Preview screen because you can see the effects of the changes you are making. Changing margins in the Print Preview screen is described earlier in this hour, in the "Print Preview" section.

The Header/Footer Tab

The Header/Footer tab of the Page Setup dialog box is shown in Figure 11.6. Use this tab to create a header or footer as described in Hour 5, "Navigating and Manipulating Excel Documents."

Figure 11.6.

The Header/Footer tab of the Page Setup dialog box.

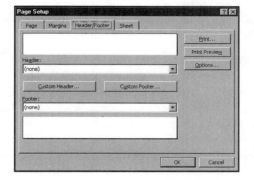

The Sheet Tab

The Sheet tab of the Page Setup dialog box is shown in Figure 11.7. Use this tab to control various options affecting the look and layout of your documents.

Figure 11.7.

The Sheet tab of the Page Setup dialog box.

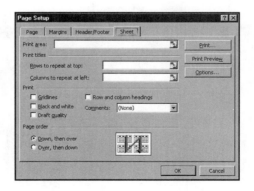

Change or input a range in the Print Area box if you want to print a smaller or larger default area of the worksheet. For example, if you want to print the range with the upper-left corner of A3 and the bottom-right corner of D11, enter **A3:D11**. (Another way of setting the print area is discussed in the section "Selecting a Print Area," later in this hour.)

You can have titles for the text labels of your data in your worksheet appear on every printed page. Suppose that you have sales figures for Product A, Product B, and so forth, and that these text labels appear at the top of your worksheet. When the worksheet is printed, it would be very helpful if these text labels were in place at the top of every worksheet. To do this, click one of the Collapse Dialog icons in the Page Setup dialog box so that the dialog box moves out of the way. Select the row or column in the worksheet that you want to use as the titles on the printed page (usually, the titles are the labels in the topmost row or leftmost column). Click the Expand Dialog icon to display the dialog box again and click OK when finished.

Look through the remaining options to decide whether you want gridlines, comments, and so forth.

Note that dark backgrounds and color graphics generally do not print attractively (unless you have a high-resolution laser printer or other high-end printer product). If your worksheets use dark backgrounds or color graphics, you can adjust your worksheets for black-and-white printing by selecting the Black and White checkbox. This option prints the worksheets with a white background and black text. You also save ink or toner with this option because you do not have to print the colored background as a continuous shade of gray. However, the graphics themselves are shaded gray/black/white when printed with this option.

Using the Print Dialog Box

Once you have set up your pages the way you want and put the page breaks in the right places, you are ready to print. Select File | Print from the main menu to display the Print dialog box (see Figure 11.8).

Figure 11.8.
The Print dialog box.

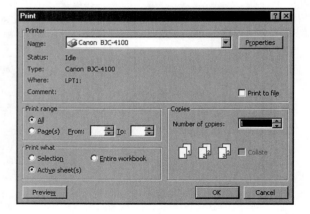

11

The Name drop-down list allows you to choose which of the printers installed on your system you want to use (in most cases, you will have only one).

Click the Properties button to display a dialog box similar to the one in Figure 11.9. The dialog box you see depends on the type of printer you have. Changing the printer properties in this dialog box changes them for other applications as well, so be aware that you may have to make changes again later.

Figure 11.9.

A typical Printer Properties dialog box.

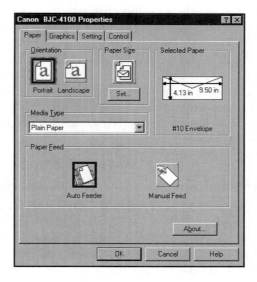

Here are some of the options in the Print dialog box you should consider:

- [ ] The Status line tells you whether or not the specified printer is currently printing.
- [ ] The Type line specifies the type of printer that is selected.
- [ ] The Where line identifies the port to which the printer is connected.
- [ ] The Comment line identifies the selected printer (if your computer is hooked up to more than one).
- [ ] If you select the Print to File checkbox, the document does not print to the printer, but to another file (you can specify the filename you want to use).
- [ ] Use the Print Range options to set the pages of the worksheet you want to print. For example, if you want to print only pages 3 through 5 of your workbook, type **3** in the From box and **5** in the To box.
- [ ] Use the spin buttons to change the number of copies you want to print.
- [ ] The Print What options let you choose to print a selected area, the entire workbook, or just the active worksheet.

☐ Click the Preview button to display the Print Preview window, described earlier in this hour.

Selecting a Print Area

Here's how to print a particular area of your worksheet:

1. Select the area of the worksheet you want to print.
2. Choose File|Print Area from the main menu, and choose Set Print Area.

Printing Objects

If you are printing a worksheet, you may or may not want to print the accompanying graphics, maps, and charts. To make an object (such as a map, some clipart, or a drawing object) printable or not, right-click the object and select Format Object from the popup menu to display the Format Object dialog box. Select the Properties tab and check or uncheck the Print Object box. When you later print the worksheet, the selected object won't be printed with the document.

Summary

Printing worksheets with Excel is simple. You can place the page breaks where you need or want them to be. You can choose selected areas to print, rather than printing the entire worksheet. Remember that, when you are performing any task within Excel, online help is but a keystroke away: Click the Office Assistant tool and enter your query. Chances are, you will find an answer to your problem.

Workshop

Term Review

page   An Excel worksheet (if it is large enough) can be divided into pages both horizontally and vertically. If the worksheet is too wide horizontally to fit onto one page, there is a vertical page break. If the worksheet is too long to fit onto one page, there is a horizontal page break. You can control where the page breaks are placed.

Q&A

Q How do you print within Excel?

A Click the Print tool to print instantly.

Q How do you change the type of paper you are printing on?

A Choose File | Print from the main menu to display the Print dialog box. Click the Properties button to display the Properties dialog box. Select the Paper tab and change the settings to agree with the paper you want to print on. You can also change the orientation to Portrait or Landscape.

Q How do you set up pages for printing within Excel?

A Display the Page Setup dialog box by choosing File | Page Setup from the main menu. Use this dialog box to make any changes to the way the printed page is set up.

Q How do you print only a specific area of a worksheet within Excel?

A Select the area in the worksheet and choose File | Print Area | Set Area from the main menu.

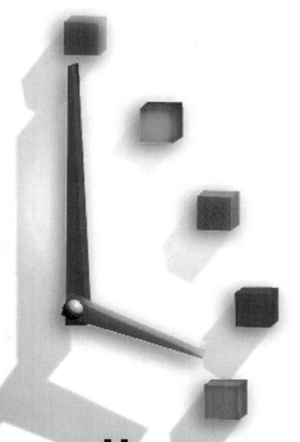

PART

III

Excel and Interactive Data

Hour

Hour 12

Using Formulas in Excel

Excel is great for entering, storing, and presenting data, as you learned in Part I, "Excel: The Preliminaries," and Part II, "Graphical Manipulation and Display of Data," of this book. The heart and soul of the spreadsheet, however, is its capability to use these data values to calculate new data values. Excel allows you to use *formulas* that use arithmetic and algebraic operations to calculate values.

You are probably familiar with formulas from mathematical studies. For example, distance = rate × time is a *formula*. In Excel, a formula performs a mathematical operation on one or more values or variables. The values or variables can be specified numbers—or they can be cell references. Excel has a specific syntax for entering formulas, as described in the next section and throughout this hour. The term *equation* is sometimes used as a synonym for *formula* in Excel.

Using Excel as a Calculator

If you want to use Excel as a calculator, just enter an equation into a cell. Begin with an equal sign (=) so that Excel can recognize that what you are entering is a formula. If you type **=35-48** into a cell and press Enter, Excel does the calculation (see Figure 12.1) and places the number -13 in the cell. Notice that the *result* is what you see in the cell instead of the actual formula you entered. However, the actual data in the cell is still the formula (as you can see by looking at the cell contents in the white bar above the column labels).

Figure 12.1.

Using Excel as a calculator.

Contents of cell

Results of formula displayed in cell

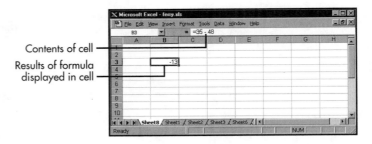

This type of equation has a fairly limited application because it does not make direct use of values from other cells. Nevertheless, these straightforward calculations do have their uses.

Excel allows you to use certain operators when you are creating mathematical formulas. You have more options when you use the built-in functions described in Hour 13, "Using Functions in Excel." The arithmetic operators you can use with Excel formulas are listed in Table 12.1.

Table 12.1. Excel's arithmetic operators.

Operator	Name	Description
+	plus sign	Addition
–	minus sign	Subtraction (or to indicate a negative number)
*	asterisk	Multiplication
/	slash	Division
%	percent sign	Percent
^	caret sign	Exponentiation ("to the power of")

Most formulas you create include one or all of these arithmetic operators. Here are a few examples of simple formulas and the results they return. Remember that every formula must begin with an = sign.

Formula	Result
=2+4	6
=8*3	24

Formula	Result
=35%	0.35
=14/7	2
=8^2	64

Your formulas can also include at least one of the *comparative operators* (also called *logical operators*) listed in Table 12.2. Formulas that use logical operators are evaluated to be either TRUE or FALSE, as described in the next section, "Evaluating Logical Expressions."

Table 12.2. Excel's logical operators.

Symbol	Meaning
=	equals
<	less than
>	greater than
<=	less than or equal to
>=	greater than or equal to
<>	not equal to

Evaluating Logical Expressions

Excel can evaluate whether certain mathematical statements are true or false. If you enter =56 < 57 in a cell, Excel returns the value TRUE because 56 is less than 57. If you enter =58 < 57 into a cell, Excel returns the value FALSE because 58 is not less than 57.

Try entering expressions like the following into cells to see the results:

```
= 1000*9 <(2000+2000+3000+1000+500+500)
= 2800 >= 1800*2/(1/2)
```

The first expression gives you the value TRUE; the second expression gives you the value FALSE.

Using AutoSum

The AutoSum tool is very convenient and is probably one of the most useful functions available in Excel.

 Figure 12.2 shows a column of figures in the range C6:C8. If you highlight C9 and click the AutoSum tool in the Standard toolbar, the sum of all the cells appears in cell C9.

You can use the AutoSum tool in the same way when all the data is displayed in a row. Just highlight the first empty cell in the row and click the AutoSum symbol. The sum of all the preceding cells is displayed in the last cell.

Figure 12.2.

Using the AutoSum tool to add a column of figures.

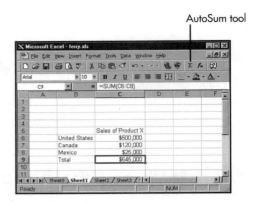

You can even use the AutoSum tool to add more than one column and row together. In the screen shown in Figure 12.3, select the entire region in the range C6:E9 and click the AutoSum tool. You will get totals in each of the blank selected cells. Here is what happens with the worksheet shown in Figure 12.3 if the AutoSum tool is used as shown:

☐ Cell C9 contains the sum of the cells C6, C7, and C8 (for a total value of $645,000)

☐ Cell D9 contains the sum of the cells D6, D7, and D8 (for a total value of $349,000)

☐ Cell E6 contains the sum of cells C6 and D6 (for a total of $750,000)

☐ Cell E7 contains the sum of cells C7 and D7 (for a total of $200,000)

☐ Cell E8 contains the sum of cells C8 and D8 (for a total of $44,000)

☐ Cell E9 contains the sum of cells C9 and D9 (for a total of $994,000)

Figure 12.3.

Using the AutoSum tool to add a range of figures.

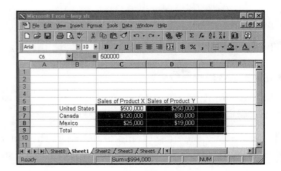

12

Creating Formulas

A more complicated formula refers to cells by their cell references. In Figure 12.4, the formula in cell E8 is supposed to calculate total sales; the formula in that cell is =C8+D8. Cell C8 contains the sales for the Eastern region, and cell D8 contains the sales for the Western region. Adding the two together gives the total.

Figure 12.4.

*A formula for calculating
total sales.*

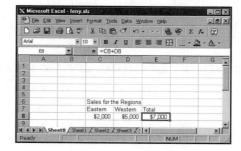

If a cell contains a formula, its value changes if the value in one or more of the cells referenced by the formula changes.

Entering a Simple Formula

Figure 12.5 shows the data for a simple worksheet. Notice that the formula in cell C9 calculates the total sales of Product X for the U.S., Canada, and Mexico. The formula adds cells C6, C7, and C8 together.

Figure 12.5.

*Calculating the total sales
for a range of values.*

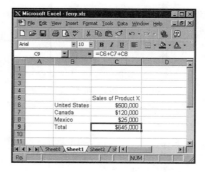

When you enter this formula in a cell, begin the entry with the = sign. This sign indicates that what follows is a formula. Remember that this rule was also in effect when you entered a calculation, earlier in this hour. Then type **C6** in the formula cell, then the + sign, then **C7**, then the + sign again, and finally **C8**. Press Enter when finished to enter the formula into the cell and calculate the result.

TIME SAVER

To view all the formulas in a worksheet at once, press Ctrl+' (apostrophe) to switch back and forth between viewing the formulas. Alternatively, you can choose Tools | Options from the main menu to display the Options dialog box. Select the View tab, select or deselect the Formulas checkbox, and click OK.

With either method, you can also make the formulas visible or not when you print the worksheet, as well as when you view the worksheet on the screen.

Entering a Formula by Pointing

You don't have to type the cell reference directly into a formula. You can enter the cell references by pointing to them with the mouse. To enter the formula =C6+C7+C8, here is one way to do it:

1. Select the cell in which you want to enter the formula. Start by typing the = sign. This character appears in the formula bar at the top of the window. Even when you are using the mouse to enter the cell references used in a formula, you must still type the preceding equal sign.

2. With the mouse, point to cell C6 and click; the cell name C6 appears in the formula bar.

3. Type the + sign. Even though you are entering cell names by pointing to them, you must still type the operators used to join the cell values.

4. Point to cell C7 and click; type the + sign again; point to cell C8 and click.

5. Press the Enter key to complete the formula and calculate the results.

TIME SAVER

You can calculate time differences with formulas just as you can calculate other differences. For example, if you type **3:30** in one cell, **2:15** in another cell, and then enter a formula in a third cell that subtracts the second cell from the first cell, you end up with 1:15 (meaning 1 hour and 15 minutes).

Editing Formulas

To edit a formula, select the cell containing the formula you want to modify. Place the cursor in the cell and start typing. You can use the Backspace and Del keys as needed.

Changing the Values in the Formula

You can change the result of a formula by changing the values in the cells that the formula references. In the example shown in Figure 12.5, try changing the value for U.S. sales in cell C6 from $500,000 to $400,000. The formula result in cell C9 instantly changes to $545,000.

You can also have a formula in which the cell references themselves contain formulas. Suppose that you want to add the total sales for a number of regions. Each of these regions has a sales total that is compiled by adding together the sales totals of various products. In this scenario, the grand total is calculated by adding together the results of other formulas.

Understanding the Order of Operations and Nesting

Excel performs mathematical operations from left to right, but multiplication and division are done before addition and subtraction.

The formula =B5 + C6*C7/C8 - D10 is calculated like this: C6*C7/C8 is calculated and added to the value in cell B5. The value in cell D10 is subtracted from that result.

You can use parentheses to change the prescribed order, or you can use parentheses simply for clarity. You should include parentheses in formulas even if you're not sure they are needed but if including them makes the formula easier to read.

Here's an example of a formula containing parentheses:

=A2 - (B2*B3 - C2)/C3

Here's how to calculate the result:

> The value in cell B2 is multiplied by the value of cell B3; the value of C2 is subtracted from that result. That quantity is then divided by the value in cell C3. This value is then subtracted from the value in cell A2.

In the example shown in Figure 12.6, the formula just described is located in cell C4. The result is 9.25, given the values shown in cells B2, B3, C2, C3, and A2.

Figure 12.6.

Using parentheses to change the order of operations.

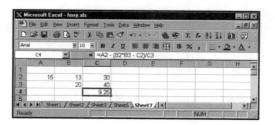

Using Absolute and Relative References

Suppose that the formula =C6+C7+C8 (intended to calculate the total sales for a product) is in cell C9. (Try entering the formula on a worksheet.) If you copy and paste the formula in cell C9 to cell D10, the new formula in cell D10 is D7+D8+D9. Each of the cell references in the new formula is changed to correspond to the position it was in relative to the original formula cell.

The formula is calculated by looking at the relative position of the cells. With the formula =C6+C7+C8 located in cell C9, cell C6 is three cells to the left of cell C9. When you move the formula to cell D10, cell D7 is three cells to the left of C10. Similarly, cell C7 is two cells to the left of C9; cell D8 is two cells to the left of D10. Cell C8 is one cell to the left of C9; cell D9 is one cell to the left of D10.

Thus, entering the formula =C6+C7+C8 in cell C9 is equivalent, in relative terms, to entering the formula =D7+D8+D9 in cell D10. Therefore, the cell references within the formula are called *relative references.*

Here is another example: If you enter the formula =B2*4 in cell C2 and then copy cell C2 to cell E5, the new formula is =D5*4. Because cell C2 is one cell down from B2, the relative reference changes during the move to refer to cell E5, which is one cell down from D5.

The results of the formula calculations differ, of course, depending on the values of the variables used.

Relative references are useful in conjunction with the AutoFill tool. Suppose that you want to calculate the area of a square, based on its side length, as shown in the table in Figure 12.7. You know that Area = s², where s is the length of the side. Type the formula =D7^2 in cell E7. You can then copy the formula to each of the other cells in E8 and E9 by using the AutoFill tool. Because the references are relative, the formula automatically adjusts to calculate the area based on the value in the cell to the left of the cell in which the formula is located.

However, *absolute references* are sometimes necessary. Suppose that a formula in cell G8 refers to cell D6. If you move the formula to cell E10, the new reference is to cell B8. In each instance, the referenced cell is two cells to the left and two up from the cell in which the formula resides. But what if cell D6 holds a constant (for example, an interest rate) that you want the formula to use regardless of where it is copied in the worksheet? You must then refer to cell D6 *absolutely*; that is, you must make Excel realize that it cannot change the reference to cell D6.

To refer to a cell absolutely, you use a dollar sign ($) before the column letter and before the row number, like this: $A$5. When a formula refers to a cell in this fashion, even if you move the cell containing the formula, the reference is still to cell A5.

12

Figure 12.7.

Using the AutoFill tool for a formula.

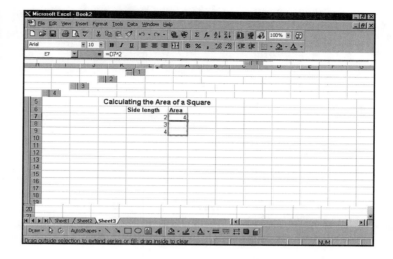

If you aren't going to move cells around, using absolute references is not necessary. Relative references work very well in almost all cases—particularly so if you move the table and formula to different locations. When you use relative references, the formulas still work in their new locations.

An absolute reference works well for a constant that you use in your formulas and that is stored in a cell with a location that isn't going to change.

Using Circular References

A *circular reference* in a formula is one that refers directly or indirectly to the formula itself. Suppose that you enter the formula =A1+A2 in cell A1. The formula requires the value of cell A1 to complete the calculation, but it cannot get the value of cell A1 unless the calculation is complete. . . . The formula has a circular reference.

Most of the time, circular references are accidental. If you try to create a circular reference, you see the message box shown in Figure 12.8. Most of the time, you don't want to have a circular reference in your formula and want to fix the formula so that the circular reference is eliminated. If you click OK, the Circular Reference toolbar appears; you can use it to find the circular reference.

If you click Cancel, the circular reference remains in the formula. Excel *can* use circular references in formulas by iterating the values over and over again. The default number of iterations is 100. By default, the formula stops calculating before finishing the default number of iterations if the values in the circular reference change by less than 0.01 in a single calculation. Circular references are used only for some scientific and engineering functions; they are not used for the type of simple arithmetic formulas described in this chapter.

12

Figure 12.8.

The circular reference
message.

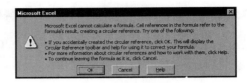

TIME SAVER

You can change the number of iterations and the interval of change by
displaying the Options dialog box, selecting the Calculation tab, and
making changes to the Maximum Iterations and Maximum Change boxes.

Naming Cells and Ranges

Naming cells and ranges is a way to make formulas more understandable. For example,
instead of referring to a range of cells as E7:E13, you can name the range and then refer to
it in other formulas by its range name.

To name a cell or a range, select it and then click the name box (the box above the column
letter A). Enter a descriptive text value in place of the standard alphanumeric value.

Here are the rules for creating names:

☐ A name can contain the uppercase and lowercase letters A through Z, the digits 0
through 9, the period (.), and the underscore (_) symbol.

☐ The first character must be a letter or an underscore.

☐ Names must be less than 256 characters long.

☐ A name cannot be the same as a cell reference, whether absolute, relative, or mixed.
For example, you cannot give the range C5:D10 the name B52.

Because you can't have spaces in a name, you can use the underscore character (_) to serve
the same purpose.

Here are some acceptable range names:

```
_1997
Georgia_State
Interest
MyVeryOwnSpecialName
```

Here are some names that do not work:

```
25December   (It starts with a digit.)
Interest Rate   (It contains a space.)
A2   (It is the same as a cell reference.)
```

12

Naming cells and ranges helps clarify the purpose of a formula. For example, if you name one cell Velocity and one cell Time, you can write a formula for calculating distance in this way: =Velocity*Time—which makes much more sense than =A2*B15!

In Figure 12.9, the formula for calculating interest earned is written as =Principal*Interest_Rate. Cell B3 is named Principal, and cell B4 is named Interest_Rate.

Figure 12.9.

A formula using name references.

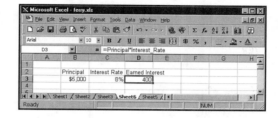

Naming a Constant

A numeric or text value that is not a formula is a *constant*. There are lots of reasons you might want to use a constant repeatedly and name it. For example, the acceleration caused by gravity is 9.8 meters per second per second. You can enter the value 9.8 in a cell and name the cell g. Then you could use the physics formula d = 0.5*g*t*t to calculate the distance traveled by an object in a particular length of time dropped from a height (in the absence of air resistance). Many mathematical expressions use constants.

If you have a group of constants you are using in your worksheet or workbook, you may find it helpful to place them all in one place away from the rest of your work. You can lock this area of the worksheet to prevent the constants from being changed. Constants you may need or want to use in your worksheets include scientific values like the speed of light or sound, mortgage rates, specific dates and times, and so forth.

Freezing Formula Values

After you have entered your formulas and obtained results for them, you may want to preserve the calculated values. Suppose that you have calculated the result of a formula that depends on cells in other worksheets. You know that the cells in the other worksheets are subject to change, and you may or may not have control over those worksheets. You may want to preserve the results of the formula based on the values of the cells in the other worksheets at a particular time. Or suppose that you are calculating the payroll for a specific week and are using a list of employees' wages in another worksheet. You know that the list will change, but for your purposes, you are interested only in the current values of the employees' wages list. You may want to preserve the results of the payroll formula based on this week's employees' wages list.

12

To "freeze" a formula's value or values, select the cell or range containing the formulas and the results you want to preserve. Choose Edit | Copy from the main menu. Move the insertion point to a new location, select Edit | Paste Special from the main menu, choose the Values button, and click OK.

Troubleshooting Formulas

When you create formulas, you must make sure that what you create is mathematically valid and that it actually means what you want it to mean. Here are a few basic tips:

☐ Make sure that you nest your parentheses correctly.

☐ Make sure that you specify a range using the : (colon) symbol, not the ¦ (pipe) symbol.

☐ Use unformatted numbers in formulas. Do not use date format, currency format, or other numerical formats directly.

Error Messages

Table 12.2 lists the basic error messages you may see when you work with formulas in Excel.

Table 12.2. Error messages.

Symbol	Meaning
#####	The cell is too narrow for the value produced by the formula. Resize the cell as necessary.
#DIV/0!	In one way or another, you have tried to divide by zero. Make sure that the divisor (whether you have entered it into a cell manually or it results from another formula) is not zero.
#N/A	One of the values needed to complete a formula is not available.
#NAME?	You have used a range name in your formula that Excel does not recognize. If you have misspelled the name or referred to a range with a name that you forgot to actually assign to the range, the formula won't work. Fix it, and the formula should work (unless there's another error, of course).

Summary

Doing calculations and using formulas is the basic reason you are using Excel. You can use formulas to take your data and make sense of it. Excel is good for both storing and processing data. Functions, described in Hour 13, allow you to do more complex mathematical calculations and other operations on text and numbers than formulas do.

Workshop

Term Review

absolute reference   A cell reference that does not depend on a cell's position in regard to other cells; it stays the same no matter what cell the formula that uses it is located in.

argument   A value or variable used in a formula.

constant   A numerical value that remains the same; a constant is not determined by a formula.

equation   As used in Excel, the term *equation* is synonymous with *formula*.

formula   A calculation or evaluation of particular values or variables.

formula bar   The strip near the top of the Excel worksheet just above the column labels, in which you can see the data you are entering in the active cell.

relative reference   A cell reference that refers to the horizontal and vertical distance of one cell relative to another.

Q&A

Q What are formulas used for?

A Formulas make a spreadsheet come alive because they take the various data values and use them in equations at your command.

Q Why would you use absolute references?

A You use absolute references when you want to refer to a specific cell. Relative references are the default; using them allows the formulas to remain valid if a table is moved as a whole.

Q Why are names used for some cells and ranges?

A It is easier to understand a formula if its elements have names instead of cell references. It's easier to understand a formula such as =Yearly_Salary/12 than it is to understand a formula such as =B5/12.

12

Exercise

Create the worksheet shown in Figure 12.10, with the Quantity, Price, and Tax values in place.

To calculate the totals for each column, type the formula =B7*C7*1.97 in cell E7. Use the AutoFill tool to copy the formula into cells E7 through E11. Because the formula uses relative references, it automatically adjusts to create the right formula for each.

Use the AutoSum tool to calculate the Grand Total in cell E12. If you do so, you may get the ###### error, indicating that column E is too narrow to fit the result of the formula. Select Format | Column | AutoFit to make the column wide enough to display the result of the formula.

Figure 12.10.

The sales figures exercise.

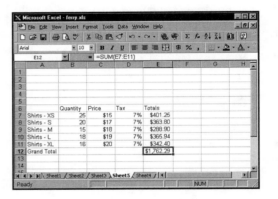

12

Hour **13**

Using Functions in Excel

Functions are prebuilt formulas for evaluating data. If you want to do trigonometric functions, for example, you need either a calculator or a program such as Excel (assuming that you have progressed beyond the use of mere pencil, paper, and your brain). Similarly, if you are calculating interest for a T-bill or figuring out a standard deviation in an experiment, you will probably want some sort of calculating aid. Excel includes hundreds of functions that handle all sorts of different situations, many of which you probably have never considered.

How and Why to Use Functions

If you want to perform operations on your data, there likely exists a function for your purposes. Excel offers several hundred functions that perform a variety of different tasks. These functions are subdivided into the following categories:

☐ Financial
☐ Date & Time
☐ Math & Trig
☐ Statistical
☐ Lookup & Reference

☐ Database

☐ Text

☐ Logical

☐ User-defined

☐ Engineering

Using the Paste Function Button and Entering Functions

 Although you can enter a function directly into a cell, it's often easier to use the Paste Function button. Click this button, located on the Standard toolbar, to display the dialog box shown in Figure 13.1. Alternatively, you can choose Insert | Function from the main menu to get the same dialog box.

Figure 13.1.

The Paste Function dialog box.

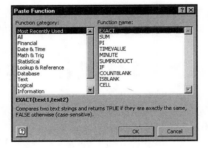

Every function has one or more arguments. *Arguments* are the values on which the formula operates. Depending on the formula, these values can be cell references, named cells, cell ranges, specific numeric values, logical values, or text values. Some functions take no arguments. For example, the PI function simply returns the value of the numerical constant π—3.14159... to 15 decimal places. Its syntax looks like this:

```
=PI()
```

From the Paste Function dialog box, you select the category of function from the left panel and then a specific function from the right panel. Notice the syntax of the function and the brief description at the bottom of the dialog box. If this is the function you want to use, click OK to display a dialog box in which you can enter the arguments for the particular function you have selected. Figure 13.2 shows the dialog box for the SUM function. The text boxes provide a convenient place to enter the arguments for the function. If you want to add the values in cells C2 and C3, for example, enter those cell names in the relevant boxes.

13

Figure 13.2.

*Entering arguments in
the dialog box for the
SUM function.*

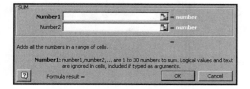

Of course, you don't have to use the Paste Function dialog box to enter a function in your worksheet. You can enter the SUM function with the arguments C2 and C3 by typing the following directly into a cell:

=SUM(C2,C3)

When you enter a function in a cell, you always begin by preceding the function name with the = sign—just as you do when you enter formulas, as described in the last hour (see Figure 13.3). The following sections describe some of the many functions available in Excel.

Figure 13.3.

*Entering a function
directly into a cell.*

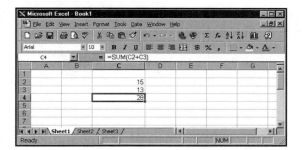

Finding the Function to Use

More than 300 functions provided by Excel, and you still can't find the one you want? Here's help: Click the Paste Function button to display the Paste Function dialog box. Click the Office Assistant button in the lower-left corner of the dialog box and choose Help with this Feature. The dialog box shown in Figure 13.4 appears; you can use it to search for the function you want. You can also access a list of functions from the Index tab on the Help Topics dialog box.

13

Figure 13.4.

Searching for the function you want with Office Assistant.

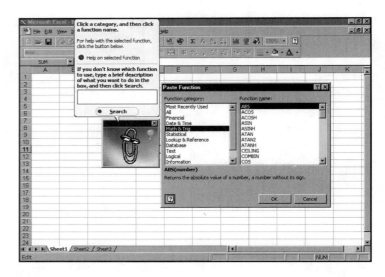

Financial Functions

Excel includes several dozen financial and accounting functions. For more information and a list of these functions, use Office Assistant to search or use the Help Topics dialog box. Suppose that you want to calculate the straight-line depreciation of an item. You use the SLN function, of course. Its syntax looks like this:

```
=SLN(initial_cost,salvage_value,number_of_depreciation_periods)
```

For this example, assume that you purchased a piece of office furniture for $500, you want to depreciate it over a period of 10 years, and it is to have a salvage value of $100 at the end of that time. The SLN function for this scenario looks like this:

```
=SLN(500,100,10)
```

The result of this function is a depreciation allowance of $40 for each year. (See your tax guidelines for the appropriate depreciation periods, of course.)

You can see a list of all the financial functions available: Select Help | Contents and Index from the main menu. Click the Index tab, and search for `financial functions`.

Date and Time Functions

Microsoft uses serial numbers to represent dates, beginning with January 1, 1900. The date and time for January 2, 1900, at 12:00 P.M. is represented as `1.5`. The date and time for January 30, 1900, at 6:00 A.M. is represented as `30.25`. The serial numbers simply look at how many days and fractions of days have elapsed since January 1, 1900.

13

As an example, the TIMEVALUE function takes a specific time of day and converts it into a fraction of a 24-hour day. The function =TIMEVALUE(3:36) gives you the result 0.15 because at 3:36 A.M., 15 percent of the day has elapsed.

Excel offers many different functions to assist you in getting the date and time. To see all the available data and time functions, select Help | Contents and Index from the main menu. Click the Index tab, and search for date functions.

Mathematical and Trigonometric Functions

Although Excel does not divide the mathematical and trigonometric functions into separate subcategories, there are three basic types of these functions: arithmetic, algebraic, and trigonometric. To see a list of the several dozen math functions available, select Help | Contents and Index from the main menu. Click the Index tab, and search for math functions.

Arithmetic Functions

Arithmetic functions use the mathematical operations of adding, subtracting, multiplying, and dividing.

The SUM function does the same thing you can do with the + sign or the AutoSum tool. Suppose that you want to add the values contained in the ranges A1:A3, B2:C9, and D1:D4. Using the SUM function, the formula looks like this:

```
=SUM(A1:A3,B2:C9,D1:D4)
```

You can use single cells, arrays, or names for the arguments of the SUM function. The generic syntax looks like this:

```
SUM(argument1,argument2, . . .)
```

The SUM function ignores any logical values, text values, or empty cells it may encounter in the ranges you specify.

Another useful function is QUOTIENT. This function returns the integer portion of the division operation and discards the remainder. Here is the general syntax:

```
=QUOTIENT(dividend, divisor)
```

The function =QUOTIENT(55,8) gives a result of 6. The remainder of 7 is discarded.

Algebraic Functions

Algebraic functions can calculate logarithms, exponents, square roots, and more.

13

The FACT function gives you the factorial of a number. Remember that the factorial of the number 5 is 5*4*3*2*1. The factorial of a whole number *N* is given as follows:

```
N*(N-1)*(N-2)*...1
```

If the number includes a fraction, the number is rounded to the nearest whole number. If you try to take the factorial of a negative number, the #NUM! error is returned.

Trigonometric Functions

Excel offers various trigonometric functions, including SIN, COS, TAN, and others.

A typical trigonometric function works like this:

```
=COS(0)
```

Text Functions

Text functions are used to compare character strings, evaluate text, change cases, and so forth.

Suppose that you want to convert a character string to all lowercase characters. Just use the LOWER function:

```
=LOWER("CHARACTER String")
```

This function results in the value character string.

You can use this function to convert a bunch of values to lowercase characters. If you want to convert a value to uppercase characters, use the UPPER function.

The PROPER function capitalizes the first letter of each word in a value. Suppose that the values in your worksheet are written in mixed case, and you want to convert them to all uppercase characters. You can do this by editing the cell contents and inserting =UPPER(" in front of the actual value and a ") at the end of the actual value. Once the change is made and all the values are converted, you can freeze the values as discussed in Hour 12, "Using Formulas in Excel."

TIME SAVER

> To freeze values in a group of cells, first select the cells. Select Edit I Copy from the main menu. Move the insertion point to a new location in the worksheet (or leave the original range of cells selected if you want to replace the original values with the new values) and select Edit I Paste Special. Select Values from the resulting dialog box and click OK.

If you process text in this way extensively, you may want to use macros to make the process easier. Macros are discussed in Hour 22, "Creating and Running Macros."

13

Logical Functions

The logical functions are IF, AND, OR, NOT, TRUE, and FALSE. You use these functions to evaluate a condition and determine whether it is true or false. TRUE and FALSE can also be the *results* of logical conditions (if a logical condition is evaluated, its result is either TRUE or FALSE). The AND, OR, NOT, and IF functions evaluate the logical conditions and determine the value for the cell.

TRUE and FALSE Results

A logical condition, a function, or a formula, can return the value TRUE or FALSE. A *logical condition* is a statement that can be either true or false. Here are some examples:

```
C5>50
D1=D2
D5=D4 - D3
F8=B2*B3 - B1
B2<=101
```

These are just a few of the possible conditions you can have. The condition involves a comparison of values.

Suppose that you enter the value 3 in both cell C3 and cell C4. If you enter the condition =C3=C4 into another cell, that cell returns the value TRUE because cell C3 (with a value of 3) does indeed equal cell C4 (with a value of 3). If you enter the condition =C3>C4 into another cell, that cell returns the value FALSE because cell C3 (with a value of 3) is not greater than cell C4 (with a value of 3).

TRUE and FALSE can also be used as functions by themselves. If you enter =TRUE() into a cell, the cell has the value TRUE. If you enter =FALSE() into a cell, the cell has the value FALSE.

The AND Function

The general syntax for the AND function is given here:

```
=AND(logical_condition1, logical_condition_2, . . ., logical_condition_N)
```

You can have up to 30 logical conditions within a single AND function. All these conditions must be satisfied for the value in the cell to be TRUE. Otherwise, the value is FALSE.

Suppose that you have the function =AND(C3=50,C4=60). If the value of C3 is 50, and the value of C4 is 60, the value of the function is TRUE. If either or both of the conditions are false, the result of the function is FALSE. Both conditions must be satisfied for the AND function to return TRUE.

13

The OR Function

The OR function is similar to the AND function, but only one of the logical conditions must resolve to TRUE for the result of the OR function to be TRUE. If all the conditions are false, the value of the cell will be FALSE. As with the AND function, the OR function can have up to 30 conditions.

Any of the logical functions can make use of nested functions, as in this example:

```
=OR(SUM(C1:C8)<25,SUM(C1:C8)>50,20,30)
```

The NOT Function

The NOT function reverses the value of TRUE or FALSE for the given condition. For example, the function =NOT(2+3=5) gives a value of FALSE and =NOT(3+4=8) gives a value of TRUE.

The generic syntax for the NOT function is as follows:

```
=NOT(condition)
```

The IF Function

With the IF function, you can evaluate from 1 to 30 logical conditions and return a different numeric or text value depending on whether the conditions are TRUE or FALSE.

The syntax for the IF function looks like this:

```
IF(logical_test,value_if_true,value_if_false)
```

You can use the IF function when you want a cell to contain the value Yes if a condition is true; if the condition is false, you want the cell to contain the value No. The "condition" might be the value of a specific cell. Such a function might look like this:

```
=IF(C10>50,"Yes","No")
```

In this example, the value in cell C10 is compared to the value 50; if the value in cell C10 is greater than 50, the condition (C10>50) is true and the cell containing the IF function is assigned the value Yes. If the value in cell C10 is less than 50, the condition (C10>50) is false and the cell containing the IF function is assigned the value No.

JUST A MINUTE

If you want a text value to be placed in a cell as the result of a logical condition, place the text value in quotation marks—refer to the example just presented and notice the text values "Yes" and "No". If you omit the quotation marks, you get an error message and the function does not work.

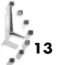

13

You can use the IF function if you want a certain discount to kick in after a certain quantity of merchandise is sold, for example. You can set up your worksheet so that if your bank balance drops below a certain point, a warning message shows up. In the following example, BANKBALANCE is a named cell reference. What happens if the value in that named cell drops below 100?

```
=IF(BANKBALANCE<100,"Your balance is low","Your balance is fine")
```

Information Functions

Information functions determine the type of data stored within a cell. You can determine the formatting of a cell, decide which cells in a range are blank, and pinpoint other characteristics.

Suppose that you want to find out how many cells in the range B2:C9 are blank (see the spreadsheet in Figure 13.5). The formula you enter in a cell to determine the number of blank cells in that range is =COUNTBLANK(B2:C9). In this example, the value returned is 11 because 11 of the cells in the indicated range are blank.

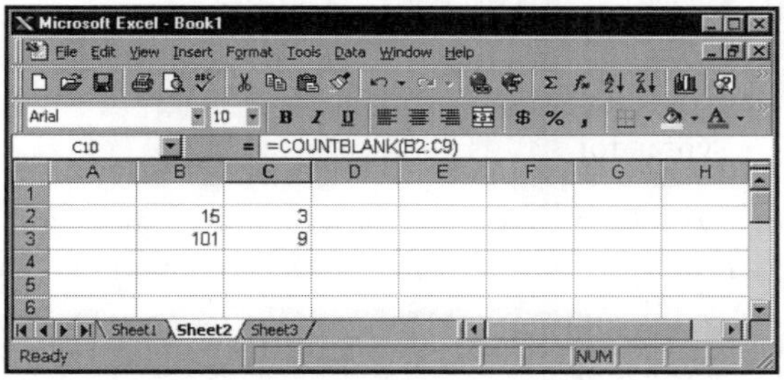

Figure 13.5.

Counting the empty cells with the COUNTBLANK function.

JUST A MINUTE

Excel includes tools you can use to analyze data. Some of these tools are described in Hour 16, "Using Excel to Analyze Data." The statistical analysis, regression analysis, and forecasting functions are not discussed in this book, although all those functions are very helpful if you want to do that type of work. You can create your own functions with Visual Basic for Applications, but extensive discussion of that topic is outside the scope of this book. For more information about Visual Basic for Applications, look at Hour 22, "Creating and Running Macros."

13

Engineering Functions and the Analysis ToolPak

Engineering functions are powerful tools for manipulating numbers and data. Functions are available for many different purposes. To see whether you have access to these functions, select Tools | Add-ins from the main menu to display the Add-ins dialog box. This dialog box contains a list of possible add-ins for Excel. If the Analysis ToolPak box is checked, you have the engineering functions installed. If not, check the box and click OK to install the add-in.

As an example, Excel allows you to express complex numbers with the COMPLEX function. The standard syntax for this function is COMPLEX(a,b), which means a + bi (where i is the square root of -1). For example, the function COMPLEX(5,6) means 5 + 6i.

The DELTA function tests whether two numbers are equal. Its syntax is as follows:

DELTA(number1,number2)

If the two numbers are equal, the value of the cell containing the function is 1. If the two numbers are different, the value of the cell is 0.

Every complex number has a conjugate. If the complex number is a + bi, its conjugate is a - bi. Entering the function =IMCONJUGATE(a + bi) returns the value a - bi.

The HEX2BIN function converts a hexadecimal (base 16) number to a binary (base 2) number. For example, the function =HEX2BIN("E3") gives you the result 11100011. With the HEX2BIN function, you can also include an argument for the number of places you want to return. You include this argument if you want the result to be returned with leading zeroes; without this argument, HEX2BIN returns a number with the minimum number of places.

The standard syntax of this function is as follows:

HEX2BIN("numerical_value",number_of_places)

numerical_value is written in base 16 and is always surrounded by quotation marks. number_of_places is written as an ordinary base-10 number.

These are just some of the engineering functions you may find helpful. If you are mathematically inclined, you can learn a lot by studying the different engineering functions included in Excel.

13

Using Functions as Part of a Formula

You can use a function as part of a formula. Suppose that you want to calculate twice the absolute value of a number. The absolute value of a number is its magnitude—for example, ABS(-3) = 3.

To create a formula that takes the absolute value of cell D8 and doubles it, you enter =2*ABS(D8) in another cell. In Figure 13.6, this formula is entered in cell E8. In this example, the result is 16 because the value in cell D8 is -8.

You can use any of the arithmetic and comparative operators combined with any function when you create your special-purpose formulas.

Figure 13.6.

Using a function as part of a formula.

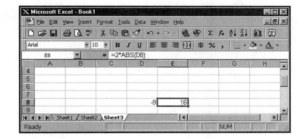

Concatenating Text and Mathematical Expressions

You can combine text values with other values. The text operator & combines two text values. For example, if you enter the formula ="value1"&"value2", the result is value1value2.

If you want to include a space between the various text values, include the space within the quotation marks that surround the character strings. In the following example, notice that a space follows the characters value1, within the quotation marks:

="value1 "&"value2"

This formula results in the string value1 value2 (notice the space separating the two words).

You can also use the CONCATENATE function to join strings. The formula =CONCATENATE("Days ", "of Our Lives") results in the value Days of Our Lives (again, notice the space that follows the string Days).

13

You can use the CONCATENATE function or the & operator in conjunction with a value from a cell. Suppose that the final grade for a course is located in cell E8. You can enter a formula like this one to print out a sentence that specifies the final grade:

```
="Your final grade is" &E8
```

If the value in cell E8 is 90%, the final result looks like this:

```
Your final grade is 90%
```

Reference Operators

Reference operators are used to combine ranges of cells for the purpose of doing calculations on them. There are three reference operators: the colon (:), the comma (,), and the single space.

The colon (:) is used to indicate a cell range, as described in Hour 3, "Introduction to the Excel Environment." For example, C3:F4 indicates that cell C3 is the upper-left cell of the range, and F4 is the bottom-right cell of the range.

The comma (,) is used to combine multiple references into one reference, as shown in this function, which adds the value of cell B3 to the number 4:

```
=SUM(B3,4)
```

A single space is used to refer to the intersection of cells common to two ranges. Consider this function:

```
=SUM(B3:D6 D2:D5)
```

This function adds the values in cells D2, D3, D4, and D5 together because those are the cells common to both ranges.

Nesting Functions

You can *nest* functions. That means you can place one function inside another function. The result of one function is used as an argument for another function. You can nest functions up to seven levels deep. However, you must make sure that you keep your parentheses matched and balanced.

Suppose that you want to add quotients. A typical equation would nest the two QUOTIENT functions within the SUM function, like this:

```
=SUM(QUOTIENT(25,3),QUOTIENT(27,4))
```

This equation results in the value 14 because QUOTIENT(25,3)=8 and QUOTIENT(27,4)=6.

Suppose that you want to calculate the sine of 80 degrees. Before you can use the SIN function, you must convert 80 degrees into radians with the RADIANS function. You can nest the two functions together into a single equation, like this:

```
=SIN(RADIANS(80))
```

You can have up to seven levels of nested functions in a formula.

Referencing Cells in Other Workbooks

When you are using formulas and functions, you may want to refer to cell values located in other worksheets of the same workbook or in other workbooks.

Suppose that you want to refer to cell D4 in Sheet3 of a workbook called Book2. You place the name of the workbook inside square brackets, for example, [Book2]. The name of the worksheet comes next, followed by an exclamation mark, for example, Sheet3!. You then refer to the cell absolutely, by using the $ character before the cell letter and a $ character before the cell number. The reference to cell D4 in Sheet3 of a workbook called Book2 looks like this:

```
[Book2]Sheet3!$D$4
```

If you want to refer to Sheet3 in the active workbook, the reference looks like this:

```
Sheet3!$D$4
```

Suppose that you want to add cells D2 and D3 in Sheet2 of the active workbook. The formula to accomplish this feat looks like this:

```
=SUM(Sheet2!$D$2,Sheet2!$D$3)
```

Suppose that you want to refer to a workbook called jansales.xls and a worksheet called ProductA. If you want to refer to cell D4 in that worksheet and workbook, the reference looks like this:

```
[jansales]ProductA!$D$4
```

13

This approach to referencing workbooks and worksheets works if you are dealing with workbooks in the same directory. However, if you want to refer to a workbook in a different directory, you must use the full pathname. Suppose that you want to refer to cell D4 in Sheet2 of a workbook called febsales.xls in a directory called sales on a network drive that is called drive E in your office. You reference the cell like this:

```
E:\sales\[febsales]Sheet2!$D$4
```

When you use these complex cell references in a formula, they are used in the same way as any other cell reference. For example, if you want to add cell C3 in the active worksheet, and cell C3 in the worksheet called Sheet2 in the workbook called febsales.xls on drive E, the formula to do so looks like this:

```
=C3+E:\sales\[febsales]sales!$C$3
```

Using Arrays

Arrays are a way to represent a group of variables in a single unit. An array is commonly a range, but it can be a group of noncontiguous cells as well.

An array has dimensions. If you want a single variable to list the grades for 28 students, you would make that variable an array with the dimensions 1×28 (one value—the grade—and 28 different occurrences of it). If you want a single variable to list sales for four quarters of one year for two products, you would make that variable an array with the dimensions 4×2 (4 quarters and 2 products).

You can perform operations quickly and efficiently with arrays. Suppose that you want to use the SUMPRODUCT function. SUMPRODUCT adds the products of 1 to 30 arrays. It multiplies the corresponding elements of each array within itself, and then adds the products. In Figure 13.7, the different arrays are B2:B9, C1:C8, and D3:D10. The arrays do not have to be lined up, but it is easier to follow what is being done if they are. Each array *does* have to be of the same dimensions, however.

In this example, the formula is =SUMPRODUCT(B2:B9,C1:C8,D3:D10). This formula adds the following products, like this:

```
(B2*C1*D3) + (B3*C2*D4) + (B4*C3*D5) + (B5*C4*D6) + (B6*C5*D7) + (B7*C6*D8) +
(B8*C7*D9) + (B9*C8*D10)
```

The result is 783.

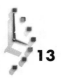

Figure 13.7.
The SUMPRODUCT
function.

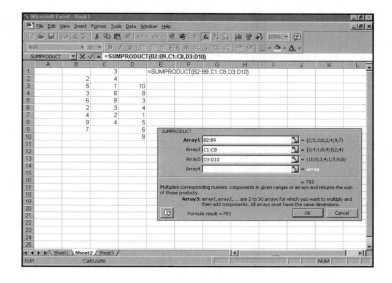

Customizing Calculations

By default, when the underlying values in a formula change, Excel recalculates all the affected values. You can control how Excel does this by selecting Tools | Options to display the Options dialog box; then select the Calculation tab to see the options shown in Figure 13.8.

Figure 13.8.
*The Calculation tab of
the Options dialog box.*

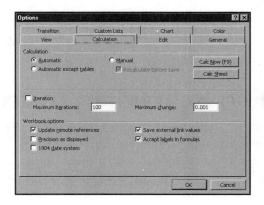

13

If you select the Manual option and click OK, Excel does not recalculate your functions and formulas automatically. To recalculate all open worksheets manually and update any associated charts, press the F9 key or click the Calc Now button in the Options dialog box. To calculate only the active worksheet, click the Calc Sheet button on the Calculation tab in the Options dialog box.

You can change the iteration options for functions and formulas that contain circular references, as described in Hour 12.

The Workbook Options at the bottom of the Calculation tab apply to the entire workbook. The Update Remote References option causes cells in other workbooks and worksheets to be updated if a value in the active worksheet changes and affects values in another worksheet.

If you select the Precision as Displayed option, the values are converted to the same number of decimal places they are displayed with. For example, if the actual value in a cell is 3.12345 but the cell has been formatted to display numbers with 2 decimal places, the number is displayed as 3.12. The Precision as Displayed option converts the number 3.12345 so that it is actually 3.12. You can format the cell to display the desired number of decimal places by selecting Format | Cells and changing options in the Format Cells dialog box.

The 1904 Date System option refers to the date calculation system used with Excel for Macintosh. Check this box if your worksheets have to be compatible with that system.

The Save External Link Values option saves copies of the values from external worksheets within your active worksheet. Selecting this option means that you will generally save time because Excel does not have to look at the external data source to get the values every time you need them. However, if you have a lot of these values, the worksheet may take up a considerable amount of disk space because it has to save these values separately, and it will take longer to open. In general, checking the Save External Link Values box is the appropriate choice, but pay attention to what happens with your particular documents.

Selecting the Accept Labels in Formulas option means that you can use label names in formulas if the ranges in your worksheet have row or column labels.

Click OK to close the Options dialog box when you have made your calculation selections. In general, the defaults work very well.

Getting Help when Entering a Function

When you are entering a function, Excel helps you if you have it wrong by displaying a troubleshooting dialog box. To get help with general troubleshooting, click Help. To get help with the specific function, click OK and then select Insert | Function from the main menu (or click the Paste Function button). If you use the Paste Function dialog box to enter the function in the first place, you can avoid many common errors encountered when entering functions manually.

Summary

Excel's functions are built-in formulas. You can use them together and nest them to evaluate data in different ways. Excel includes functions for a variety of purposes: accounting, science, engineering, statistical analysis, and more. Subsequent chapters in this book discuss certain types of functions in more detail.

Workshop

Term Review

argument   A variable that a function evaluates to get a result.

array   A way to arrange a group of values or variables so that a function can act on all of them at once.

comparison operator   Used to compare two values and return a value of TRUE or FALSE. The six comparison operators are < (less than), > (greater than), = (equals), <= (less than or equal to), >= (greater than or equal to), and <> (not equal to).

function   A built-in formula. Functions can operate on numbers, text, or other information.

logical condition   A statement that evaluates to either TRUE or FALSE.

nested function   A function that relies on the result of another function to return a result. That is, a function that uses another function as one of its arguments. Functions can be nested to seven levels.

reference operator   Reference operators combine ranges of cells so that you can do calculations on them. There are three reference operators: the colon (:), the comma (,), and a single space.

Q&A

Q What can functions do?

A Functions can process data values in a particular way. There are mathematical, accounting, scientific, and engineering functions available in Excel.

Q What is the difference between a formula and a function?

A Functions are prebuilt formulas. Excel includes several hundred functions as part of the software package.

Q Can you nest functions?

A Yes. You can use functions as arguments for other functions.

13

Exercises

In these exercises, find the applicable function and then apply it. Try experimenting with different functions, just so that you can get an idea of what is available.

1. What function would you use to compare text strings to determine whether they are exactly the same?

   This would be a text function; you can search through the text functions listed in the Paste Function dialog box, or you can use Office Assistant to search for the appropriate function, as described in the section "Finding the Function to Use," earlier in this hour.

   Suppose that you want to test whether cells D5 and Z1 contain the exact same character string. The function you use looks like this:

   =EXACT(D5,Z1)

   You can compare only two text strings at once with this function.

2. What function would you use to round up a number to the nearest even number?

   The EVEN function is the appropriate one to use. It is used like this:

   =EVEN(*number*)

   If you want to apply this function to the number 24.8, you use the function =EVEN(24.8), which returns the result 26. If you use nonnumeric values with this function, the function returns the #VALUE! error. Negative numbers are rounded *down* to an even number, so that the function =EVEN(-3) returns the value -4.

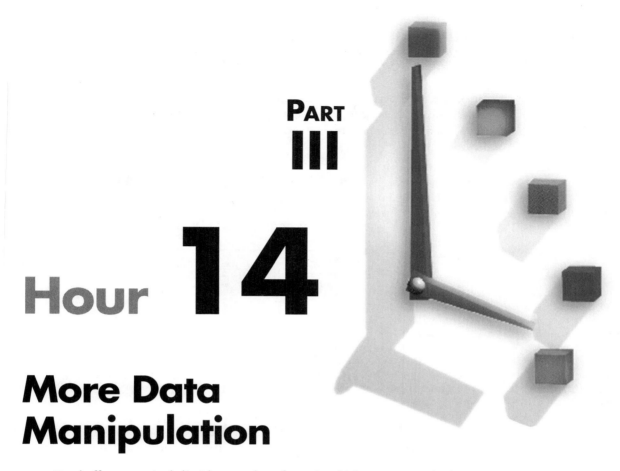

Hour 14

More Data Manipulation

Excel offers a seemingly limitless number of ways in which you can manipulate data. In this hour, you learn how to create Excel internal databases and how to filter and sort the data.

You can use Excel to store data; the program has many of the capabilities that full-powered database programs have. For example, Excel has excellent features for filtering and processing data. However, Excel cannot hold nearly as much data as database programs such as Microsoft Access, Oracle, SQL, or others, and it can be inefficient in comparison to "real" database programs, particularly those with large amounts of data. Excel loads an entire database into memory, no matter how large it is; database programs load data only as necessary.

Creating and Filtering Lists

A *list* is an internal database within Excel. A list is not really anything more than what you have seen in many of the preceding chapters: Information is stored in rows and columns.

In database terminology, a *field* is equivalent to a column within Excel. The labels describing the fields are called *field names*. A *record* is equivalent to a row within Excel. In Figure 14.1, there are four fields: Students, Test1, Test2, and Average. There are nine records: one for each of the student names.

Figure 14.1.

A typical list in Excel.

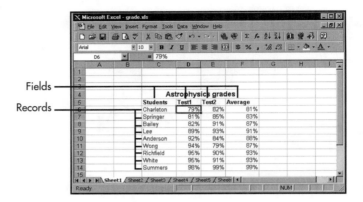

Here are a few simple tips for creating lists:

☐ Have only one list in a worksheet. This tip simplifies matters and makes it easier for Excel to see the data to be filtered.

☐ Keep the list consolidated. Don't leave blank spaces in the list.

☐ Don't put important data to the right or left of the list because Excel may consider it part of the list when you filter the list.

Filtering Data

Filtering a list means that you hide certain rows according to specific criteria or rules. Suppose that you have a list containing all your customers in 50 states; you can filter the list to show only those customers who live in Tennessee. Or suppose that you have a customer list but you want to filter it so that you see only the customers in the top 15 percent of purchases made. There are many other possible ways to filter data—and many other criteria.

Using the AutoFilter Tool

You can use the AutoFilter tool to display specific rows of a worksheet. It has a number of specific capabilities.

Choose Data | Filter | AutoFilter from the main menu to see the AutoFilter arrows shown in Figure 14.2. If you click one of the AutoFilter arrows, you get a drop-down list; the drop-down list in Figure 14.2 provides various filtering options. You can filter the list in several ways:

☐ By specific records

☐ With the Top-10 filter

☐ With a custom filter

Figure 14.2.

A typical list with AutoFilter arrows and a choice of options.

AutoFilter arrows

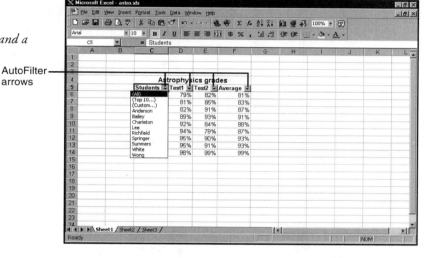

Filtering by Specific Value

The filtering options are appropriate to the type of data you are working with. You can sort numerical data by percentages or by whether particular data points are in the top or bottom of the distribution. If you select a specific percentage from the scroll-down menu, only those records with that percentage value are displayed. For example, if you choose Data | Filter | AutoFilter from the main menu, select the Test2 list control, and then select 91%, all the records are hidden except for the records for Bailey and White, because 91% is the Test2 value for those two students.

Similarly, you can filter by a specific value for either numerical or textual data. For example, if you have a column of data in which two of the values are 823, and you filter by 823, those two records are displayed. If you have a column in which four of the entries are Smith, and you filter by the name Smith, those four entries are displayed and the rest of the column is hidden.

Thus, if you select the Students list control and then choose one of the names from the drop-down menu, only the record with that name is displayed; all the rest of the records are filtered out.

The AutoFilter arrows for each field in your list show the various entries in the column so that you can filter by any of the specific entries.

14

Filtering with the Top-10 Filter

If you choose Data | Filter | AutoFilter from the main menu and select the Top-10 filter, you see a dialog box similar to the one in Figure 14.3. You can specify whether you want to see the Top 10, Top 5, or some other number of the items in your list by changing the value in the second text box. The top value in the list is the one with the highest numerical value; the bottom value in the list is the one with the lowest numerical value. You can use the spin buttons or type the number of items in your list that you want to see.

You can also change the filter so that it shows the Bottom values in the list. Click the arrow button next to the first text box in the Top 10 AutoFilter dialog box and select the filter option you want to use.

If you click the Items drop-down menu (the third text box in the dialog box), you can choose whether the Top or Bottom entries shown are in terms of numbers of items or in terms of a percentage of the whole list.

For example, if you use the Astrophysics Grades data shown in Figure 14.1 and choose to show the Top 20 for the Test1 field, specifying that the Top 20 is to be in terms of percentage (and not items in the list), you see the record for Summers, but none of the others.

When you filter a column, the cell addresses stay the same. However, there are missing rows and columns. For example, if rows 6 and 7 are filtered out, the row numbers you see on your worksheet jump from 5 to 8.

Figure 14.3.

The Top 10 AutoFilter dialog box.

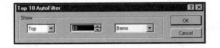

JUST A MINUTE

> If you want to see how many records of the total are displayed, look at the status line at the bottom of the worksheet. The status line shows the following information after you have filtered the data:
>
> X of Y records found
>
> In this syntax, X is the number of records displayed, and Y is the total number of records.

To remove an AutoFilter, simply select Data | Filter | AutoFilter again from the main menu to deselect the option. All the data is once again displayed.

Filtering with a Custom Filter

What if you want to filter your records by a specific criteria? Perhaps you want to include all records within a particular range of numerical values. Or perhaps you want to include all records in the alphabetical range *A* through *M*.

14

Here's how to filter a column with a filter that you design yourself: Choose Data | Filter | AutoFilter from the main menu and select the Custom option. The dialog box shown in Figure 14.4 appears. In this example, the cell selected was in the Test1 column.

Using the Astrophysics Grades data list, suppose that you want to see only the records for students whose names begin with the letter *A*. First display the Custom AutoFilter dialog box. Select begins with from the drop-down list and type **A** in the top text box on the right. Click OK. For this example, only the student record for Anderson would be displayed.

If you want to see all the student records for which the student's name does *not* begin with the letter *W*, you select does not begin with from the drop-down list on the left, type **W** in the text box on the right, and then click OK. All the records *except for* White's and Wong's show up.

Figure 14.4.

The Custom AutoFilter dialog box.

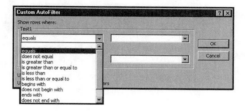

The drop-down list on the left side of the dialog box shows a number of different filtering options:

```
equals
does not equal
is greater than
is greater than or equal to
is less than
is less than or equal to
begins with
does not begin with
ends with
does not end with
contains
does not contain
```

For example, if you want to display all student records in which the entries in the Students column begin with the letter *A*, you first select a cell in that column. Then click the AutoFilter arrow and choose Custom. When the Custom AutoFilter box appears, choose begins with from the list on the left in the dialog box and enter **A** in the right text box in the dialog box. Then click OK.

Using Two Custom Filter Options

You can easily use two custom filter options to further narrow a search. Suppose that you want to display all the records for which the student name begins with a *W* and ends with an *e*. You select a cell in the Students column of the data list, display the Custom AutoFilter dialog box, and enter criteria so that it looks like the dialog box in Figure 14.5.

Figure 14.5.

The Custom AutoFilter dialog box used to filter with two criteria.

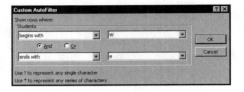

COFFEE BREAK

Using Multiple Custom Filter Options

If there are more than two filtering criteria you want to use on a data list, you can first perform a sort with two of the criteria using the instructions just provided. Then you can repeat the sort on the filtered list using the other criterion or criteria.

Using Advanced Filters

Advanced filters allow you to use an essentially unlimited number of criteria to filter your data.

To make what is known as a *criteria range*, copy the labels for the columns into an area at least three rows above the actual list. Suppose that you want to show only those students who have more than 90 percent in both the Test1 and Test2 fields. (As it turns out, you can filter this data using the AutoFilter tool, but many worksheets require criteria that examine more than two fields.) Enter the conditions for each field you want to filter by in the row directly beneath the appropriate column labels, as shown in Figure 14.6. Because this example does not filter by criteria for the Students and Average labels, these labels were not copied to the criteria range. If you want to have criteria for those fields also, place them in the same row as the others, with the criteria you wanted in the corresponding cell underneath.

Once you have the criteria range in place, select a cell of the data and choose Data | Filter | Advanced Filter from the menu. Enter the range of cells you want to filter. In the example shown in Figure 14.6, the entire table of data is specified in the List Range box. In the Criteria Range box, enter the range of cells in which the criteria is located. In this example, the criteria range is C1:D2. You can make the references relative or absolute, depending on your purposes.

14

Figure 14.6.

Entering advanced filter criteria.

Criteria range ——

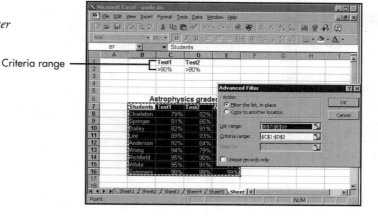

You can then choose from one of two options:

- [ ] **Filter in place.** The default option is Filter the List, In-Place. The column labels at the top of the data table stay in place but some rows may disappear, based on the filtering choices.

- [ ] **Copy the list to another location.** If you select the Copy to Another Location checkbox on the Advanced Filter dialog box, the filtered cells are copied to a new location. If you select this option, enter the cell range to which you want to copy the filtered data in the Copy To box (alternatively, you can point to and click the cell that is to be the upper-left corner of the copied range).

If you select the Unique Records Only checkbox, any duplicate rows are filtered out of the results. Of course, most of the time, your database will not contain two rows that are exact duplicates.

Once you have made your selections from the Advanced Filter dialog box, click OK; the filtering takes place, just as you specified.

TIME SAVER

> If you create a range named `Criteria` in your worksheet, Excel looks there for the Advanced Filter criteria. Place the labels and conditions in the `Criteria` range as described at the beginning of this section if you want to use this option.

14

Sorting Data

You can use the sort feature to organize data according to particular criteria. Excel can take some guesses about how you want the data organized, depending on what type of data it is. In comparison to filtering data, sorting data does not eliminate any of the data from view. You still see all the data, but it is organized in a particular way.

 Suppose that you have entered several names of American states in an Excel worksheet. You can use the Sort Ascending tool to alphabetize these names beginning with the letter A. To sort the list of state names in ascending order, select the column containing the data you want to sort and click the Sort Ascending tool in the Standard toolbar; the names in the column are automatically alphabetized.

For a numerical list of data, the Sort Ascending tool sorts the data beginning with the smallest numerical entry and progressing to the largest numerical entry.

If you click the Sort Descending tool, the state names are sorted in reverse order (that is, beginning with the letter Z and progressing to the letter A). For a numerical list of data, the Sort Descending tool sorts the data beginning with the largest numerical entry and progressing to the smallest numerical entry.

JUST A MINUTE

> If you have a list of dates, the Sort Ascending tool arranges the dates from earliest to latest; the Sort Descending tool arranges the dates from latest to earliest.

You can do the same kind of sorting if the data is organized in a row. Just select the data and use the Sort Ascending or Sort Descending tool.

Figure 14.7 shows a list with two fields: Customers and amount of Product Purchased. You can sort this data by either field. If you do an ascending sort by customer names, the list appears in alphabetical order beginning with the letter A. If you do an ascending sort by product purchased, the customer who has purchased the least is first in the resulting list. The opposite occurs if you do a descending sort.

JUST A MINUTE

> When the sort tools are arranging data, they use the *actual value* of the data within the cells, not the data's formatted appearance. Although you can display numbers with only a specified number of decimal places, they contain up to 15 decimal places. Excel sorts data based on its actual value.

14

Figure 14.7.

Sorting a list by one of the fields.

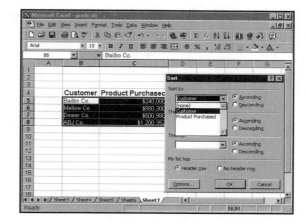

Creating a Custom AutoFill List

With Custom AutoFill, you can create a list and then save it for later use. For example, you can create a list of countries and make it a Custom AutoFill list. Then, when you enter the names of two of the countries in the list, you can use Custom AutoFill to fill in the rest of the list. Or you may have a list of the months of the year or days of the week in another language. The default Excel AutoFill feature recognizes months of the year and days of the week in English; you might want to expand this feature to include other languages.

Here's how to use the Custom AutoFill feature:

1. Create the list you want to use later for Custom AutoFill. One simple possibility is to enter abbreviations for the days of the week: S, M, Tu, W, Th, F, and Sa.

   Enter the list in a sequential row or column in your Excel worksheet, just as you would any other data.

2. Select the list.

3. Select Tools | Options to display the Options dialog box; select the Custom Lists tab, as shown in Figure 14.8.

4. Click the Import button.

5. Click OK.

Instead of selecting the list in the worksheet before you open the Options dialog box and click the Import button, you can type the range of cells in which the list is located in the Import List from Cells box in the Options dialog box.

14

Figure 14.8.

The Custom Lists tab of the Options dialog box.

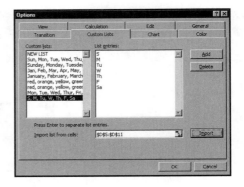

Once you have created the AutoFill list, you can use it in any of your Excel worksheets. Just enter the first two terms of the series in your worksheet and then use the AutoFill tool to fill in the rest of the series. For example, if you save a list with the entries S, M, Tu, W, Th, F, and Sa, you can later enter S and M in two adjacent cells and AutoFill will recognize the pattern. You can also enter any two adjacent entries from the list, such as Th and F, and use the AutoFill tool to complete the series. With a custom AutoFill list—just as with a default AutoFill list— the series repeats as necessary to fill all the cells selected. Thus, if you start this custom AutoFill series with S and want to fill 10 cells in a row, the 10 cells are filled in the following order from left to right:

S M Tu W Th F Sa S M Tu

You can also display the Options dialog box, select the Custom Lists tab, and create a new list directly in the dialog box, without first having to enter one in the worksheet. From the Customs List tab, click the Add button and then enter the entries you want in the List Entries pane. Click OK when you are finished with your list.

The lists you add to the Custom Lists tab of the options dialog box are available not just to the worksheet; they are available globally.

Sorting by an AutoFill List

If you have data that corresponds to the entries in an AutoFill list, you can sort the data according to the AutoFill list. Consider the worksheet shown in Figure 14.9; you can sort the list using the AutoFill option that lists the days of the week in order. The result of such a sort is that your data list is sorted in order by days of the week.

14

Figure 14.9.

Sorting by an AutoFill list.

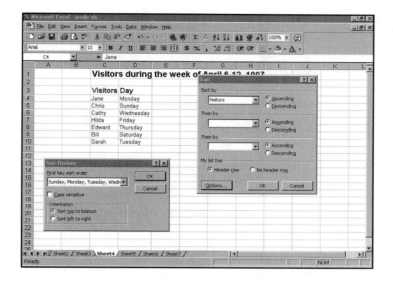

Here's how to sort a list of data using the order of elements in an AutoFill list:

1. Select a cell of the data you want to sort.

2. Choose Data | Sort from the main menu and click the Options button to display the Sort Options dialog box.

3. Click the arrow next to the drop-down list and choose the list by which you want to sort. In this example, choose the option to sort by the days of the week. Click OK on the Sort Options dialog box and click OK on the Sort dialog box.

The records are then sorted by the days of the week.

Sorting from Left to Right

Most sorting is usually done by rows (that is, entire records, or rows, of data are shuffled in the table). However, you can also sort by columns (that is, you can rearrange columns within a row). Consider the worksheet in Figure 14.10; you can sort the data in this worksheet either by name (in alphabetical order) or by hourly wage.

Here's how to sort from left to right using the Sort dialog box:

1. Select the cells in the range B7:H8. Don't include the row labels or they will be sorted with the data.

2. Select Data | Sort from the main menu to display the Sort dialog box; click the Options button to display the Sort Options dialog box.

3. Click the Sort Left to Right button at the bottom of the dialog box.

4. Click OK to close the Sort Options dialog box.

14

5. In the Sort dialog box, make sure that Row 7 is specified in the Sort By list box if you want to sort by name; make sure that Row 8 is specified in the Sort By list box if you want to sort by hourly wage.

6. Click OK to close the Sort dialog box and execute the sort.

Figure 14.10.

Sorting from left to right.

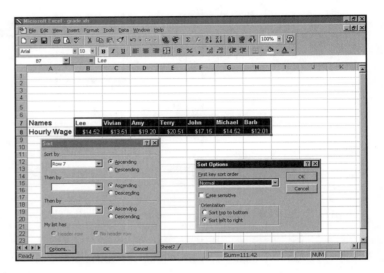

JUST A MINUTE

You can make searches case sensitive by selecting the Case Sensitive checkbox on the Sort Options dialog box.

Automatic Outlining

Outlining is a way to emphasize the important data in your worksheet, just as an outline for a word processing document shows all the headings. This section discusses how to do *automatic outlining*, in which Excel makes the decisions about to what to do. You can also do *manual outlining* if the automatic option does not suit your worksheet. For more information about manual outlining, search for Outline in Excel's online help.

If you collapse an outlined worksheet, the worksheet is reduced so that it shows only the leftmost column, the top row, and any summary columns or rows. Of course, any worksheet on which you want to use Auto Outline must be well organized. The summary columns and summary rows must use consistent formulas for each of the entries. In Figure 14.11, for example, the summary column is the one labeled Average, and the same formula is used for each row to calculate the average.

14

Creating an Outline

You can create an outline for your worksheet by choosing Data | Group and Outline from the main menu. Choose Auto Outline from the submenu. Figure 14.11 shows the Astrophysics Grades worksheet from earlier in the hour with the Auto Outline feature applied. Notice the wide bar just above the column labels. If you click the – symbol in this wide bar, the worksheet collapses to show only the Students and Average fields. Excel recognizes that the Average column consists of formulas and must therefore contain summary information. You can similarly expand or collapse the worksheet by choosing Data | Group and Outline | Hide Detail, or Data | Group and Outline | Show Detail.

Figure 14.11.

A worksheet with the Auto Outline feature applied.

Click here to collapse the worksheet

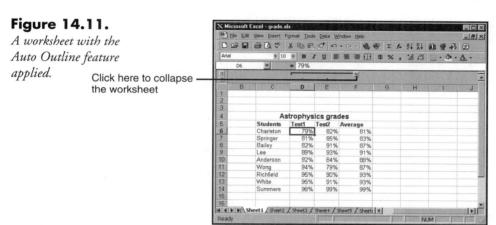

If you have laid out your data in a logical manner, Excel can discern an appropriate outline—most of the time. If your worksheet is more complex than the example shown in Figure 14.11, you are given more options to expand or collapse it. To find out more about the different outline options, look in Excel's online help under Outlines—expanding and collapsing.

Clearing the Outline

To clear the outline from the worksheet so that all the rows and columns are once again displayed, simply choose Data | Group and Outline | Clear Outline from the main menu.

Summary

Internal databases in Excel are called *lists*. A database has fields and records; *fields* are equivalent to columns, and *records* are equivalent to rows. With filtering tools like AutoFilter, you can hide or display all rows or columns that fit certain criteria. The Advanced Filter tool allows you more options to filter the data in lists. Outlining data is a way for you to see the

14

various parts of a list more clearly, and to zero in on the data that is important to you. You can sort alphabetically or numerically in a logical manner with the Sort Ascending and Sort Descending tools. And you can use the Custom AutoFill feature to create lists and custom sort patterns.

Workshop

Term Review

criteria range   A range in which you enter the specific filtering criteria for a list.

database   A document that stores information in an organized fashion and that is designed for retrieval of information.

field   A database term that is equivalent to a column in Excel.

field name   The label for a field (equivalent to the label for a column in Excel).

filter   With a filter, certain data is hidden or displayed in accordance with specific criteria you specify.

list   An internal database—one stored in an Excel worksheet.

outline   A summary of the data in an Excel worksheet.

record   A database term that is equivalent to a row in Excel.

sort   When you sort data, it is organized in a way that makes sense. For example, textual data can be alphabetized, and numeric data can be organized from least to greatest or vice versa. No records are hidden, as they are when you filter data. You can also choose your own sort criteria.

Q&A

Q What does Custom AutoFill do?

A You can use this feature to create lists that the AutoFill tool can recognize.

Q What is AutoFilter?

A AutoFilter is a tool for filtering rows in a worksheet (equivalent to records in a database) so that only the rows you are looking for are displayed.

Q What is Advanced Filter?

A Advanced Filter is a tool for filtering with multiple criteria in place on one or more fields.

14

Exercises

1. Create a Custom AutoFill list for the colors of the rainbow: red, orange, yellow, green, blue, violet, and indigo.

   To do this, first enter the list in a worksheet. Select the list and then select Tools | Options from the main menu to display the Options dialog box. Click the Custom Lists tab.

2. Outline some of the worksheets you have created in earlier chapters.

14

Hour 15

Using Pivot Tables

Pivot tables are mechanisms you can use to "swing" data around to get a different perspective on it. You may have a spreadsheet with masses of information on it, but no real way to make sense of it. Pivot tables can help make sense of those rows and columns. They can be used to analyze data, summarize data, prepare data for charting, and create reports. Pivot tables are suited to data that has many repeated categories and data that is reasonably complex. If your data consists of only one field, you probably won't find a pivot table to be helpful.

The PivotTable Wizard makes the process of creating a pivot table easy. Follow the steps, and you can present your data in a number of different ways based on the fields you choose to highlight or ignore.

Although a pivot table can use outside data, this chapter focuses on pivot tables created from lists. When you create the list for the pivot table, make sure that you use column labels. Because the pivot table generates totals and subtotals, you don't need to include the total information in your list.

Creating Pivot Tables Using the PivotTable Wizard

The first step in creating a pivot table is to have your data in the form of a list, as described in Hour 14, "More Data Manipulation." Figure 15.1 shows a typical list representing the sales of two products in various regions. (This example is very simple; you could complicate it by adding the names of salespersons, more products, and so forth.)

The pivot table you create in this example is really a means by which you can filter data in an advanced and efficient manner. In this example, the pivot table will summarize the product sales totals by region. You will be able to see the total product sales for any particular region, or for all the regions at once.

Figure 15.1.

A simple data list.

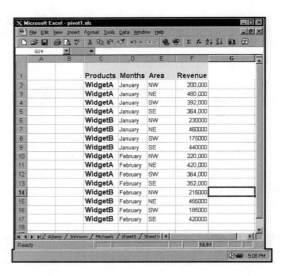

Select any cell within the list, and then follow these steps to use the PivotTable Wizard:

1. Choose Data | Pivot Table Report from the main menu to display the dialog box in Figure 15.2.

2. Because this example focuses on taking data from a Microsoft Excel list, select the Microsoft Excel List or Database option (the default). Click Next to display the second step of the PivotTable Wizard (see Figure 15.3).

15

Figure 15.2.

The first step of the PivotTable Wizard.

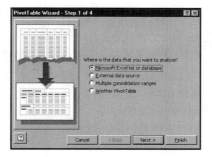

Figure 15.3.

The second step of the PivotTable dialog box.

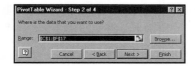

3. Verify that the default range in the Step 2 dialog box is the data list you want to use as the pivot table. Excel makes a good effort—and is usually correct—at choosing the cells that make up the pivot table. If the range Excel displays in the Step 2 dialog box is not correct, you can change it: Place the cursor inside the field and change the cell references of the range. In this example, the range is $C$1:$F$17. If you want to include only the range C1:F14, for example, type **$C$1:$F$14**.

If you want to select the range with the mouse, click the Collapse Dialog icon. You can then highlight the cells you want; click the Expand Dialog icon when you are finished selecting the range to return to the dialog box.

4. When the correct range has been specified, click Next. The Step 3 dialog box of the PivotTable Wizard appears (see Figure 15.4).

The choices you make in this dialog box determine the field around which your pivot table will pivot. You can drag the control buttons to the following areas of the pivot table: Page, Column, Row, and Data. (The best way to see the effects of different choices is by experimenting.)

Area	Description
Page	The field or fields you choose are what is used to filter the data by.
Row	The field or fields you choose are displayed in a row orientation in your pivot table.
Column	The field or fields you choose are displayed in a column orientation in your pivot table.
Data	The field or fields you choose are the fields whose data is summarized. For example, the fields dealing with numerical data are the appropriate choice for this sample pivot table.

Figure 15.4.

*The third step of the
PivotTable Wizard.*

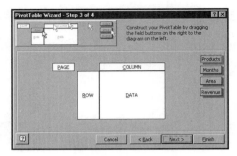

5. You can make other choices if you want, but for this example, drag the Area
   button from the right side of the dialog box to the Page area. Drag the Products button from the right side of the dialog box to the Column area. Drag
   the Revenue button from the right side of the dialog box to the Data area. Drag
   the Months button from the right side of the dialog box to the Row area.

   The result of all this manipulation is shown in Figure 15.5. If you have a complex
   list, you do not have to use all the fields. Simply choose those you want to analyze.

Figure 15.5.

*The third dialog box
with the buttons in place.*

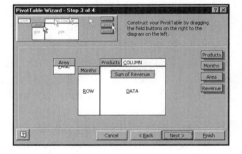

6. Click Next when you are finished. The Step 4 dialog box of the PivotTable Wizard
   appears (see Figure 15.6).

Figure 15.6.

*The fourth step of the
PivotTable Wizard.*

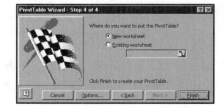

7. Select the New Worksheet option if you want to display the pivot table in a
   separate worksheet; select the Existing Worksheet option if you want the pivot
   table to be displayed in the active worksheet.

8. Click Finish to complete the wizard. The final pivot table looks like the one in Figure 15.7.

Figure 15.7.

A simple pivot table.

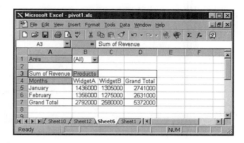

When you look at the pivot table in Figure 15.7, you may wonder what has happened to the original data. The pivot table shows summarized totals instead of each month's sales for each region, as the original data list showed.

If you want to see the total sales for a particular region, click the arrow next to the Area cell at the top of the pivot table to display a drop-down list. Note that Products is displayed as columns (remember that you placed the Products button in the Column field in the Step 3 dialog box). Months are displayed as rows (because you placed the Months button in the Rows field). Each of the fields you moved into a particular location in the Step 3 dialog box has its corresponding button.

COFFEE BREAK

Renaming Fields

Note that the field Revenue, which was put in the Data portion of the pivot field, is automatically renamed Sum of Revenue. In fact, any field you place in the Data area is automatically preceded by Sum of in the pivot table. If you don't like the Sum of XXXXXX name, you can change it within the pivot table, just as you change the name of any other cell. However, you cannot change Sum of Revenue back to Revenue; if you try to do so, you get an error message saying that the pivot table field name already exists. You can change the name to Revenues, put a space in front of the word Revenue, or come up with a similar workaround.

Similarly, you can rename any of the other field names in your pivot table. Just follow the same procedure you do for other cells in an Excel worksheet: Click the cell and type over the text you want to replace with the new information. Keep in mind that you cannot use a label that is already in use.

Using the PivotTable Options Dialog Box

You can change a number of the options that control how your pivot table appears and behaves. In the Step 4 dialog box of the PivotTable Wizard, click the Options button to display the PivotTable Options dialog box shown in Figure 15.8.

JUST A MINUTE

You can access the Step 4 dialog box even after you finish with the Pivot-Table Wizard: From the main menu of the worksheet containing the pivot table, select Data | PivotTable Report. The Step 3 dialog box appears. Click Next to display the Step 4 dialog box and then click the Options button.

Figure 15.8.

The PivotTable Options dialog box.

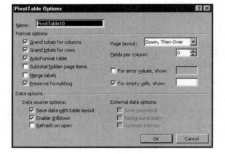

Check and uncheck the boxes as needed to get the result you want. You can choose a variety of formatting and data options, as shown in Table 15.1. Most of these options are presented as checkboxes: If you want a certain option, check the appropriate box. In general, the defaults for the options in this dialog box work very well; there is little need to change them.

Table 15.1. Pivot table options.

Option	Results
Format Options	
Grand totals for columns	Displays the grand totals for the columns of the pivot table.
Grand totals for rows	Displays the grand totals for the rows of the pivot table.

15

15

Option	Results
AutoFormat table	Formats the pivot table in the standard Excel manner.
Subtotal hidden page items	Includes the value of hidden cells in the subtotals.
Merge labels	Merges cells for the outer row and column labels.
Preserve formatting	Retains the formatting of the data in the pivot table when the layout is changed.
Page layout	Use this option to specify the order in which the page fields appear.
Fields per column	Use this option to select the number of page fields to include in a row or column before another row or column of the page layout is started.
For error values, show	Use this option to choose your own error message if you want one.
For empty values, show	Use this option to specify a message or value to display for empty cells.

Data Options

Option	Results
Save data with table layout	Saves an external copy of the data to which the pivot table is linked.
Enable drilldown	Prevents showing source data when a cell in the pivot table is double-clicked.
Refresh on open	Updates the pivot table data from the source data every time the workbook containing it is opened.

External Data Options

Option	Results
Save password	Saves the password to the external database so that you do not have to enter it again.
Save background query	Saves the query to the external database so that you do not have to enter it again.
Optimize memory	Conserves memory when you create a table from external data.

Manipulating the Pivot Table

Once the pivot table exists, you can manipulate it to see the data in a different light. In Figure 15.7, earlier in this chapter, notice the Area button in the top-left corner of the worksheet. If you click the arrow in cell B2, you see a list of the following Area options: All, NE, NW, SE, and SW. Each option provides you with a different look at the data. In this pivot table, the Area field serves as the "pivot" around which you can "swing" the data.

If you choose a particular value for Area, such as SW, the pivot table shows you the values only for the SW area. Similarly, if you choose NW, the pivot table shows you only the values for the NW area. As you can see, a pivot table is essentially a sophisticated filtering device.

Modifying Pivot Tables

You can modify pivot tables by dragging the buttons to new locations on the pivot table itself. Suppose that you do not want to "pivot" the data by the Area (refer back to Figure 15.7); suppose that you want to pivot the data by the Product instead. To see this kind of result, drag the Area button to where the Product button is located and then drag the Product button to where the Area button was located. In this version of the pivot table, you can look at the totals by product; the subtotals are given by region (see Figure 15.9).

Figure 15.9.

A reorganized pivot table.

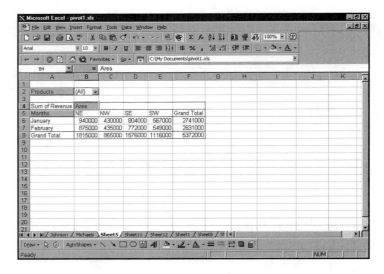

You can also change the orientation of the rows and columns. Right-click a button and select Field from the popup menu. The PivotTable Field dialog box appears (see Figure 15.10). Make your choices and click OK to return to the PivotTable Options dialog box.

Changing the way you make subtotals with the PivotTable Field dialog box is discussed later in this hour, in "Using the PivotTable Toolbar."

15

Figure 15.10.

The PivotTable Field dialog box.

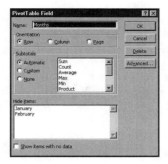

Deleting a Pivot Table

The easiest way to delete a pivot table is to delete the worksheet that contains it (unless, of course, the pivot table's worksheet contains other data you want to keep). You can also select all the cells in the pivot table and clear the contents of the cells, or delete the cells as you would any others. You can delete fields from a pivot table (as described in the following section), but you cannot delete individual cells of a pivot table.

Deleting Data or Fields from a Pivot Table

It's usually easier to *not* include data in your pivot table in the first place rather than to delete it later. However, if you want your pivot table to have less data, an easy way to do that is to use a list that itself contains less data.

You control which data from your original data list is used for the pivot table when you are asked for the range in the Step 2 dialog box of the PivotTable Wizard. Remember that you do not have to include all the fields of your original data list when preparing a pivot table; don't drag the fields you don't want to use into the pivot table in the Step 3 dialog box of the PivotTable Wizard.

You can also delete fields from existing pivot tables. To delete a field from an existing pivot table, position the mouse pointer over the field button and drag it. As the pointer leaves the pivot table, it changes to the form of a large ×. When you release the mouse, the field button and the accompanying data are gone from the pivot table.

Displaying the Wizard Dialog Boxes Again

You can display the PivotTable Wizard dialog boxes again at any time. Choose a cell or a range within the pivot table and right-click to see the popup menu shown in Figure 15.11.

Click the Wizard option and you will see the Step 3 dialog box of the PivotTable Wizard (refer back to Figure 15.4). You can use this dialog box to readjust the fields if you want. You can also go to any of the other dialog boxes by clicking the Back or Next button. Make the modifications you want for any of the dialog boxes and click Finish when you are done.

Figure 15.11.

Get this popup menu by
right-clicking the pivot
table.

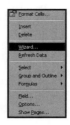

Changing the Data

If you change the data in the original list, you can update the pivot table by choosing
Data | Refresh Data from the main menu in the worksheet in which the pivot table is located.

If you add new fields or records to your original data list, you must bring up the Step 3 dialog
box of the PivotTable Wizard again. Here's how:

1. Go to the worksheet containing the pivot table.
2. Either right-click a pivot table cell and select Wizard from the popup menu or
   choose Data | Pivot Table Report from the main menu. The Step 3 dialog box of
   the PivotTable Wizard appears.
3. Click the Back button to return to the Step 2 dialog box.
4. Change the cell range in the second dialog box to include all the new data you have
   entered.
5. Click the Next button to go to the Step 3 dialog box again.
6. Drag the buttons to the various areas as you did in "Creating Pivot Tables Using
   the PivotTable Wizard," earlier in this hour.
7. Either click the Next button to continue to the Step 4 dialog box or click Finish to
   complete the wizard.

Having Two or More Pivots

You can have two or more fields serve as pivots. Just open the Step 3 dialog box of the
PivotTable Wizard and drag the buttons for the fields you want to use as pivots onto the Page
area. Figure 15.12 shows what the list originally shown in Figure 15.7 looks like with two
pivots: Products and Area.

You can also drag the buttons around in the pivot table worksheet to achieve the same effect.
For example, if you want to filter by both Product and Area, you can drag the Product button
to where the Area button is.

15

Figure 15.12.

A pivot table using two pivots.

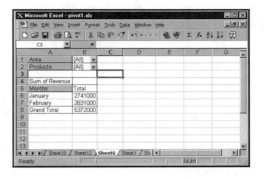

Using the PivotTable Toolbar

You can display the PivotTable toolbar, shown in Figure 15.13, by choosing View | Toolbars | PivotTable from the main menu.

Figure 15.13.

The PivotTable toolbar.

Pivot Table Field tool

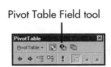

If you click the PivotTable Field tool on the PivotTable toolbar, the PivotTable Field dialog box shown in Figure 15.14 appears. The pivot table examples shown in this chapter all use the SUM function to get the totals. However, you can use other mathematical functions, instead. Suppose that you want to see the maximum for the Revenue field. Choose Max of Revenue from the Summarize By options. The other Summarize By options may or may not be applicable, depending on the type of data you have. As discussed in the section "Modifying Pivot Tables," earlier in this hour, you can also change the row and column orientation of your data with the PivotTable Field dialog box.

Figure 15.14.

The PivotTable Field dialog box.

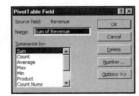

If you have selected a numeric field, the Number button appears on the dialog box, as it does in Figure 15.14. To format the cells, click the Number button to see a list of formatting options.

Summary

Pivot tables let you look at data from a number of different perspectives. You can get different subtotals for different fields, depending on how you choose to arrange your data. If you use pivot tables properly, you can get a much better insight into what your data means. The examples in this chapter are, of necessity, on a small scale. The usefulness of the summarization features is much more apparent when you have a large list with numerous fields and records.

Workshop

Term Review

pivot table   An interactive table that lets you look at relationships between the data and serves as an advanced data filtering device.

Q&A

Q What do pivot tables do?

A Pivot tables allow you to look at data in different ways. You can get different subtotals depending on the conditions you choose.

Q Are pivot tables easy to make?

A Yes, the PivotTable Wizard makes the process easy. Follow the prompts and experiment to see different possibilities.

Exercises

1. Enter the data shown in Figure 15.15 into a worksheet. This data list represents visitors to two attractions: SeaSaw and DryDock.

2. Create a pivot table with the PivotTable Wizard so that the result looks like the result shown in Figure 15.16.

   Try moving and rearranging the buttons to see different orientations.

   For more fun, create and add to the original data list some figures for visitors for a third attraction: SpaceHigh. Then refresh the pivot table to reflect the new information.

   For even more extra credit, format the pivot table. Remove the gridlines and choose the size and color options you prefer for maximum attractiveness.

15

Figure 15.15.

A worksheet data list example.

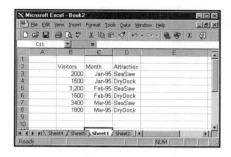

Figure 15.16.

A pivot table made from the sample data.

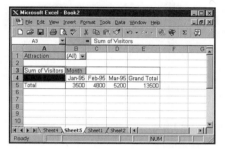

Hour 16

Using Excel to Analyze Data

Excel includes a variety of tools to use for data analysis and forecasting. You can do "what-if" scenarios to determine the best values for given variables.

So far, you have learned how to use functions and formulas in Excel. However, what you have done up until now has focused on obtaining the end result of the formula, rather than looking backward to obtain values of variables based on a particular formula result.

For example, you know that if you want to compute the income you will earn on $1,000 with an annual interest rate of 8 percent, you use the formula `0.08*1000`. Tools such as Goal Seek and Solver, which come with the Excel package, let you decide the formula value you want and then find the values of the variables needed to get that formula value. For example, if you want to know how much money you have to invest at an annual 8-percent interest rate to end up with $1,200 at the end of the year, you can do so easily with Excel's data-analysis tools.

Using the Goal Seek Tool

The Goal Seek tool can look at a formula and then determine the appropriate value of a single variable, given the formula result. Goal Seek is good for single-variable formulas. The Solver tool, described later in this hour, is designed for finding multivariable solutions.

An Example of Goal Seek in Action

In this example, you see how to use Goal Seek to determine the amount of sales Jane Smith would have to make to earn $4,000 per month. Suppose that Jane earns $2,000 per month base salary; she earns commissions of 5 percent on gross sales. Figure 16.1 shows a simple table that represents the situation. The formula in cell F4 is =C4+D4*E4.

Figure 16.1.

The pay structure for a sales commission job.

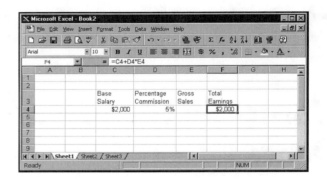

You could fiddle around with various values for gross sales to find monthly earnings to total $4,000. Although you probably can do the question in your head in a moment, this exercise is designed to show how to use Goal Seek. Goal Seek's power is most apparent when you are dealing with complicated worksheets and workbooks or repeating similar tasks over and over again.

In this example, you want to find what value cell E4, Gross Sales, has to be in order to make the value of cell F4, Total Earnings, equal to $4,000. Here's how you use Goal Seek to answer this question:

1. Select the cell that contains the formula whose value you want to control. In this example, select cell F4.

2. Select Tools | Goal Seek from the main menu to display the Goal Seek dialog box shown in Figure 16.2.

3. Make sure that the cell you want to control (that is, the cell for which you know the desired answer—cell F4 in this example), is shown in the Set Cell box.

16

4. Enter the value you want Total Earnings to be in the To Value box. For this example, enter 4,000.

5. Enter the cell whose value you want to change in the By Changing Cell box. For this example, the cell you want to change is E4.

6. Click OK when finished. Goal Seek displays the Goal Seek Status dialog box that indicates whether or not it was able to achieve the result. Goal Seek places a value in the changing cell (in this example, cell E4). Goal Seek changes the value of F4 to the result you wanted. In this example, Goal Seek calculates that the value in E4 has to be 40,000. Click OK to accept the values.

What the results of Goal Seek tell you is this: If Jane earns $2,000 per month base salary and earns 5% commission on gross sales, she must make monthly gross sales of $40,000 to achieve total monthly earnings of $4,000.

Figure 16.2.

The Goal Seek dialog box.

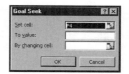

Using Goal Seek with a Chart

Suppose that you have created a table of data like the one shown in Figure 16.3 to get a better idea of the sales you need to make to reach various monthly earning targets. You can convert this data table into a chart, as described in Hour 9, "Creating Excel Charts." As you know, you can create a chart based on any formula-generated values. The chart shown in Figure 16.3 graphs total earnings against gross sales.

Figure 16.3.

A table of data and its corresponding chart.

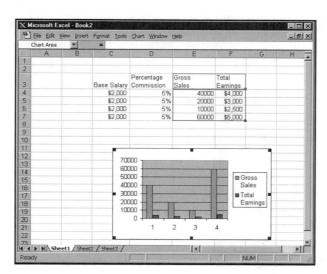

When you have a chart that includes values calculated by a formula, you can use Goal Seek to alter values. To use Goal Seek with a chart, click one of the data points for the values generated by a formula and drag it to the value you want it to be. In this example, try dragging one of the data points for Total Earnings. You will immediately see the Goal Seek dialog box. Enter the values as described in the preceding section and click OK. Goal Seek generates a solution and displays the Goal Seek Status dialog box. Click OK if you want to redraw the chart to reflect the new value.

Understanding Goal Seek Error Messages

If you select a cell that does not contain a value or enter a blank cell into the Set Cell box in the Goal Seek dialog box, you get the `Cell must contain a value` error message.

If you select or enter a cell that contains a constant rather than a formula into the Set Cell box in the Goal Seek dialog box, you get the `Cell must contain a formula` error message.

Using the Solver Tool

The Solver tool uses algorithms to solve problems with multiple variables. Most often, the solutions Solver offers are not exact; they are found by approximation.

To use Solver, first make sure that the tool is installed: Pull down the Tools menu on the main menu bar and look for the Solver option. If Solver is not there, you must install it: Choose Tools | Add-ins from the main menu to display the Add-Ins dialog box. Select the Solver Add-In box and click OK.

Excel includes an example of Solver's being used to solve a problem. If you have installed the program in the default directory, this is the path to the sample file:

```
C:\Program Files\Microsoft Office\Office\Examples\Solver\Solvsamp.xls
```

This file includes examples showing Solver applied to several unique commercial, industrial, and scientific problems. Looking at this file can give you some inspiration about when you might want to apply Solver to your data.

When you use Solver, you must be familiar with these terms:

- ☐ **Changing cells.** These are the values of the variables in the cells that the Solver utility manipulates to get the target value. You can have up to 200 changing cells.
- ☐ **Constraints.** These are the limits placed on the variables. Perhaps one or more of the variables must be a positive number, a negative number, an integer, or must fall within a given numerical range.
- ☐ **Target cells.** These are the cells that contain the values for which Solver tries to solve by changing the values in the changing cells.

16

A Solver Example

Suppose that you are developing a type of all-purpose flour that is to have between 12 and 12.5 percent gluten. You want the cheapest mix you can make, and you will be using and mixing up to three different types of flour to achieve this result. (*Gluten* is a special protein in flour that makes it possible for bread to rise, but it is also the component that can make cakes and pastries tough.) You know these things about the three types of flour you will mix together:

☐ Flour A has 10 percent gluten. It is the cheapest, at 8 cents per pound.

☐ Flour B has 14 percent gluten. It is the most expensive at 20 cents per pound.

☐ Flour C has 11 percent gluten. It costs 11 cents per pound.

Start by creating a table with headings like the ones shown in Figure 16.4.

Figure 16.4.

A simple table for calculating an optimal flour mix .

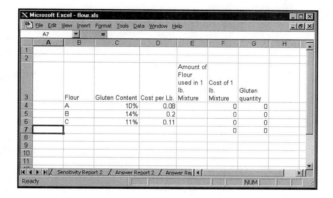

Columns C and D contain the *constants*: the percentage of gluten of each type of flour, and the price per pound of each type of flour. You are trying to solve for the values in cells E4, E5, and E6, and you want to minimize the cost of the mixed flour.

Cells E4, E5, and E6 contain the amount (in pounds) of each type of flour used in the mix. E7 must total one pound and E4:E6 are the *changing cells*.

Cell F7 is the *target cell*. It contains the total cost of one pound of flour, based on the costs of each component of the mix. Cells F4, F5, and F6 contain the cost of each component. You calculate the cost of each component with reference to the values in columns D and E. The formula to place in cell F4 is =D4*E4, which is the cost per pound (cell D4) multiplied by the amount of flour used in pounds (cell E4). Drag this formula to cells F5 and F6. Cell F7 contains the sum of cells F4, F5, and F6. Place the formula =F4+F5+F6 in cell F7.

Cells G4, G5, and G6 show the amount of gluten contributed by each type of flour used in the mix. The formula to enter in cell G4 is =C4*E4, which is the gluten content multiplied by the amount of flour used in the one-pound mixture. Drag this formula to cells G5 and G6. Cell G7 contains the total amount of gluten in one pound of flour; therefore, enter the formula =G4+G5+G6 in cell G7. Because you know that the gluten content must be between 12 and 12.5 percent, you know that the value in cell G7 must be no less than 0.12 and no greater than 0.125; you will set this constraint accordingly later.

Now you are ready to use the Solver tool. Choose Tools | Solver from the main menu to display the Solver Parameters dialog box shown in Figure 16.5. Make sure that the target cell for this example is F7 (the cost per pound). Type E4:E6 in the By Changing Cells box. From the Equal To options, select Min. You choose Min in this example because you want the minimum price of flour. If you had set up a different scenario in which you wanted to maximize the result cell, you would choose Max. If you had a particular value in mind, you would select Value Of.

Figure 16.5.

The Solver Parameters dialog box.

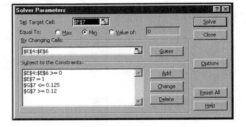

Now you must set up the constraints. You know that cell E7, which contains the sum of cells E4 to E6, must equal 1 because we are considering one pound of flour. Click the Add button to display the Add Constraint dialog box shown in Figure 16.6. Choose the appropriate values for the Cell Reference (in this case, the cell is E7), the comparison operator (in this case, the operator is =), and the Constraint (the value you want to set the cell to is 1). Click OK when finished.

Figure 16.6.

Setting constraints in the Add Constraint dialog box.

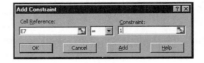

16

There are other constraints as well. You know that none of the values in column E can be negative. To add this particular constraint, click Add from the Solver Parameters dialog box to display the Add Constraint dialog box again. Enter E4:E6 in the Cell Reference box, choose >= as the comparison operator in the middle box, and enter 0 in the Constraint box. Click OK.

You also want to place a constraint on cell G7 so that its value is less than or equal to 0.125 and greater than or equal to 0.12. Each of these constraints must be added separately. Click Add from the Solver Parameters dialog box to display the Add Constraint dialog box again, and enter the constraint G7 <= 0.125. Click OK and then add the constraint G7 >= 0.12.

Note that if you want to change or delete constraints, you can do that from the Solver Parameters dialog box. Highlight the constraint and click Change or Delete.

When you are finished adding constraints, click OK to close the Solver Parameters dialog box. If you have done everything right, the Solver program works out a solution and shows you the Solver Results dialog box (see Figure 16.7). The values Solver comes up with are shown in the empty spaces in the data table. Click OK if you want to keep the values, or click Cancel if you do not. The Save Scenario button is discussed in the next section.

JUST A MINUTE

As you can see in Figure 16.7, Solver may provide you with answers that use more decimal places than you want or need. You can control the numeric display by formatting the cells with the Format Cells dialog box, as you ordinarily do, so that only a specified number of decimal places are shown.

Figure 16.7.

The Solver Results dialog box and the values calculated by Solver.

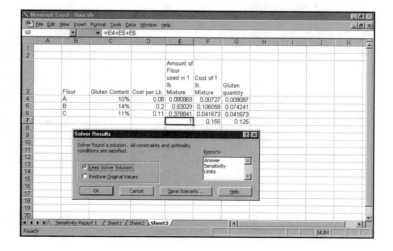

JUST A MINUTE

This example of the use of Solver started with no values entered in the target cells E4:E6. However, if you enter guesses in the target cells, you can make it easier and quicker for your computer to come up with the answers, particularly for complicated situations. When you enter guesses in the target cells, you give Solver "hints" about what values it can start experimenting with. Even if your guesses are way off base, Solver still finds a correct answer; if your guesses are reasonable, Solver can find an answer more quickly.

Making Use of Solver's Options

From the Solver Parameters dialog box, you can click Options to display the Solver Options dialog box (see Figure 16.8). You can change any or all of the options in this dialog box. If you are doing a complicated problem, you may want to increase the maximum iterations and the maximum time. Solver works by plugging numbers into the changing cells and then adjusts the values by looking at whether the result cell is close to the result you wanted. The next numbers Solver chooses in its effort to get the appropriate result are based on the previous numbers. Each separate set of numbers that Solver tries is called an *iteration*. In general, the more iterations you do, the closer the final result is to what you want. This is particularly true if you have a complicated problem you want Solver to solve. If you specify a maximum time, you limit the amount of time Solver can spend on the problem. Clearly, the greater the time, the more iterations Solver can perform.

You can also set the precision level you want for the final result. In general, real-world problems are never solved precisely; they are solved to a specified number of decimal places. You can determine how precise you want the final result to be.

Figure 16.8.

The Solver Options dialog box.

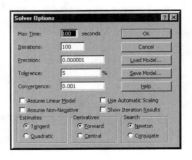

Solver is a relatively easy tool to use to crunch difficult numerical problems.

16

Obtaining Solver Reports

After you obtain a result from Solver, you see the Solver Results dialog box, which you can use to generate reports. Choose the report option you want from the Reports list in the Solver Results dialog box and double-click it. Three types of reports are available:

Report Type	Description
Answers	This report shows the target cell, the changing cells with their original and final values, and the constraints.
Sensitivity	This report looks at how small changes in the formula affect the values Solver provides.
Limits	This report indicates the upper and lower limits for the target cell and the changing cells, their initial values, and their target values.

Each report you create is placed on a separate worksheet.

Changing Scenarios

A *scenario* is a particular set of values for the changing cells. You can alter these values and save each separate altered set as a different scenario.

When you finish running Solver for a set of data and get the values it produces, you can click the Save Scenario button at the bottom of the Solver Results dialog box. Choose a name for the scenario and click OK.

To create a scenario manually, choose Tools | Scenario from the main menu to display the Scenario Manager dialog box shown in Figure 16.9. Click the Add button to display the Add Scenario dialog box. Enter the name of the scenario you are going to create and enter the cell references for the changing cells. You can choose whether or not you want to protect the scenario, and whether or not to hide the scenario.

Figure 16.9.

The Scenario Manager dialog box.

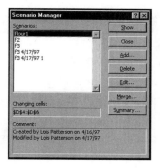

16

If you want to use a particular scenario again, simply select its name from the Scenario Manager dialog box and click Show. The values in the changing cells change to correspond to the selected scenario.

Obtaining a Scenario Report

To create a summary of different scenarios, first select the scenario you want to summarize from the Scenario Manager dialog box. Then click Summary to display the Scenario Summary dialog box. From this dialog box, you can select either Scenario Summary or Scenario Pivot Table. You can accept the default cell reference (Excel chooses the target cell Solver calculates for you) or you can change the cell references in the Result Cells box if necessary. If you have multiple result cells, enter the cell references separated by commas. Click OK.

If you choose the Scenario Summary option, a new worksheet is added to your workbook called Scenario Summary. This new worksheet lists the changing cells, their associated values, and the result cells.

If you choose the Scenario Pivot Table option, a worksheet called Scenario Pivot Table is added to your workbook. You can edit this pivot table in the same way you can any other pivot table, as discussed in Hour 15, "Using Pivot Tables."

Merging Scenarios

You can merge scenarios from different worksheets into the active worksheet. If you have scenarios in two or more worksheets and want to merge them, click Merge from the Scenario Manager dialog box to display the Merge Scenarios dialog box. The various scenarios must refer to the same changing cells, including the changing cells on the active workbook.

Using the Report Manager Tool

The Report Manager is used to create and define custom reports. You can use specific worksheets, views, and scenarios in your reports. You generally create reports so that you can print only the information you require, rather than the entire worksheet or workbook.

Creating a Report

To create a report, select View | Report Manager from the main menu to display the Report Manager dialog box shown in Figure 16.10.

Click Add to display the Add Report dialog box shown in Figure 16.11. In the Report Name box, enter a name for the report you are going to create.

16

Figure 16.10.

The Report Manager dialog box.

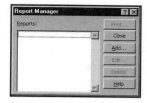

Figure 16.11.

Add Report dialog box.

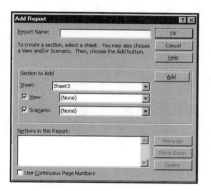

Click the Sheet drop-down list to add a worksheet to your report. Click Add when you have selected the worksheet you want. Similarly, you can use the View and Scenario drop-down lists to select any views or scenarios you want to include in the report. Add as many worksheets, views, and scenarios as you want. Each is added to the box titled Sections in this Report.

Once you have selected the sections you want to include in the report, you can rearrange them for printing. Select a section from the pane at the bottom of the dialog box and click Move Up or Move Down to change its location in the list of sections.

Check the Use Continuous Page Numbers box if you want your report's page numbers to be continuous throughout the different sections.

When you have made all your report choices, click OK to close the Add Report dialog box.

Printing a Report

To print a report, start with the Report Manager dialog box. Select the report you want to print and click the Print button.

Editing a Report

To edit a report, start with the Report Manager dialog box. Select the report you want to edit and click the Edit button to display the Edit Report dialog box. With this dialog box, you can add or delete sections from the report and change whether or not a view or scenario is added.

Deleting a Report

To delete a report, start with the Report Manager dialog box. Select the report you want to delete and click the Delete button. Click OK when prompted.

Performing Data and Statistical Analysis: The Analysis ToolPak

Excel comes with the Analysis ToolPak add-in for doing statistical and other data analysis. If the Data Analysis option does not appear on the Tools menu, install it using the instructions for installing add-ins in Hour 2, "Installing Excel 97." You can see the various tools available in the Analysis ToolPak by selecting Tools|Data Analysis from the main menu. Scroll through the dialog box shown in Figure 16.12 to see the various options available.

Figure 16.12.

The data analysis tools available in the Analysis ToolPak.

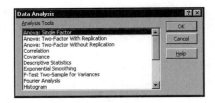

You must be familiar with the scientific or engineering significance of these functions to know what they are and how to use them. For more information about how to use these analytical tools, use the Help menu.

Summary

Excel offers a number of different tools for analyzing data and for solving for variables if given the result of the formula. You can solve simple linear equations in one variable, and you can also solve complex multivariable problems. Excel uses various algorithms to find the best possible "fit" for a problem. You can save sets of values for different variables as scenarios.

Workshop

Term Review

changing cells   The values of the variables in the cells that the Solver utility manipulates to get the target. You can have up to 200 changing cells in a problem.

constraints   The limits placed on the variables.

result cell   The cell that holds the final result calculated by the Solver or Goal Seek tool.

16

scenario   A group of constraints and assumptions made about the variables in a worksheet. You can have more than one scenario per worksheet and can use the different scenarios as appropriate.

target cells   The cells that contain the value for which the Solver tool tries to solve by changing the values in the changing cells.

Q&A

Q What's the best tool for determining the optimum value for a single variable?

A Goal Seek is the best tool for problems that have only one variable.

Q What's the best tool for determining the optimum values for more than one variable?

A Solver is an excellent tool for determining optimum values for a combination of variables, given constraints on these variables.

Q How can you do statistical analysis and Fourier analysis with Excel?

A You can do statistical, Fourier, and other types of data analysis in Excel by using the Analysis ToolPak add-in.

Exercise

Tim is paid $15 per hour for the first 40 hours per week he works; he is paid $30 per hour for the next 20 hours he works each week. Tim can work no more than 60 hours per week. Use Goal Seek to find out how many overtime hours Tim has to work to make a total of $4,000 in four weeks. Figure 16.13 contains several hints to help you solve this problem.

Figure 16.13.

Using Goal Seek to solve a wage-earning problem.

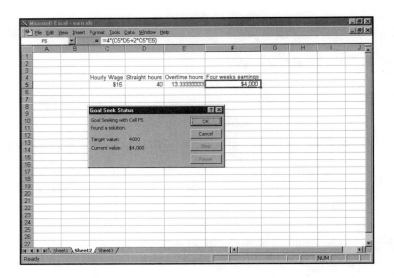

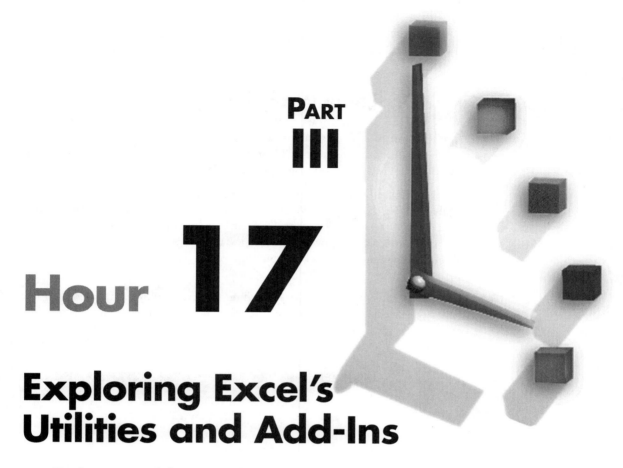

Hour **17**

Exploring Excel's Utilities and Add-Ins

Excel 97 uses wizards for a variety of processes. A *wizard* guides you through the steps of a process—you don't have to worry about missing anything as long as you carefully follow the instructions. In previous hours, you learned to use the Chart Wizard and the PivotTable Wizard. In this hour, you look at wizards designed to facilitate the creation of certain types of formulas, and wizards designed to facilitate the file conversion and file import processes. Excel also includes several wizards for use with databases; these are discussed in Hour 19, "Using Excel with Databases."

Using Wizards for Formulas

Excel has two wizards you can use to construct formulas: Conditional Sum and Lookup. You can create the same formulas without these wizards, but most of the time it's easier to use the automated wizard process. With both the Conditional Sum Wizard and the Lookup Wizard, you get the option of which cell you want to place the resulting formula in.

The Conditional Sum Wizard

The Conditional Sum Wizard is used to sum certain columns and ranges—provided that specific conditions are met. You can sum specific entries from a particular column of data—provided that certain conditions are met. These conditions can be for the entries themselves, or the conditions can be placed on other columns of data.

The following example is very simple. Another situation in which you might want to use the Conditional Sum Wizard is if you make a table showing the salaries of all of your company's employees and want to total the salaries for all employees who earn more than a given amount, or to total the salaries for all employees who earn less than a specific amount. Undoubtedly, you can think of other examples in which you want to sum only certain entries of a column, depending on the data.

Figure 17.1 shows a table in which the overtime hours of five employees are listed. Suppose that you are a management consultant measuring productivity and want to find out how many total overtime hours were worked in a given week by employees who worked more than 10 hours overtime.

Figure 17.1.

A simple table of data.

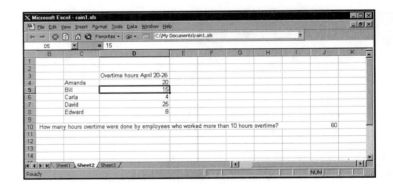

Here's one way to solve the consultant's dilemma:

1. Start by selecting the range D3:D8—the cells containing the hours of overtime worked.

2. Choose Tools|Wizard|Conditional Sum from the main menu to display the first dialog box of the Conditional Sum Wizard (see Figure 17.2). If you selected the range before you invoked the wizard, you don't have to change anything in this dialog box. If you did not select the range before invoking the wizard, enter the range that contains the values you want to add (including the column label).

17

Figure 17.2.

Step 1 of the Conditional Sum Wizard.

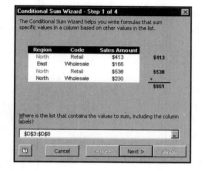

3. Click Next to display the second dialog box of the Conditional Sum Wizard (see Figure 17.3).

   In this dialog box, you want to set up a formula that sums the total hours of overtime for only those employees who worked more than 10 hours of overtime.

Figure 17.3.

Step 2 of the Conditional Sum Wizard.

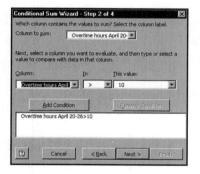

4. Set up the condition that limits which overtime hours you are adding together. The value in the Column to Sum box is `Overtime hours April 20-26` (the label in cell D3 of the worksheet range). The Column value box should also contain the value `Overtime hours April 20-26`. Choose > from the Is drop-down list. For the This Value box, specify `10`. The condition you have specified is this: For values in the `Overtime hours April 20-26` column, choose only those that are greater than `10`. Click the Add Condition button.

   If you want, you can also choose other conditions. Remember that the conditions do not have to be based on the column on which you are doing the sum.

5. Click Next to display the third dialog box of the Conditional Sum Wizard (see Figure 17.4). You can put only the formula in its own cell by choosing the Copy Just the Formula to a Single Cell option. Alternatively, you can place the formula and conditional value or values in their own cells by choosing the Copy the Formula and Conditional Values option.

Figure 17.4.

Step 3 of the Conditional Sum Wizard.

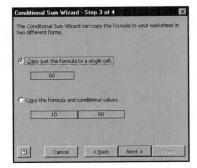

6. When you have decided how you want the formula inserted into your worksheet, click Next to display the fourth dialog box of the Conditional Sum Wizard.

   If you chose to show only the formula, you see the dialog box shown in Figure 17.5. The cell in which you want the formula placed is D10 (cell D10 is positioned as an answer to the question in cell B10 in Figure 17.1). Click Finish. The formula appears in cell D10. Select the cell and press Enter to see the result. In this case, the result is 60, meaning that those employees who worked more than 10 hours of overtime did 60 total hours of overtime.

   If you chose to show both the formula and the conditional values, you must enter the cell address in which you want the conditional values placed and the cell address in which you want the formula placed.

Figure 17.5.

Step 4 of the Conditional Sum Wizard.

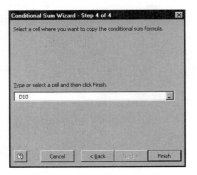

17

Note that you can move the formula to any other empty cell in the worksheet. The Conditional Sum Wizard creates the formula, and you can do with the formula as you like afterwards.

The Lookup Wizard

The Lookup Wizard program is another add-in. If you do not see it on the Tools | Wizard submenu, you can install it as an add-in using the instructions in Hour 2, "Installing Excel 97." The Lookup Wizard helps you write the formulas you need to look up the values of specific cell references in a worksheet. The wizard creates the formula, and you can then move the formula to another part of the worksheet or a different worksheet or workbook as needed. The LOOKUP, VLOOKUP, INDEX, and MATCH functions (in addition to other lookup and reference functions) are also used to locate particular values in a worksheet.

If you have a large Excel worksheet, or if you are working with a group of worksheets, you may want to look up a particular value automatically and copy that value to another cell. The Lookup Wizard creates a formula that automatically looks up a specified cell and then copies it to another cell.

The following example shows how to use the Lookup Wizard to find the cell at the intersection of a particular column and row. In this example, the formula developed by the Lookup Wizard looks up the cell at the intersection of the column Bayville and the row April. Follow these steps to use the Lookup Wizard:

1. Select a cell in the range for which you want to look up the value.
2. Choose Tools | Wizard | Lookup from the main menu to get the dialog box shown in Figure 17.6. Excel makes a fair guess at the range of data you want to search. If you want to change the range to search, enter the new range reference in this dialog box.

Figure 17.6.

Step 1 of the Lookup Wizard.

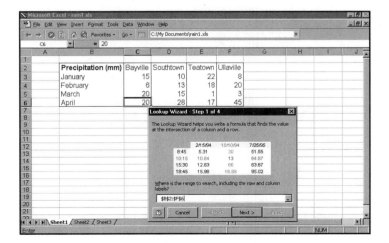

3. Click Next to display the second dialog box of the Lookup Wizard.

4. Choose the column and row you want to look up and enter the labels for the column and the row. In this example, the reference is to the cell at the intersection of the column `Bayville` and the row `April`.

5. Click Next to display the third dialog box of the Lookup Wizard. This dialog box gives you the choice between copying just the formula to a single cell and copying the formula and the lookup parameters to separate cells.

6. When you have decided how you want the formula inserted into your worksheet, click Next to display the fourth dialog box of the Lookup Wizard.

   If you chose to copy just the formula to a single cell, the fourth dialog box lets you choose the cell in which you want to paste the formula. Click Finish when you are done.

   If you chose to copy the formula and the lookup parameters, you are prompted to enter the cells in which you want to paste the formula and the lookup parameters. Click Finish when you are done.

The formula the Lookup Wizard created to look up the cell at the intersection of the column `Bayville` and the row `April` is shown here:

```
=INDEX($C$5:$G$9, MATCH("April",$C$5:$C$9,), MATCH("Bayville",$C$5:$G$5,))
```

Opening, Using, and Converting Different File Types in Excel

You can open a variety of different file formats in Excel. Choose File | Open from the main menu and select the file you want to open. Excel can open the following types of files:

- ☐ Excel 97/7.0/5.0
- ☐ Excel 4.0 macros, charts, and workbooks
- ☐ Text
- ☐ Lotus 1-2-3
- ☐ Quattro Pro/DOS
- ☐ Microsoft Works 2.0
- ☐ dBASE
- ☐ SYLK
- ☐ Data Interchange Format
- ☐ HTML
- ☐ Quattro Pro 1.0/5.0 (Windows)

17

If you are trying to import a text file, Excel guides you through the conversion steps with the Text Import Wizard, described in the following section.

You use the File Conversion Wizard to convert batches of files from one of a variety of formats to Excel format. This wizard is explained in the section, "The File Conversion Wizard," later in this hour.

You use the Convert Text to Columns Wizard to copy data from another program to Excel without converting the other file. This wizard is explained in the section, "The Convert Text to Columns Wizard," later in this hour.

The Text Import Wizard

Suppose that you have a text file containing columns of data, and you want to deal with this data in Excel. You can import a text file into Excel as-is—with a little help from the Text Import Wizard. This process opens a new workbook with a single worksheet.

This example starts with the simple text file shown in Figure 17.7. This file was created in the Notepad applet.

Figure 17.7.

A simple text file that contains data you want to use in Excel.

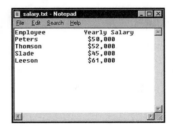

Follow these steps to import the file into Excel:

1. Choose File | Open from the menu to display the Open dialog box.
2. Locate the text file you want to open and attempt to open it. Because Excel recognizes the file as a text file, the first dialog box of the Text Import Wizard appears (see Figure 17.8).

Figure 17.8.

Step 1 of the Text Import Wizard.

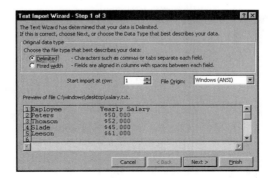

3. Choose the category in which the text file best fits. In this example, the columns are fixed width, so choose that option.

4. Determine whether you want to begin your text import at the first line or elsewhere. Specify the line or row number at which you want to start the conversions by entering the appropriate value in the Start Import at Row box.

   In the File Origin box, specify what kind of system the text file originated on. The default choice is Windows(Ansi), but you can choose from the other options if your file comes from a different system.

5. If you chose Delimited as the file type and clicked Next, the second dialog box of the Text Import Wizard appears as shown in Figure 17.9. Specify which type of delimiter your text file uses. Some text files use tabs between the data fields—this is the most common choice. Other text files use spaces, commas, semicolons, or other delimiters to separate the data in the columns. Select the option that is valid for your text file.

Figure 17.9.

Step 2 of the Text Import Wizard—for delimited data.

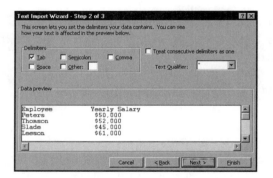

If you chose the Fixed Width option in the Step 1 dialog box and clicked Next, the second dialog box of the Text Import Wizard appears as shown in Figure 17.10. Set the columns to the width you want by dragging the vertical divider in the pane at the bottom of the dialog box. You can also add dividers by clicking at the desired position. Remove dividers by double-clicking them.

17

Figure 17.10.

Step 2 of the Text Import Wizard—for fixed-width text.

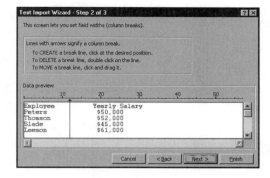

6. Click Next from either Step 2 dialog box to display the third and final dialog box (see Figure 17.11). In this dialog box, you set the format for each column in the text file. You can also skip a column altogether. In the Data Preview pane at the bottom of the dialog box, highlight each column in turn and select the data format you want to apply to that column. The default format is General. Click Finish when you are done applying formats to the columns.

Figure 17.11.

Step 3 of the Text Import Wizard.

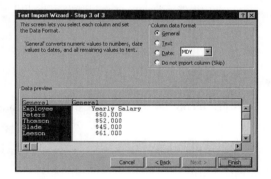

The data from the text file appears in a workbook with a single worksheet, with the upper-left cell being A1. By default, the worksheet and the workbook have the same name as the text file from which the workbook was generated. If you choose File | Save from the main menu, the file is saved as a text file. If you want to save it in standard Excel format, choose File | Save As from the main menu, and change the default extension under Save As Type in the Save As dialog box.

You can now interact with the data just as you would any other data in an Excel worksheet. You can save it as a text file when you are finished manipulating it in Excel, or you can save it in any other format supported by Excel.

JUST A MINUTE

The Text Import Wizard tries to convert just about any type of file—even if the file is not in text format. If you try to convert a graphics file, a word processing document, or some other type of file that is not a text file, the wizard goes through the steps just described but produces garbled nonsense.

The File Conversion Wizard

It's easy to save a single Excel 97 file in another format without using a wizard: You select File | Save As from the main menu, choose the desired option from the Save As Type list in the Save As dialog box, enter the filename in the File Name text box, and click OK. The Save As Type list includes several different text options, options for versions of dBASE and Excel, and other choices. However, if you have a batch of files you want to convert in a few easy steps, you will find the File Conversion Wizard a handy aid.

TIME SAVER

You may have a situation in which you have to share your Excel files with another user who has an earlier version of Excel. Using Excel 97, you can save your files in the desired file format by choosing the correct option from the File Save As dialog box.

You can use the File Conversion Wizard to convert a batch of files from one of a number of possible formats to Excel 97 format. Follow these steps to use the wizard:

1. Choose Tools | Wizard | File Conversion from the main menu to display the first dialog box of the File Conversion Wizard (see Figure 17.12).

Figure 17.12.
Step 1 of the File Conversion Wizard.

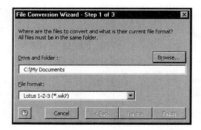

2. In the Drive and Folder text box, enter the directory in which the files you want to convert are located. You can use the Browse button to simplify the entry of the appropriate drive and directory.

17

3. From the File Format drop-down list, choose the file format of the original files (for example, if the files you want to convert are in Lotus 1-2-3 format, select Lotus 1-2-3 (*.wk?) from the list). Click Next to display the second dialog box of the File Conversion Wizard.

4. Select the files you want to convert. You can click the Select All button to highlight all the files in the directory. Remember that all the files you select must be in the same format.

5. Click Next to display the third and final dialog box of the File Conversion Wizard.

6. Select the directory in which you want Excel to place all the converted files. You can click the Browse button to find the directory you want, or you can type the directory name directly in the text box.

   You can also click the New Folder button to create a new directory for the files. When you click New Folder, you see a dialog box in which you can enter the name of the new folder.

7. Click Finish to convert the files.

When the files have finished converting, you see the File Conversion Wizard Report dialog box. This report tells you whether the conversions have been successful. The original files are left in place and unchanged.

COFFEE BREAK

What if Excel Doesn't Support Your File Format?

You may have a file or files in a format that Excel does not support. Don't give up hope! Maybe you can open the files in the original program and then save them in a format that Excel does support. If you can save the files as text, for example, you can convert them into Excel worksheets. You will lose some formatting in this conversion process, but the data should transfer intact. Maybe the company for the other application offers a conversion program of its own that you can obtain to convert the file into Excel format—it is worth checking out the possibilities if you don't want to reenter all the data by hand!

The Convert Text to Columns Wizard

What if you don't want to convert a whole text file? What if you want to convert only some of the data? You can convert parts of the original data into Excel columns with the aid of the Text to Columns Wizard. The original file does not have to be a text file; the data just has to be in alphanumeric format. You may want to use data that appears in a Microsoft Word document, a file from some other word processing program, or a document created in any of a variety of Windows programs that can store numbers and text.

To convert data from another program into columns in Excel, follow these steps:

1. Open both Excel and the program that created the file from which you want to convert the data. Make sure that the second application has loaded the file that contains the data you want to bring into Excel.

2. Copy (or cut) the data from the second program using the Edit | Copy or Edit | Cut command (alternatively, you can use the Cut or Copy tool from the Standard toolbar).

3. Switch to Microsoft Excel and select the cell at the upper-left corner of the area in which you want to paste the data from the other application.

4. Click the Paste tool in the Standard toolbar or choose Edit | Paste from the main menu. The text you copied from the other application appears in your Excel worksheet—but it is only one column wide.

5. Select the portion of this data that you want to convert into Excel columns. Select Data | Text to Columns from the main menu to display the Convert Text to Columns Wizard dialog box, shown in Figure 17.13.

    This wizard uses dialog boxes that are almost identical to those used by the Text Import Wizard. Refer to "The Text Import Wizard," earlier in this hour, if you need help following the directions in the Text to Columns Wizard.

Figure 17.13.

Step 1 of the Convert Text to Columns Wizard.

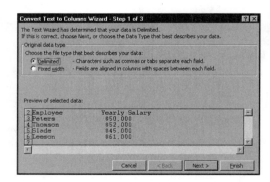

Summary

Excel wizards are a very helpful innovation when you want to learn how to do different tasks. Excel has wizards for charts, pivot tables, databases, and more. In this hour, you learned how to use wizards that create complex formulas and that convert files and import data into Excel.

17

Workshop

Term Review

file conversion   The process of converting a file from one format to another.

wizard   One of a number of small programs included with Excel and used to automate a particular process—at least to some extent. Wizards are used to create charts and maps, to do file conversion, to turn worksheets into Web pages, and many other tasks.

Q&A

Q What can you do with the Conditional Sum Wizard?

A You can create a formula with the Conditional Sum Wizard that sums particular entries of a column—if certain specified conditions are met.

Q What can you do with the Lookup Wizard?

A You use the Lookup Wizard to find the value of a specific cell reference, which you indicate by the column and row names.

Q What does the Text Import Wizard do?

A The Text Import Wizard converts text files into Excel worksheets.

Q What does the File Conversion Wizard do?

A The File Conversion Wizard converts a specified batch of files from one of a variety of formats into Excel 97 format.

Q What does the Convert Text to Columns Wizard do?

A The Convert Text to Columns Wizard converts copied textual data from another program (such as Microsoft Word) into columns of data in Excel. It does not convert an entire file.

Exercise

Create the following table of data in Microsoft Notepad and convert it to an Excel worksheet with the Text Import Wizard.

Company	Yearly Net Earnings
ABCDE Inc.	$1,201,250
BCDEF Inc.	$1,304,020
CDEFG Inc.	$500,300
DEFGH Inc.	$2,020,400

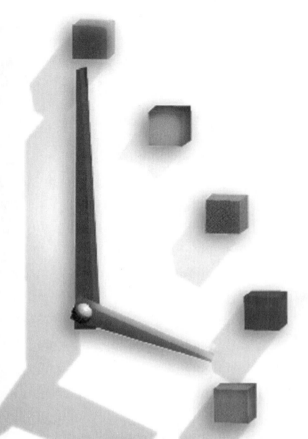

PART
IV

Using Excel with Other Applications

Hour

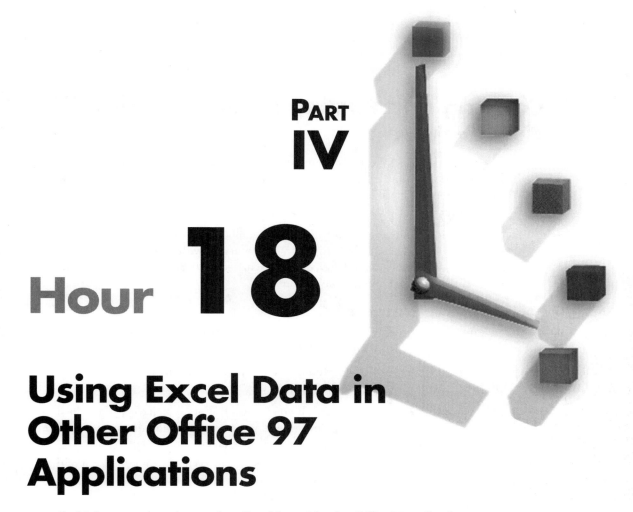

Hour 18

Using Excel Data in Other Office 97 Applications

In this hour, you learn how to share Excel data with other Office 97 applications, and how to share data from other applications with Excel. This chapter does not discuss Microsoft Access; Hour 19, "Using Excel with Databases," explains how you can use databases with Excel. Hour 20, "Excel and the World Wide Web," explains how to link Excel documents to and from the World Wide Web and with each other.

This hour does not give you all the information you need to use Microsoft Word, PowerPoint, and Outlook. Refer to the companion *Teach Yourself in 24 Hours* volumes for more information about how to use these programs. In this hour, you learn some ways to use these applications, with a focus on using other Office 97 applications with Excel.

Copying and Pasting between Office 97 Applications

Although Office 97 applications are designed to facilitate sharing of information, you can also share information between Excel and other Windows applications. If you're not sure whether copying and pasting data between applications will work, you can always try it and see what happens. Of course, it's a good idea to save your documents first.

This discussion about using Excel with other applications focuses on Microsoft Word, PowerPoint, and Microsoft Exchange. In Word, you deal with documents; in PowerPoint, you deal with presentations; and in Microsoft Exchange, you deal with e-mail. The principles for working with other applications are similar.

Copying a Range of Cells

You can copy the contents of a range of cells (or just one cell) from Excel to another application and vice versa. Here are the easy steps to follow:

1. Select the range just as you would if you were manipulating it within Excel.
2. Choose Edit | Copy from the Excel main menu.
3. Switch to the other application. If you are using Word, you have a Word document open; if you are using PowerPoint, you have a presentation open; if you are using Microsoft Exchange, you are composing an e-mail message.
4. Place the cursor in the other document where you want the upper-left cell of the range you copied in Excel to go. Now you have several options about how you want to paste the range into the application. These options are described in the following sections.

Pasting Excel Cells in their Formatted State

You can choose Edit | Paste from the main menu of the other application to copy the contents of the cells in their formatted state. The gridlines of the Excel cells remain, as do the color and style of the fonts.

Pasting a Range of Excel Cells as an Object

To copy the range of Excel cells as a link or as an object, choose Edit | Paste Special from the main menu of the other application to see the dialog box shown in Figure 18.1.

TIME SAVER

Compatible Windows applications have a main menu bar similar to the main menu bar available in Excel. Most Windows applications have the Edit menu option and the Cut, Copy, Paste, and Paste Special suboptions.

18

Figure 18.1.

The Paste Special dialog box for a range of cells.

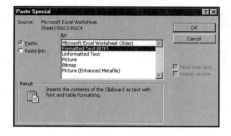

You can choose from any of the options shown:

☐ You can copy the range of cells into Word (or whichever application you are using) as a `Microsoft Excel Worksheet Object` so that you can edit the cells in Word using the E xcel toolbars.

☐ If you choose the `Unformatted Text` option, the information from the range is placed in the other document without any formatting whatsoever except for spaces between the words and numbers.

☐ If you choose the `Formatted Text` option, the range appears similar to how it does within Excel, complete with the gridlines (if present) and the font color and style. This option achieves the same effect as described in "Pasting Excel Cells in their Formatted State," earlier in this hour.

☐ If you choose the `Bitmap`, `Picture`, or `Picture (Enhanced Metafile)` option, the range of cells is pasted into the other application as a graphic image. After pasting it, you can double-click the object to edit it using the tools on the Picture toolbar. Choosing the `Picture` option produces better print quality for your images than does the `Bitmap` option; the `Picture` option also takes up less space on disk. However, choosing the `Bitmap` option gives you exactly what you see on-screen. Choosing the `Picture (Enhanced Metafile)` option inserts the contents of the Clipboard as a metafile.

Copying the Results of a Formula to Another Application

You can copy the results of an Excel formula to Microsoft Word or another program. Follow these steps to copy the results of a formula and then paste them to another application:

1. Select the Excel cell containing the formula you want to copy.

2. Choose Edit | Copy from the Excel main menu.

3. Switch to the other program.

4. Click in the document for the other application where you want to paste the result of the Excel formula.

18

5. Choose Edit | Paste Special from the menu to display the Paste Special dialog box.

   Decide whether you want to paste the formula result as an object or as text. If you paste the formula result as an object, you can manipulate it as you can any other graphic object, and you can adjust it with the tools on the Picture toolbar. If you paste the formula result as text, you can edit it as you want and you can also format it as text.

   ☐ Choose Unformatted Text if you don't want the result formatted. Choose Formatted Text (RTF) if you want the text formatted.

   ☐ Select Microsoft Excel Worksheet Object if you want the result to be inserted as an object.

   ☐ If you just want to paste the results without linking them back to Excel and the values that make up the formula, select the Paste radio button.

   ☐ If you want to paste the formula with a link back to Excel, and therefore have its value change when the corresponding values in the Excel worksheet change, click the Paste Link radio button.

If you choose Microsoft Excel Worksheet Object, you can choose either to have the pasted object float over the text in its new location (the default) or have it display as an icon. Select the Display as Icon checkbox if you want the result of the formula to be displayed as an icon. You are then given the option of choosing what type of icon you want. When you click your choice of icon, you then see the result of the formula. If you choose to have the object float over the text, it is separate from the text, just as any other graphic object or picture is separate from the text.

If you choose to paste the formula as text, you can also paste the formula as a link by selecting the Paste Link radio button. If you choose to paste the formula as a link, you can also select the Display as Icon checkbox.

JUST A MINUTE

> If you want to copy the actual formula itself, place the cursor inside the cell containing the formula, select the formula, copy it, and paste it into the other application.

Copying Charts and Maps into Other Applications

If you are creating a document in Microsoft Word or a presentation in PowerPoint, you may find that a chart created from data in an Excel worksheet can add just the right touch. Here's how to copy an Excel chart to another program:

1. In Excel, click the border of the chart to select it.

 2. Click the Copy tool in the Standard toolbar or choose Edit | Copy from the main menu in Excel.

3. Switch to the other program and place the cursor in the document where you want the upper-left corner of the Excel chart to be.

4. Click the Paste tool or choose Edit | Paste from the main menu in the other program. The Excel chart is pasted into the second application.

You can also choose Edit | Paste Special to display the dialog box shown in Figure 18.2. Using this dialog box, you can paste the chart as a link or as an embedded object, and you can determine whether the chart should float above the text or have an icon indicate its presence.

Figure 18.2.

The Paste Special dialog box for an Excel chart.

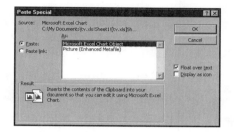

Similarly, you can copy maps generated by Microsoft Map from your Microsoft Excel worksheet. Click the border of the map to select the map, and follow steps 2 through 4 just presented. You can paste the map as a graphical image, or you can link to it.

Note that you can use the Object dialog box to insert and create maps and charts in other programs, as discussed in "Inserting, Embedding, and Linking Objects," later in this hour. The pros and cons of linking and embedding are discussed in "Linking versus Embedding," later in this hour.

Copying a File Shortcut to an Excel Document

If you have used Windows 95 for any length of time, you are likely familiar with shortcuts. *Shortcuts* are represented by icons that are frequently placed on the Windows 95 desktop. When you click a shortcut icon, a particular program or file opens up.

To create a shortcut to a file, locate the file within Windows Explorer. Right-click the file and choose Add Shortcut from the popup menu. A shortcut icon appears.

You must have both Windows Explorer and Excel open to less than their full window size if they are both to appear on-screen at once. Drag the shortcut icon from Windows Explorer to your Excel document. If the file is in a format Excel can recognize (such as a text file or an Excel file), Excel opens up the file represented by the shortcut icon.

Copying Objects to Excel

In Hour 17, "Exploring Excel's Utilities and Add-Ins," you learned how to copy and import textual data and text files into Excel with the Text Import Wizard. Here's how to copy an object from another program to your Excel worksheet:

1. In the other application, click the border of the object to select it and choose Edit | Copy from the main menu.
2. Switch to Excel and place the cursor where you want the upper-left portion of the object to be.
3. Select Edit | Paste or Edit | Paste Special from the main menu. If you selected Edit | Paste Special, make the appropriate choices from the Paste Special dialog box as described earlier in this hour.

Inserting, Embedding, and Linking Objects

Microsoft Windows applications are based on the concept of OLE (Object Linking and Embedding). In short, OLE means that you can share data between programs in the form of *objects*. You can either embed data objects from other programs within the current application, or you can link to the data objects in other applications. The following sections describe the use of the Object dialog box for inserting Excel objects into other programs and for inserting other types of objects into Excel worksheets. Although this section focuses on working with Office 97 applications, the same principles apply to any application that supports OLE.

Which Application Should Act as the OLE Client?

Excel is a great spreadsheet program, Word is an excellent word-processing program, and PowerPoint is terrific as a presentation program. What if you want to use features and capabilities from all three programs? Which one of these should serve as the *host program*— or as it is called, the OLE *client*?

Microsoft Word is most often the preferred OLE client, particularly if you are creating reports that involve a lot of formatted text in addition to numerical data, charts, and maps. The Excel objects will fit in nicely, and you can work around them and edit them in place.

However, you can also copy text and objects from Microsoft Word into Excel. In this situation, Excel is the OLE client. If you have mostly data and only a little text, this arrangement may be your best choice.

For some situations, such as when you are creating overhead transparencies, PowerPoint is the only feasible choice as the OLE client.

18

You can avoid the problem of choosing which application should be the client to some extent if you use Microsoft Binder (described in "Using Microsoft Binder," later in this hour). The Binder application is part of Office 97; it allows you to group documents together that have been created by various Office 97 applications. However, the documents remain separate, and their components are not integrated into one unit.

Example: Using Word as the OLE Client

If you insert a Microsoft Word object into Excel, you get a result similar to the one shown in Figure 18.3. It can be awkward to try to create a Word document when you lack access to all the features of the Word program. However, if you want to type only a few words or lines, creating a Microsoft Word object from within Excel works fine. When you are finished typing, click outside the object; the Microsoft Word toolbar disappears, leaving only a text box. The process of inserting a Microsoft Word object into Excel is discussed in the following section.

Figure 18.3.

Editing a Microsoft Word object within Excel.

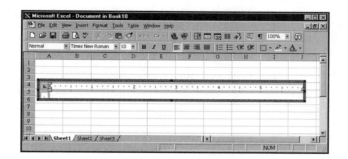

18

Inserting an Embedded Object into an Excel Worksheet

You may want to insert into an Excel worksheet a Microsoft Word object, a video clip object, a music clip, or any other object supported by Excel. Here's how to insert objects from other applications into an Excel worksheet:

1. From the Excel main menu, select Insert | Object to display the Object dialog box. Click the Create New tab (see Figure 18.4).

2. Choose the kind of object you want to create and click OK; the appropriate program opens to allow you to create the object of the selected type. The creation of graphical and multimedia objects within Excel was discussed in detail in Hour 8, "Adding Graphics and Multimedia to Your Excel Documents."

   For example, you can insert a Microsoft Word object into your Excel worksheet (refer back to Figure 18.3). The type of object you can embed depends on the programs you have on your machine. Your Object dialog box may differ from the one shown in Figure 18.4 because you may have different programs on your system than I do on mine.

Figure 18.4.

The Object dialog box.

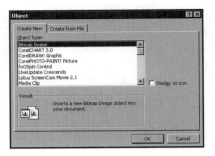

Embedding an Excel Object in Another Application

Just as you can create or incorporate an object from another program into Excel, you can insert an Excel object into another program. You can create Excel objects (or other kinds of objects) from within other Office 97 applications such as Word, PowerPoint, and Exchange, as well as other non-Microsoft applications that support OLE.

This section gives two examples: inserting an Excel object into Word and inserting an Excel object into PowerPoint.

From Word's main menu, choose Insert | Object to display the Object dialog box; select the Create New tab. Then select the type of object you want to create and click OK.

If you choose to create and insert an Excel worksheet within Word, you get the toolbars and worksheet shown in Figure 18.5. You can then enter and manipulate data in the Excel worksheet as you normally would.

Figure 18.5.

Inserting an Excel worksheet within Word.

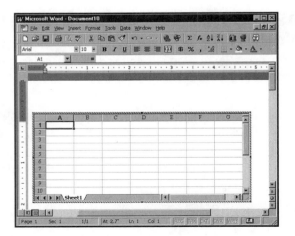

Similarly, you can choose Microsoft Map from the Object dialog box, and the Microsoft Map program opens up within Microsoft Word. You can also use the Insert | Object menu choice from within PowerPoint to include Excel objects within a presentation. From Microsoft Exchange or Microsoft Mail, you can embed Excel objects by choosing Insert | Object from the main menu when composing an e-mail message. If the recipients of your e-mail have a Microsoft e-mail program, they see your e-mail as you intended—complete with Excel data. If the recipients do not have a Microsoft e-mail program, they will likely receive the Excel files as coded e-mail attachments, which many e-mail users find annoying.

In the second example, suppose that you want to create an Excel object from within PowerPoint 97. Open PowerPoint as usual and start developing the presentation you want to make. If you want to create an Excel object from within PowerPoint, choose View | Insert Object from within PowerPoint (see Figure 18.6). You can create an Excel worksheet, chart, graph, or Microsoft Map. Select your choice. Make sure that the Create New option is selected and click OK. The object you chose—whether it is a worksheet, chart, graph, or map—appears. Once the object appears, you have rudimentary editing capability: You can make some alterations to the object, but not as many as if you were actually working within Excel.

Figure 18.6.

Inserting an Excel object in a PowerPoint presentation.

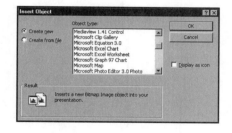

18

Creating an Object from an Existing File

The previous section indicated how to create a new Excel object in an Office 97 application. You can also place an Excel object that already exists into another application such as Word or PowerPoint.

From the other application's main menu, choose View | Insert as Object. The Insert dialog box appears (as just shown in Figure 18.6). Select the Create from File radio button. Browse through the directories to find the file you want, or enter its pathname.

As described in the previous section, you can choose the Float Over Text checkbox or the Display as Icon checkbox, depending on how you want to display the object.

Editing an Embedded Object

When you use the OLE technology (as you have been doing throughout this hour), you can do in-place editing of the object. *In-place editing* means that you do not have to leave Excel to perform modifications of the data from other applications. If you have embedded an Excel object in another Office 97 application, you can edit the Excel object in place. Simply click the border of the object, and you will get toolbars that allow you to edit the object in some way. If you click an Excel worksheet that you have inserted as a Microsoft Excel object in a Microsoft Word document, for example, you get the Excel toolbars.

You can also right-click the embedded object to get a variety of options. If you right-click an Excel Worksheet object where it is located in another application, you see the popup menu shown in Figure 18.7. Choose Worksheet Object | Edit to edit the data. You can also edit and manipulate the object as a picture by selecting Show Picture Toolbar, which gives you the Picture toolbar. If you manipulate the object as a picture, you can alter image shading, contrast, brightness, and other characteristics using the various tools on the Picture toolbar.

Figure 18.7.
The Excel Worksheet Object popup menu.

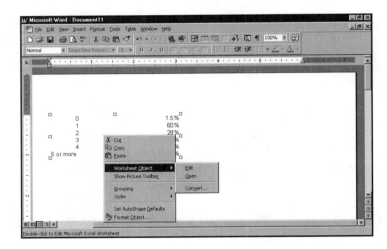

Linking versus Embedding

When should you create a link to an object, and when should you embed an object? If you create a link to an object rather than embedding it in a file, you must be sure that the object will still exist the next time you open the file containing the link. However, linking saves disk space because you do not have to save the object within the file.

If the linked-to object changes, your file is also altered automatically. Suppose that you create a link from a Microsoft Word document to an Excel chart that shows monthly sales figures. When the next month's sales are added to the chart, you do not have to make any changes to the original Word file.

If you want a specific object only, and *do not* want it to change, you should embed the object instead of linking to it. For example, if you want to show the Excel chart for January's sales figures in your Word document, but do not want that chart to be updated to show February's sales figures, you should embed the Excel chart object. Now, even if you change the Excel chart to show February's sales figures, the embedded copy of the chart in the Word document is not affected.

18

You should embed objects instead of linking to them particularly if you do not have control over the object. Some examples include situations in which someone else uses your computer, or when the object is located on a network.

If you move your file to a different computer system and do not also move the linked-to object, the link will no longer work. If you are copying a file to a floppy disk to give someone, you probably should embed the objects instead of linking them. Similarly, if you are sending a file with e-mail to someone, you should embed the objects rather than linking them.

Capturing an Excel Worksheet as an Image File

You can use an image-capture program to capture an Excel worksheet as a graphic. Then you can insert the image file into other applications, just as you would any other image file.

To capture a graphic image of an Excel worksheet, you need a program such as HiJaak! or Paint Shop Pro. You can download Paint Shop Pro from its Web site at http://www.jasc.com. Follow the screen-capture instructions for the program and save the image in your preferred image format.

You can then embed or link this graphic object just as you would any other graphic object, as discussed in Hour 8, "Adding Graphics and Multimedia to Your Excel Document."

Using Microsoft Binder

Microsoft Binder allows you to create and group documents from various Office 97 applications. It is installed with the typical installation of Microsoft Office. If it is not installed on your computer, run the Setup program again as described in Hour 2, "Installing Excel 97."

A typical set of documents you may want to group in a binder could include an Excel workbook representing the Annual Report and a Microsoft Word document for the annual letter to shareholders. You may also want to include two or more Excel workbooks (or two or more documents from some other application). The following sections give only a brief introduction to the Binder program; for more information, consult the online help files.

Opening a Binder

Open Microsoft Binder from the Start | Programs menu from the Windows 95 taskbar. To open an existing binder, choose File | Open Binder from the main menu and enter the filename you want to open in the Open Binder dialog box. You see a screen like the one shown in Figure 18.8.

18

Figure 18.8.

A Microsoft binder.

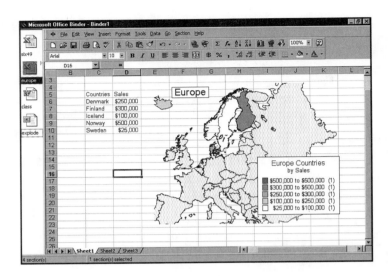

Adding Files to the Binder

The binder you create will contain the files you want to group together. The choices you make usually have a particular connection.

To add a file to the binder, choose Section | Add File from the Binder main menu. Search through the Add from File dialog box to find the file you want to add, or enter the filename in the File Name text box. Repeat as necessary to add more files to your binder.

You can also drag files from Windows Explorer to the binder. Open Windows Explorer and find the file you want to include in the binder. Highlight the icon for the file and drag it to the left edge of the Binder window, as shown in Figure 18.9. Similarly, you can drag files from the My Computer window or from the desktop and drop them on the left edge of the binder window.

Figure 18.9.

A binder with file icons along the left border.

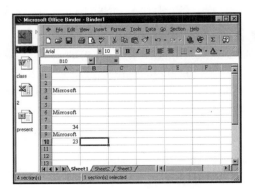

18

A shortcut way to add files to the binder is to right-click the left side of the binder window; a popup menu appears, allowing you to add sections or files to the binder.

Editing Files in the Binder

To edit a file that has been placed in a binder, double-click its icon on the left side of the binder window. The application associated with the file opens and the file itself is loaded; you can work with the file just as if the binder was not present.

Moving Files around in the Binder

You may want to change the order in which the file icons on the left side of the Binder appear. You may want to rearrange the icons to indicate the files to which you want to give precedence or for other cosmetic reasons. To change the position of the documents shown in the left border of the binder, highlight the file icon. You can select multiple files at once by pressing the Shift key and then selecting the desired file icons. You can highlight nonadjacent file icons by pressing the Ctrl key while selecting the files.

Once the file icon or icons are highlighted, you can move them by dragging the icons with the right mouse button and dropping them where you want.

Saving a Binder

When you are finished adding documents to a binder, you can save the binder as you would any other document by choosing File | Save or File | Save As from the Binder main menu. The binder saves the changes you have made to any files inside of it. However, it is important to note that *the files are not saved with these changes if you open the files independently of the binder.* The binder saves a separate copy of the files; the files of the same name that you open in their respective applications are not changed.

Deleting Files from the Binder

To delete a file from the binder, highlight the file icon in the left border of the binder window. Right-click the icon to display the popup menu and choose Delete.

Printing a Binder

To set up a binder for printing, choose File | Binder Page Setup from the main menu and make the choices you want in the resulting dialog box. You can choose whether to print all the visible documents or just the selected items in the left pane. For example, you can choose to select and print just one of the files in the left pane. Each document prints the same as if you were printing directly from the original application.

To see a preview of the binder before printing, choose File | Binder Print Preview from the main menu. You can also change the printing settings from within the Print Preview window.

To print all the documents in the binder directly, choose File | Print Binder from the main menu.

18

Using Outlook and Excel

Outlook is a scheduling and task management program included with Office 97. You can use Outlook to remind yourself to add or modify data in your Excel workbooks at a specific time. Outlook has a task list you can use to keep track of the work you need to do.

If you do not have Outlook installed, run the installation program to install it as described in Hour 2, "Installing Excel 97."

These instructions explain how to add an Excel document to your Outlook task list. With Outlook, you can track your work and your progress on an Excel document.

1. Display the Reviewing toolbar by choosing View | Toolbars | Reviewing from the main menu in Excel.

2. Open the Excel workbook you want to add to the Outlook task list.

3. Click the Create Microsoft Outlook Task tool on the Reviewing toolbar (the third tool from the right; it looks like a check mark). You see a screen similar to the one shown in Figure 18.10.

4. Choose the options you want from the Task tab on the dialog box. Here are some of the options you can specify:

   ☐ You can enter the title of the task.

   ☐ You can set a due date if that is applicable. Choose the date from the drop-down calendar you get by clicking the Due arrow.

   ☐ You can indicate the status of the task from the drop-down Status list. You have several options: Not Started, In Progress, Completed, Waiting on someone else, Deferred.

   ☐ You can indicate the priority of the task: Low, Normal, or High.

   ☐ You can check the Reminder box and arrange for a particular sound to be heard at a certain time to remind you of a task.

   ☐ You can click the Categories button at the bottom to characterize the task as belonging to a particular category.

   If you select the Status tab, you can enter information about the status of your project: the number of hours you have done on the project, mileage, billing information, and other comments.

5. Click the Save and Close button in the main menu bar to exit.

For more information about how to use Microsoft Outlook, consult *Teach Yourself Microsoft Outlook 97 in 24 Hours* (published by Sams Publishing, 1997).

18

Figure 18.10.
*Adding a task to
Microsoft Outlook.*

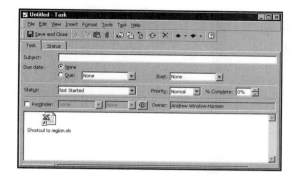

Using Excel Viewer

The Excel Viewer program is for people who have Windows 95 but do not have Excel. People can view your Excel workbooks using the Viewer, but they cannot make any editing changes to the workbooks. You can download this program from `http://www.ftp.com/product/keyv2.html`. The Excel Viewer is particularly useful if you are serving Excel documents over the World Wide Web, as discussed in Hour 20. You may also want to use the Viewer if only some of the employees in your company have Excel on their computers (and you want to buy software licenses only for those who use Excel), but you have other employees who want to be able to see the data.

Summary

You can use the Office 97 applications so that they work together as a team to process and display information. You can embed Excel worksheets, charts, and maps in other Office 97 and Microsoft applications such as Microsoft Word, PowerPoint, and Exchange. You can also create links to objects within Excel, or create links to Excel objects from other applications. Linking to an object ensures that your files are updated without having to edit the file whenever the object changes. Embedding an object ensures that it remains a permanent part of the file.

You can use Microsoft Binder to group together Office 97 applications, regardless of type. You can use this program when you want to place related documents with each other in a single unit. You can use the Outlook scheduling program, included with Office 97, to remind you to perform certain tasks, such as updating an Excel workbook.

18

Workshop

Term Review

OLE client   The application into which other types of objects are inserted. For example, if you insert a Microsoft Excel object into a Microsoft Word document, Word is the OLE client and Excel is the OLE server.

host   Same as *OLE client*.

object   A discrete item—such as a picture, graph, chart, or worksheet—you can copy, move, and manipulate at will.

OLE   Object Linking and Embedding. Refers to a set of technologies developed by Microsoft for integrating various applications.

OLE server   The application from which an object originates. *See* OLE client.

Q&A

Q Why would you want to use Excel with other applications?

A If you are creating a Microsoft Word document, for example, you may want to include data from an Excel worksheet to emphasize a point, or you may want to include a chart, graph, or map created within Excel. Office 97 allows you to create integrated documents so that you can take what you need from various applications and put them together into one document.

Q Can you insert Excel objects into other applications?

A Yes, you can insert Excel objects into documents created by applications that support OLE, as do Office 97 applications. You can also copy and paste text from Excel worksheets into any application that supports the copy-and-paste technology.

Q Can you insert other objects into Excel worksheets?

A Yes, you can insert OLE objects—such as those created by Office 97 applications or other applications—into Excel worksheets.

Exercise

In this exercise, you group several Office 97 documents together into a single binder.

1. Start Microsoft Binder from the Start menu on the Windows 95 taskbar.

2. Right-click the left pane of the Binder window and select Add from File from the popup menu. Because this is just an exercise, can choose the file you want to add from the Add from File dialog box. If you use the default C:\My Documents directory to save your Office 97 files, you will see a number of files you can use.

18

3. Add more files to the binder by repeating step 3. (As an alternative to the popup menu, you can select Section | Add from File from the main menu.)

   You should have several file icons along the left side of the Binder window.

4. Open a file by double-clicking its icon. You can make editing changes to it just as you would in its native application.

5. Save the binder by choosing File | Save Binder or File | Save Binder As from the Binder main menu. Enter a filename and click OK.

6. Exit the Binder program by choosing File | Close.

18

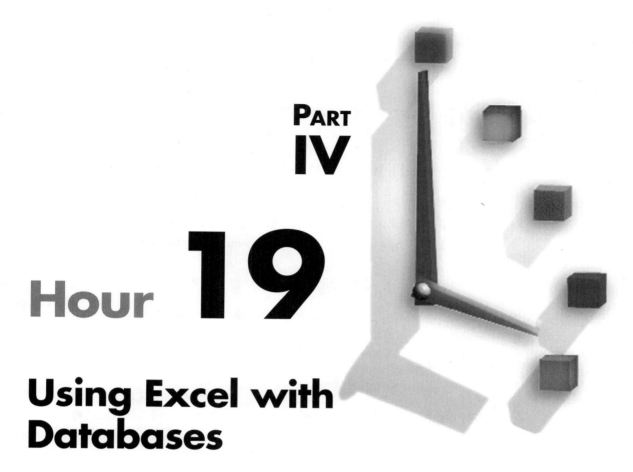

Hour **19**

Using Excel with Databases

Many offices require multiple programs to manage, process, and store their data. Excel has many capabilities, but it is not a full-fledged database program. To have full database capabilities, you need a program like Microsoft Access. This hour focuses on using Excel with Microsoft Access. Because both programs are created by Microsoft and are part of the Office 97 suite, they are specifically designed to work well together. However, you can also use other database programs—such as FoxPro, dBASE, and many others—with Excel.

Your main concern when using Excel and Access together is to find efficient ways to share information between the programs—and to convert information from one format to the other. This chapter does not explain how to use Microsoft Access—refer to the program documentation for more information.

Copying Data from Microsoft Access to Excel

Copying data from Microsoft Access to Excel is much the same as any copy-and-paste operation:

1. Open Microsoft Access and load the database that contains the records you want to copy to Excel. Select the records you want to copy to Excel.

2. Select Edit | Copy from the Access main menu to copy the records to the Clipboard.

3. Switch to Microsoft Excel and open the worksheet to which you want to copy the Access records.

4. Click the cell in the upper-left corner of the area in which you want to copy the Access records.

5. Choose Edit | Paste from the main menu in Excel. Any contents of the current cells are overwritten by the Access data.

   If necessary, adjust the height and width of the cells.

Converting an Excel List to an Access Database

Why would you want to convert a Microsoft Excel list to a Microsoft Access database? Perhaps your list is getting too large to fit comfortably within Excel. With Excel, the entire database is loaded into memory, which can tax your computer if your database is large. With Access, however, only the parts of the database that you need are loaded. Maybe you need the ability to allow more than one user at a time to save information to a database—a trick Access can do. You can use either Excel or Access for certain tasks—look at both programs if you are unsure which is best for your particular needs.

JUST A MINUTE

> All the subsequent examples of how to use various database wizards in Excel—except for the Web-based queries at the end of the hour—rely on the data shown in Figure 19.1.

Here's how to convert an Excel data list to an Access database:

1. Open the Excel worksheet containing the list you want to convert. Select any cell in the list.

2. Select Data | Convert to MS Access from the main menu in Excel. The dialog box shown in Figure 19.1 appears. You can choose either to convert the list to a new database or to convert it to an existing database. If you choose an existing database,

19

you can enter the pathname in the blank, or browse through the directories to find
the pathname you want. (If you are creating a new database, you can save it within
Access when you are finished with the conversion process.)

Figure 19.1.

*The Convert to Microsoft
Access dialog box.*

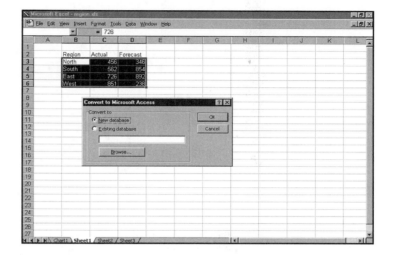

3. Click OK to close the dialog box and start the Import Spreadsheet Wizard within
    Microsoft Access (see Figure 19.2).

Figure 19.2.

*The Import Spreadsheet
Wizard dialog box.*

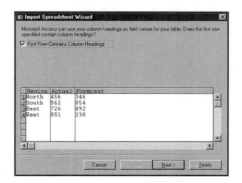

4. In this example, the First Row Contains Column Headings box should be checked
    because the column labels in the Excel data list (Region, Actual, and Forecast) are
    displayed in the first row of the list. If you have no column headings, leave the box
    unchecked. Click Next when finished to advance to the next dialog box.

5. From this dialog box, choose whether to store the data in a new table within the Access database or an existing table. If you choose an existing table, you must enter the name of the table. (In Access, a *table* is a collection of data about a specific topic.) It makes sense to add the data to an existing table if the data is related. Click Next when you have made your choice. The dialog box in Figure 19.3 appears.

Figure 19.3.

Choosing the fields for the Access database.

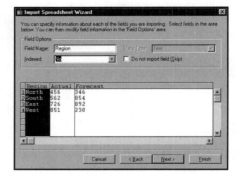

6. Specify whether or not each field in the Excel data list should be incorporated into the Access database. To do this, select each field and either check or uncheck the Do Not Import Field (Skip) box.

   You can also determine whether each field should be indexed.

   Click Next when you have finished selecting fields to display the next wizard dialog box.

7. Decide whether or not to use a primary key. (A *primary key* uniquely identifies each record so that a record can be retrieved more quickly. For more details about using or creating a primary key, see the Access documentation.) The default option usually works fine. Click Next when finished to display the final wizard dialog box.

8. In this example, Sheet1 is the worksheet that contains the list. The appropriate worksheet name usually appears, but you can change the default if needed. Click Finish when you are done.

   When you are finished, you return to the Access screen, and a new database (named after the Excel file from which you got the data) appears.

   Excel and Access work together to create an Access database from the Excel data. You can manipulate and save this new database as you would any other Access database. If you want to rename the table (which, in this example, is named Sheet1), you can do so by right-clicking the icon and choosing Rename from the popup menu.

19

Access saves changes to the database automatically. If you want to save the database under another name, select File | Save As from the main menu in Access and enter the pathname you want.

You can return to the original Excel worksheet by clicking the Excel icon on the Windows 95 toolbar. Once back in Excel, you can see that a comment has been automatically inserted to indicate that the list has been turned into a database. Because no links are kept between the worksheet and the database, you must be aware that a "split-source" problem may develop. This means that the data in the Excel list and the data in the Access database will differ if data is later added or changed in only one of the two files. If you do make changes to the Excel worksheet, it's usually easiest to generate the Access database all over again.

Using the AccessLinks Add-In

The AccessLinks add-in is designed to facilitate sharing between Excel and Microsoft Access. You can choose MS Access Form or MS Access Report from the Data menu on the main menu bar. If you do not see these options, you must install the add-in. Choose Tools | Add-ins from the main menu, click the AccessLinks add-in box, and click OK.

Once the add-in is installed, you can select either MS Access Form or MS Access Report from the Data menu on the main menu bar. Choosing Microsoft Access Form allows you to edit an Excel worksheet database. Choosing MS Access Report guides you through the creation of an Access report.

Using the Microsoft Access Form Wizard

Suppose that you want to use Microsoft Access to add entries to an Excel list. The Microsoft Access Form Wizard creates a form in Access that you can use for data entry—and the new data is placed in the Excel list. The form created is inside an Access database; the form has blanks you use for new information or to edit the data needed for each record of the Excel list. To create a Microsoft Access form for an Excel list, follow these steps:

1. Open the Excel worksheet containing the list for which you want to create the Access form.

2. Select a cell in the list.

3. Choose Data | MS Access Form from the main menu.

4. Save the workbook if prompted to do so. You will see the dialog box shown in Figure 19.4.

5. Specify whether you want to create the form in a new database or an existing database. If you choose to create the form in an existing database, you can either enter the filename or browse through the directories to find the file. The filename is generated automatically if you are creating a new database.

19

Figure 19.4.

*The Create Microsoft
Access Form dialog box.*

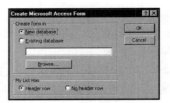

6. Specify whether or not your Excel data list has a header row. Click OK to display
   the Form Wizard dialog box shown in Figure 19.5.

Figure 19.5.

*The Form Wizard dialog
box.*

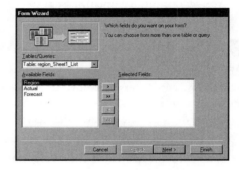

7. Select the fields from the Excel data list you want to include in your form. To
   include a single field, highlight it and click the > button. To include all the fields at
   once, click the >> button.

   You can exclude a selected field from the Selected Fields box by selecting the field
   in the right pane and then clicking the < button; you can move all the selected
   fields out of the right pane by clicking the << button. Click Next when you have
   made your selections to display the next wizard dialog box.

   The fields you choose to include will be in the form generated by this wizard. For
   example, if you want the form to include a blank for each of your column headings
   (Region, Actual, and Forecast), include each of those fields in this dialog box.

8. The next wizard dialog box offers a variety of layout options: Columnar, Tabular,
   Datasheet, and Justified. To see how each option lays out the form, select its radio
   button. Choose the one you want for your form and click Next to display the third
   wizard dialog box. The layout is rather inflexible—you can't choose the margins,
   offsets, or other features.

9. In the next dialog box, you get to choose the style of background you want for the
   form. When you select a background choice, you see a sample of how the form
   appears with that choice. Click Next to display the final dialog box.

19

10. In the final dialog box, you can specify a title for the form. If you want to view the form when you are finished, select the Open the Form to View or Enter Information radio button (which is selected by default). If you want to modify the design, select the Modify the Form Design radio button. Click Finish to see the form.

Figure 19.6 shows a sample form created using the MS Access Form Wizard. This example could be a form that represents the membership of a particular organization in a particular region, and the forecasted membership in that region. You can scroll through the various entries to see the record you want. Using this form, you can add more entries to the database or edit the ones that already exist. Because the Region, Actual, and Forecast fields were entered in the form, the form allows you to enter a value for Region, a value for Actual, and a value for Forecast.

Figure 19.6.

The Microsoft Access form created with the Form Wizard.

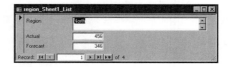

Back in the original Excel worksheet, a View MS Access Form button is placed on the worksheet so that you can view the MS Access form by clicking the icon.

Entering Data with the Access Form

To enter data with the MS Access form that you have created, click the View MS Access icon on your Excel worksheet. If the form can't be found, you see a dialog box asking whether you want to create a new form for the data in the worksheet. Otherwise, Access opens up, and the form you have created appears again.

You can use the form to change the data for any of the records or to add new records. When you switch back to Excel by clicking the Excel icon on the Windows 95 taskbar (usually located at the bottom of your screen), you will find that the changes have been made automatically within the worksheet.

Using the Microsoft Access Report Wizard

If you have an internal database in Excel, you may want to use the power of Access to make a report of it. A *report* organizes and formats the data. To create a Microsoft Access report from a list in an Excel worksheet, follow these steps:

1. Open the Excel workbook and select one of the cells in the data list for which you want to create an Access report.

2. Select Data | MS Access Report from the main menu to display the dialog box shown in Figure 19.7.

19

Figure 19.7.

*The Create Microsoft
Access Report dialog box.*

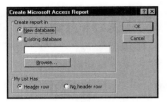

3. Specify whether you want to create the report in a new database or an existing
   database. If you choose to create the report in an existing database, you can either
   enter the filename or browse through the directories to find the file. A filename is
   generated automatically if you choose to make a new database.

4. Click OK close the dialog box. Microsoft Access opens, and the Report Wizard
   dialog box shown in Figure 19.8 appears.

Figure 19.8.

*Choosing the fields to be
included in the report.*

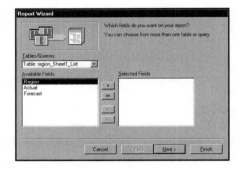

5. Select the fields from the Excel data list you want to include in your report. To
   move a single field, highlight it and click the > button. To move all the fields at
   once, click the >> button. You can move a selected field out of the Selected Fields
   box by selecting the field in the right pane and then clicking the < button; you can
   move all the selected fields out of the right pane by clicking the << button. Click
   Next when you have made your selections to display the next wizard dialog box.

   If you don't include a field on this dialog box, that field is not included in the final
   report. Depending on the list from which you are making the report and the
   purpose of your report, certain fields undoubtedly should not be included.

6. Use the next dialog box to group the fields from the Excel data list so that they fall
   in a specific hierarchical order (see Figure 19.9).

   Click Next to display the Sorting dialog box of the Report Wizard.

7. Choose the sort order for your records and specify whether the records should be
   sorted in ascending or descending order. Click Next when you are done to display
   the Layout dialog box of the Report Wizard.

19

Figure 19.9.

Grouping the fields.

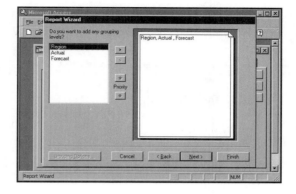

8. Choose the layout of your report. Select different options and look at the preview of what your report will look like with that option. Determine whether you want all the fields in the report to fit on one page. Click Next when you have made your choices to display the Title Options dialog box of the Report Wizard.

9. Choose how you want the title of the report to be displayed and specify the title for the report. Click Finish when you are done.

For the simple Excel list used in this example, and the options chosen, the final report looks like Figure 19.10.

Figure 19.10.

A report generated by the Report Wizard.

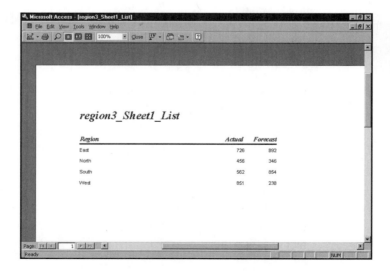

Once you finish the report, you can return to Excel. When you do, you will see a View MS Access Report button, which you can click at any time to open Access and bring up the report.

If you change the data in the Excel data list, you can update the report by clicking the View MS Access Report button. The report is then automatically updated.

Analyzing Microsoft Access Data with Microsoft Excel

You can analyze data in Microsoft Access with tools provided by Microsoft Excel. To do so, follow these steps:

1. Open Microsoft Access to the database containing the data you want to analyze. Highlight the table, form, query, or report you want to analyze in Excel.

2. Choose Tools | Office Links | Analyze It with MS Excel from the main menu in Access.

Microsoft Access saves the contents of the table, form, query, or report as an Excel workbook and saves it in the current working directory. The default working directory is C:\My Documents, unless you have changed it. If the table is named All Titles, for example, the workbook is saved, by default, with the name All Titles.xls.

You can then open the workbook in Excel as you would any other workbook and analyze it using Excel's tools, as described in Hour 16, "Using Excel to Analyze Data."

Using the Template Wizard with Data Tracking

The Template Wizard with Data Tracking allows you to create a worksheet that automatically gets the data from Excel and places it in the database you specify, thus saving a number of keystrokes and a great deal of time.

To use this wizard, start by opening the workbook, or creating a workbook, from which you want to create a template. Enter the text labels for the data you want to enter in the worksheet. Then follow these steps:

1. Select Data | Template Wizard to display the dialog box shown in Figure 19.11.

2. Make sure that the name of the workbook you want to use for the template is listed in this dialog box. If you want to use a different workbook, enter or select that filename. Also name the template, or accept the default (which is the same as the workbook name). Click Next to display the second dialog box of the Template Wizard.

19

Figure 19.11.

*Step 1 of the Template
Wizard with Data
Tracking.*

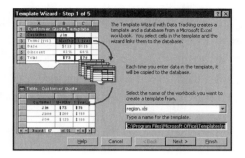

3. Select the type of database to which you want to transfer the information from the Excel template. If you are using an Excel list as the database, choose the default, Microsoft Excel Workbook. If you are using an Access database or other database, choose the appropriate option.

4. Enter or locate the pathname for the database to which you want to add the data. If the database does not already exist, it will be created. Click Next to display the next dialog box of the Template Wizard.

5. Enter the cell reference for each cell that you want to link to the specified database. As you enter a cell reference for each cell, the blank field below it opens up, and you can continue to add cell references as necessary. The references must be to individual cells, not ranges.

   The Template Wizard suggests a default field name based on the cell references you enter. You can accept this default or change it. Click Next to display the next dialog box in the Template Wizard.

6. You can also add data from any other existing workbooks to the database. However, the data in those workbooks must be organized in the same way as the template. If you select Yes, select the files from which you want to include data.

   Click Add Routing Slip if you want other people to look at your template. Your e-mail program opens so that you can enter the addresses for those people you want to review the template. Although this choice does not send the template off immediately, every time a workbook is created based on the template, it is sent to the specified address.

   Click Next to go to the final dialog box of the Template Wizard.

7. Click Finish when done.

You now return to the Excel worksheet, which appears as if nothing has happened. However, you have created a new template. The next section, "Using a Template with Data Tracking," explains how to use this template.

19

Using a Template with Data Tracking

To use the template you have generated with the Template Wizard with Data Tracking, follow these steps:

1. Select File | New from the main menu in Excel and double-click the icon for the template you have created. A new workbook based on the template opens. Because the template has interactive features built into it, it includes macros. Because you yourself have created the template and it is therefore free of viruses, it is safe to click the Enable Macros option. (Macros are discussed in greater detail in Hour 22, "Creating and Running Macros.")

2. Enter data or edit the data in the appropriate cells, as you would with any other workbook.

3. Choose File | Save from the main menu. In contrast to what happens with an ordinary workbook when you select this menu option, the Template File—Save to Database dialog box appears (see Figure 19.12). You can choose to create a new record in the associated database, or you can continue without updating and save the file as an ordinary workbook.

Figure 19.12.

Saving a template file to a database.

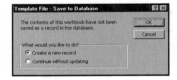

4. Click OK to close the Template File—Save to Database dialog box and to display the usual Save As dialog box.

5. Enter the filename for your new workbook and click Save.

Using the Microsoft Query Wizard

You can get data from an external database with the Query Wizard. Much of the data you need when creating reports is inside external databases, and you need to somehow access this information. Manually copying and pasting the data is time consuming. You can speed up the process by creating an automated query by following these steps:

1. Select Data | Get External Data from the main menu in Excel.

2. Select Create New Query from the submenu to display the dialog box shown in Figure 19.13.

3. Double-click New Data Source to display the dialog box shown in Figure 19.14. This dialog box provides you with four blank fields in which you enter data; each opens up after you fill in the preceding text box.

19

Figure 19.13.

*Creating a query with
the Query Wizard.*

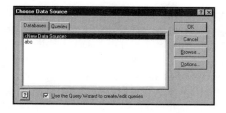

Figure 19.14.

*Creating a new data
source.*

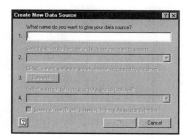

4. Enter the name you want for your new data source in the first field. Enter any reasonable name.

    Choose the driver you want from the second text box. There are several options, one for each different database format supported. Click the arrow to see a drop-down list of what is available for various database programs: Access, dBASE, Excel, FoxPro, plain text, and SQL. The database you want information from is in one of these formats (if it isn't, you can't use the Query Wizard to retrieve its data). Choose the type of database driver that is appropriate.

    Click the Connect button to set up the database driver. A dialog box appears, asking what database you want to search along with some other information, depending on the type of database driver you chose. After setting up the database driver, you return to the Create New Data Source dialog box.

    The last text box is optional; use it to enter a default table for your data source, if applicable, such as if you are using Microsoft Access or a database program that uses tables.

    You can click the checkbox at the bottom of the dialog box to save your ID and password in the data source definition. Some databases can be accessed only with a password, and by saving your password information, you won't have to enter it the next time you go to the database. However, someone else may use your computer and thus get access to the database, making your system insecure.

5. Once you have made your choices in the Create New Data Source dialog box, click OK to return to the original Choose Data Source dialog box, with the newly created data source selected.

6. Click OK to display the Choose Columns dialog box, shown in Figure 19.15, which lists the tables and columns in the database you specified in step 5. Figure 19.15 shows the available tables and columns for a database in Access named northwind, which you can get from C:\Program Files\Microsoft Office\Office\Samples\northwind.mdb (if you installed Office 97 in the default directory). If you have chosen a different database in step 4, you have different tables and columns to select. Select the tables and columns you want to include in the query. Click Next to display the Filter Data dialog box.

Figure 19.15.

A typical Choose Columns dialog box for an Access database.

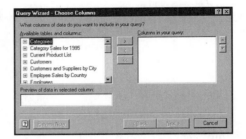

7. Use the Filter Data dialog box to filter the data according to specific conditions. Set up the filter for any or all of the columns. The purpose of most queries, of course, is to get specific data, so you will likely want to set up a filter or filters. Click Next to display the Sort Order dialog box.

8. Specify whether you want to sort the fields in ascending or descending order. Click Next to display the final dialog box of the Query Wizard.

9. Decide whether to return the data to Microsoft Excel or to view the results of the query in Microsoft Query. You can also save this query, which is a good idea if you will use it again. Click Finish when you are done.

If you have chosen to have the data returned to Excel, the Returning Data to Microsoft Excel dialog box appears to prompt you for the cell in which you want to place the upper-left corner of the data. Enter your choice of cell reference and click OK.

After creating and saving a query, you can later change the query by selecting Data | Get External Data from the main menu, and then selecting from these options: Edit Query, Data Range Properties, and Parameters. You can also choose these options from the External Data toolbar, which appears on the screen after the query is successfully completed.

If you query a database that changes, you likely have to refresh your data periodically—unless you specified a refresh time when you created the query. To refresh the data retrieved by the query you just created, you can click the Refresh Data tool on the External Data toolbar.

19

Running a Query that Has Already Been Created

To run a query you have already created, choose Data | Get External Data | Run Query from the main menu. The Run Query dialog box appears. You can select or enter or locate the filename of the query. Click OK when you have made your choice.

Running a Web Query

Microsoft Excel includes several Web queries for checking stock values and getting other data from databases on the World Wide Web. These queries have already been created, although you can edit them if you want.

To run one of these queries, follow these steps:

1. Select the cell in Excel that is to be the upper-left corner of the area in which the data you retrieve from the World Wide Web is to be placed.

2. Choose Data | Get External Data | Run Web Query to display the Run Query dialog box.

3. Select the Web query you want to run (Table 19.1 lists your options). For this example, choose `Detailed Stock Quote`. The Returning External Data to Microsoft Excel dialog box appears.

4. If you want to change the default choice (the cell you selected in step 1), enter the cell reference where you want to place the data.

   You can alter the properties of the query by clicking the Properties button to display the External Data Range Properties dialog box. You can change the query definition, refresh the data at specified intervals, and change the data layout options.

   You can alter the parameters of the search by clicking the Parameters button to display the Parameters dialog box. You can change the parameter on which the search is conducted.

5. For this query example, enter the name of the company for which you want stock information. For this example, I entered `IBM`. You can check the appropriate box if you want to use this name for later searches. Click OK to start the search.

Getting the data takes a few seconds to a few minutes. When the query is finished, your worksheet will show a table of data like the one in Figure 19.16. This query gives you a full report on the company and its recent stock history.

Table 19.1 lists the different Web queries included with Excel and the output each produces.

19

Figure 19.16.

Running a Web query.

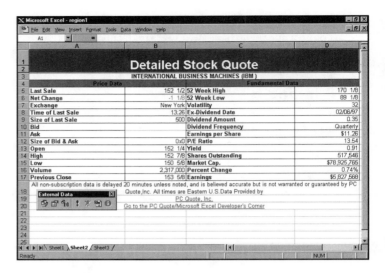

Table 19.1. External Web queries included with Excel.

Web Query	Output
Detailed Stock Quote by PC Quote, Inc.	Gives a detailed stock quote, with various details, for a specifically named stock.
Dow Jones Stocks by PC Quote, Inc.	Gives a listing of 66 Dow Jones stocks with a variety of different statistics for each.
Get More Web Queries	Brings back Web queries you can download and add to the other Web queries. These Web queries are designed for researching various financial statistics and markets.
Multiple Stock Quotes by PC Quote, Inc.	You can get multiple stock quotes (up to 20) from PC Quote with a single search.

19

Summary

Both Microsoft Excel and Microsoft Access can store data, although they differ in their functionality. Microsoft designed these programs to work together. You can copy data to and from one program to the other. You can convert an Excel list to an Access database, and you can convert an Access database—in whole or in part—to Excel. You can use tools like the Query Wizard to capture external data from a database and bring it back to your Excel workbook.

Workshop

Term Review

form   An organized method of collecting data. You use a form to enter the data for a record in specific fields; this data is then placed in a database.

primary key   In Access, if you use a primary key, every record in a database is uniquely identified, which speeds up retrieval time when you search for records.

query   A way to find particular information (of the type you specify) in another database.

report   In Access, a report is an organized compilation of data, formatted to your specifications. You can create an Access report from a Microsoft Excel list with the MS Access Report Wizard.

Q&A

Q Why would you want to use Excel with external database programs?

A External database programs may have data you need for your Excel applications. You must be able to get this information and put it into your Excel worksheets.

Q Can you get information from databases on the World Wide Web and import it into Excel?

A Yes. Excel includes several Web queries that automate the process of retrieving certain types of data from databases on the World Wide Web. You can also download more Web queries that you can use to access information.

Exercises

1. Run the Dow Jones Stock Web Query.
2. Once you have the data, convert it to a Microsoft Access database. Follow the steps described in the section, "Converting an Excel List to an Access Database."

19

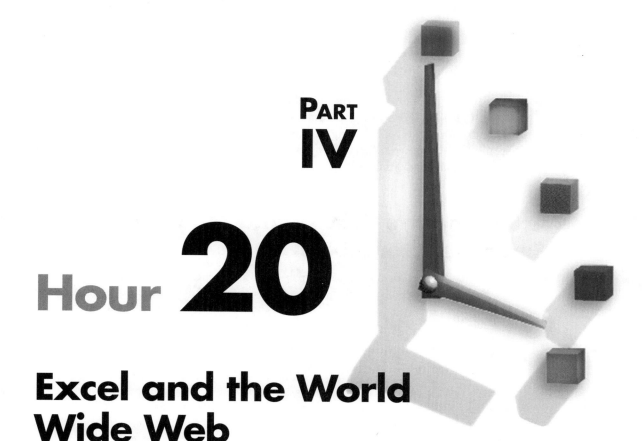

Hour 20

Excel and the World Wide Web

Microsoft Excel 97 has many new features that facilitate the process of linking to and from the World Wide Web. Microsoft is trying hard to make files from the Internet just as accessible from within Excel and other Office 97 programs as any other files from within your own computer. Microsoft Internet Explorer 3.0 and 4.0 are tightly integrated into the Office 97 suite, and you can access files from the outside world as easily as you can those files inside your own computer or on your local network. You can use Excel to access files on the World Wide Web, you can link from Excel to WWW files, and you can turn your Excel worksheets into HTML documents or portions of documents.

In short, you can access files on the Web and you can make your files accessible to other Web users. If you have an Internet connection (either a dial-up or a network connection), Excel makes the process of accessing and linking to and from the World Wide Web simple. You can even use the Web Form Wizard to make online forms, as discussed in Hour 23, "Using Custom Controls, Forms, and Data Validation."

Why would you want to use files from the Web or make your files available on the Web? The World Wide Web is the world's most accessible and largest storehouse of information. You can find information—of varying quality—on any subject in the known universe and beyond. If you make your files available on the Web, anyone in the world with an Internet connection can access your information. The business and informational opportunities are obvious.

Accessing the WWW and the Rest of Your Computer from Excel

Every Office 97 product includes the capability to access the World Wide Web. Make sure that the Web toolbar is displayed in your Excel worksheet by choosing View | Toolbars | Web from the main menu (see Figure 20.1). If you choose, you can make the Web toolbar float by dragging and dropping it someplace on the worksheet.

Figure 20.1.
The Web toolbar.

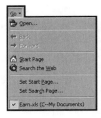

Once the Web toolbar is displayed, you can click the Favorites button to go to a Web site you have added to your list of favorite places, either from within Internet Explorer or from another Office 97 application. You can add sites to your list of favorites by right-clicking within your Web browser and selecting Add to Favorites from the popup menu.

If the site you want to visit is not listed in your favorites list—or if you don't want to look through the list—you can access different Web pages by clicking the Go button on the Web toolbar to display the submenu shown in Figure 20.2.

Figure 20.2.
The Go submenu.

Choose the option you want from the Go submenu:

☐ If you select the Open option, you can type the URL of the Internet address you want to visit. Note that you can also enter a pathname of a file instead of a URL.

20

> URL stands for Uniform Resource Locator. URL is the term used for the Web address of a file or a Web site.

- ☐ Click the Back option to move back to the previous file or item in the list of the last ten items you viewed before the present one.

- ☐ Click the Forward option to move to the next file or item in the list of the last ten items you have visited.

- ☐ The default start page for the Internet Explorer is `http://www.microsoft.com`. You can also select start page directly from the Web toolbar (its icon is the same on the toolbar and in the Go submenu). A *start page* is the page that opens by default when you open your Web browser.

- ☐ The default search page on Internet Explorer is `http://www.msn.com/access/allinone.asp`. You can also select Search the Web directly from the Web toolbar (its icon is the same on the Web toolbar and in the Go submenu).

- ☐ Use the Set Start Page option to set the default start page to your preferred URL.

- ☐ Use the Set Search Page option to set the default search site to your preferred URL.

You can also click the drop-down menu that shows the pathname of the current document, located on the right side of the Web toolbar. This drop-down list shows the files and sites you have visited recently. If the site or file you want is listed here, just click it to go to that site. Otherwise, you can type the pathname or URL at the top of the pull-down menu and press Enter.

> Most URLs on the Web begin with `http://`. However, you can both access and link to URLs with other formats, such as FTP files, Telnet sites, Gopher sites, and so forth.
>
> Some possible URL formats are shown here:
>
> | | |
> |---|---|
> | `ftp://ftp.netscape.com` | Connects to the Netscape FTP site. |
> | `telnet://fairmont.library.ubc.ca` | Connects to a specific university library site (the one at the University of British Columbia). |
> | `news://comp.apps.spreadsheets` | Connects to the Usenet newsgroup `comp.apps.spreadsheets`. |
>
> If you are unfamiliar with the Internet and HTML, there are a number of good books available on the subject. *Laura Lemay's Web Workshop: Teach Yourself HTML 3.2 in 14 Days* is an excellent resource.

20

Creating Links to the Web from a Worksheet

When you enter data into Excel worksheets, you may prefer to make the data accessible to the worksheet by creating a link, rather than by entering the data directly into the worksheet. Using links saves space and time. If you link to a Web site rather than copy the information to the worksheet, your user can access the information he or she needs without being restricted by copyright limitations, because most information available on the Web is protected by copyright. Once the hyperlink is inserted on your Excel worksheet, all the user has to do is click the link to get to the information. Of course, you have no control over the content of an external file to which you create a hyperlink. What appears to be a hyperlink to a relevant document today may be a hyperlink to a useless document tomorrow. The person in charge of the external file can change its contents at will without any input from you.

Follow these steps to create an external hyperlink:

1. Position the cursor in the cell in your worksheet where you want the hyperlink to appear.
2. Click the Insert Hyperlink tool in the Standard toolbar or choose Insert | Hyperlink from the main menu to display the dialog box shown in Figure 20.3.
3. Suppose that you want to insert a link in your worksheet to a file with the pathname C:\MyFile\explain.txt. Type that pathname in the Link to File or URL text box at the top of the dialog box and click OK. The dialog box closes and the filename appears underlined in the selected cell in the worksheet so that you can tell it is a hyperlink.

Linking to a named location is discussed in the next subsection.

Figure 20.3.

The Insert Hyperlink dialog box.

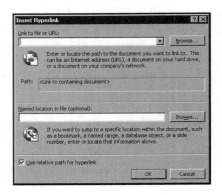

20

When you click this hyperlink in your worksheet, the specified file opens up with the associated application. Because the default application for opening a text file is Notepad, in most cases, Notepad opens with the specified file when you click the link.

If you want to specify a URL in the Link to File or URL text box in the Insert Hyperlink dialog box, just type the full URL, such as `http://www.microsoft.com/excel/`. If you click this link in your worksheet, your default Web browser opens to the specified location. Netscape and Microsoft Internet Explorer are the most commonly used Web browsers. If you are creating links to documents on the Internet, you must have an Internet connection to access them, of course.

JUST A MINUTE

> If you have a network to which your computer is linked, you can use the Insert Hyperlink dialog box to link to files on the network also. For example, if your network files are on drive F, just type the full pathname of the file in the Link to File or URL text box in the Insert Hyperlink dialog box. For example, type `F:\Our Documents\somefile.xls`—the same as you would if the file were on your own computer.

Linking to a Named Location in the File

You can link to a specific portion of a file, such as a bookmark in Word or a named range in Excel. If you want to link to the range wage in the file `C:\My Documents\earn.xls`, open the Insert Hyperlink dialog box and type `C:\My Documents\earn.xls` in the Link to File or URL box and type **wage** in the Named Location in File (Optional) box. When you click the link that appears in your worksheet, the relevant worksheet opens and the named range is selected.

If you want to link to a bookmark in a Microsoft Word document (see the Microsoft Word help system for information about creating bookmarks in Word documents), open the Insert Hyperlink dialog box and enter the pathname of the document in the Link to File or URL box and the name of the bookmark in the Named Location in Document (Optional) box. Other Office 97 applications also have ways to mark specific portions of a document in a way that Excel recognizes.

Relative versus Absolute Paths

The Insert Hyperlink dialog box has a Use Relative Path for Hyperlink checkbox you can select. If you check the box, only the relative path in respect to the active document is used, not the full pathname to the linked document. If you save the active document in another directory, its relative links no longer work. One advantage of using relative links is that they are shorter to type.

20

Whether you use relative or absolute links doesn't matter when you are dealing with documents outside your own system, such as those on the Internet. When dealing with outside documents, you *must* use the full pathname to reference the files.

Whether you use relative or absolute links, your links to files within your own system do not work if you copy the file and try to use it on another system. For example, if you copy an Excel worksheet containing links to documents in your C:\My Documents directory to a floppy disk, and then use this floppy disk with a different computer, the links do not work.

Using, Editing, and Removing Hyperlinks

You can open a hyperlink in another viewing window if you want. Select the cell containing the hyperlink and right-click to display the hyperlink popup menu; select Hyperlink to display the submenu shown in Figure 20.4.

Figure 20.4.

The Hyperlink submenu.

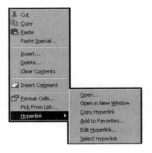

Here are the options available from the Hyperlink submenu:

Options	Description
Open	Open the linked-to file in the current window.
Open in New Window	Open the linked-to file in a new window.
Copy Hyperlink	Copy a hyperlink by selecting this option, selecting the new destination, and pressing Enter.
Add to Favorites	Add the linked-to document to a list of your favorites in Internet Explorer (IE). The Favorites files are accessible from the main menu in IE.
Edit Hyperlink	Display the Edit Hyperlink dialog box shown in Figure 20.5. If you select this option, you can change the pathname or other options. To remove a hyperlink altogether, click the Remove Link button from the Edit Hyperlink dialog box.
Select Hyperlink	Use this option when you want to select the text of a hyperlink without clicking the link.

20

Figure 20.5.

The Edit Hyperlink dialog box.

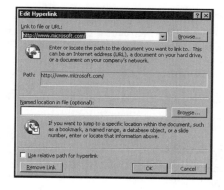

JUST A MINUTE

> Many hyperlinks are longer than the default cell width. Remember that you can easily change the width of a cell so that you can see the text of the full link. To change the column width, select Format | Column.

The HYPERLINK Function

You can also use the HYPERLINK function to create hyperlinks. The generic syntax of this function is shown here:

```
HYPERLINK(link_location,friendly_name)
```

In this syntax, *link_location* is the URL or pathname of the document to which you want to link. You can also enter a named range or cell within the current document as the *link_location* value. You must surround the value with double quotation marks.

The *friendly_name* value is the actual text that appears in the cell. This text is displayed in blue by default, or in red-violet if you have already clicked the link. You must also surround the *friendly_name* value with double quotation marks. You can use a named or alphanumerical cell reference as the *friendly_name* value if you want the text in that cell to appear.

You enter this function into a cell as you would any other function. For example, if you want to enter the hyperlink http://www.microsoft.com/excel/ into the cell with the HYPERLINK function and want the words Click to go to the Excel Web site to appear in the cell, type the following into the cell:

```
=HYPERLINK("http://www.microsoft.com/excel/", "Click to go to the Excel Web site)
```

20

If you want the text contained in cell B1 to display in another cell (to give an example), type the following into the second cell (notice that the cell name is not surrounded by double quotation marks):

```
=HYPERLINK("http://www.microsoft.com/excel/",B1)
```

If you want to link to the range wage in Sheet 1 of the Excel workbook C:\My Documents\earn.xls and have the text go to wage appear in the cell, your HYPERLINK function would look like this:

```
=HYPERLINK("[C:\My Documents\earn.xls]Sheet 1!wage]", "go to wage")
```

The pathname of the file you are referencing is placed in square brackets ([ ]), followed by the worksheet name and an exclamation mark (!). If you are referencing a particular cell or range, the name of the cell or range is placed after the exclamation mark. A square bracket is placed at the end, and the entire reference is enclosed in quotation marks.

You can edit and clear a cell containing a HYPERLINK function just as you would any other cell. Clear a cell containing a hyperlink by selecting the cell, right-clicking, and choosing Clear Contents from the popup menu. To edit a cell containing a hyperlink, place the cursor inside the cell and start typing.

Changing the Stylistic Appearance of a Hyperlink

By default, a hyperlink uses the same standard font as other text in your worksheet but is underlined. By default, hyperlinks you have followed are displayed in the color violet, and hyperlinks you have not yet followed are displayed in the color blue. This default hyperlink display is reasonable and unambiguous. However, it may not match your personal preference or design choice. Here's how to change the appearance of a hyperlink:

1. Select the cell containing the hyperlink you want to format.
2. Select Format | Cell from the main menu to display the Format Cells dialog box.
3. Select the Font tab to change the color, font face, and other features of the hyperlink text. You can also select the other tabs to change other options, as described in Hour 3, "Introduction to the Excel Environment."

Remember, however, that if you get rid of the underlining and do not otherwise distinguish the hyperlink, your reader may not be able to tell that the text is "clickable." You should include some kind of indicator that a hyperlink is present.

Changing the Appearance of All Hyperlinks in a Workbook

The previous section discussed how to change the appearance of a single hyperlink. However, you may want to change the appearance of all your hyperlinks to a single, defined style. You may want to do this if you have a particular design choice in mind.

20

Here's how to change the appearance of all your hyperlinks in the active worksheet:

1. Choose Format | Style from the main menu to display the Style dialog box shown in Figure 20.6.

2. Choose Hyperlink from the Style Name drop-down list. The Font box is selected by detail. Check the other boxes if you also want to change those features and then click Modify. The Format Cells dialog box appears. Make the modifications you want and click OK when finished. You then return to the Style dialog box. Click OK.

You now have a new default style for all the hyperlinks in the current workbook.

Figure 20.6.

The Style dialog box.

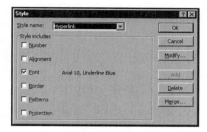

To change the style of a hyperlink that has already been clicked, open the Style dialog box and choose Followed Hyperlink from the Style Name drop-down list. Change the features for this type of text in the way just described.

Using Graphics to Link to Other Documents

You can use graphics as well as text as hyperlinks. Suppose that you want to make a graphic of a star in your worksheet link to NASA at http://www.nasa.gov. First make the graphic of a star by using the AutoShapes feature, by importing a piece of clipart, or by using whatever method you want (as discussed in Hour 8, "Adding Graphics and Multimedia to Your Excel Documents"). To make the graphic clickable, select the graphic and choose Insert | Hyperlink from the main menu to display the Insert Hyperlink dialog box. Enter the URL of the site (in this example, http://www.nasa.gov/) in the Link to File or URL box and click OK.

You can similarly use graphics as hyperlinks for pathnames of documents on your own computer system or on the local network.

20

Saving Excel Worksheets in HTML Format

To save an Excel worksheet in HTML format, choose File | Save as HTML from the main menu. If you do not see this command, you must install the Internet Assistant add-in. To install the add-in, select Tools | Add-ins from the main menu. Check the Internet Assistant Wizard box and click OK to install the wizard.

The first dialog box of the Internet Assistant Wizard appears, as shown in Figure 20.7.

Figure 20.7.

The first step of the Internet Assistant Wizard.

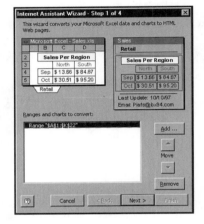

The wizard makes a reasonable effort to guess what data you want to convert. If you want to change the ranges and charts to convert or add others to the list in the pane at the bottom of the dialog box, click the Add button. Enter the range of cells you want to convert and click OK to return to the first dialog box. If you want to remove a range, select it in the pane at the bottom of the first dialog box and click the Remove button. If more than one range is listed, you can rearrange them by clicking the Move buttons.

Click Next to go to the second dialog box of the Internet Wizard (see Figure 20.8). You can choose either to have your file saved as a separate and complete HTML file, or merely to create an HTML table. An HTML table displays data with specific spacing and separation of data entries, but it is not a complete Web page. An HTML table is typically inserted inside an already existing Web page, as described in "The Just an HTML Table Option," later in this hour. Make your choice and click Next.

Depending on the choice you made in the second dialog box about whether you want to create a separate and complete HTML file or just a table, the third dialog box displays different options, as described in the following sections.

20

Figure 20.8.
The second step of the Internet Assistant Wizard.

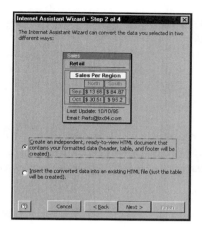

The Separate HTML File Option

If, in the Step 2 dialog box, you chose to save your file as a separate and complete HTML file, a dialog box similar to the one shown in Figure 20.9 appears. You can enter the text as you think appropriate. If you are familiar with constructing HTML documents, you may better understand what Excel is trying to do here.

Figure 20.9.
The third step of the Internet Assistant Wizard—for a separate HTML file.

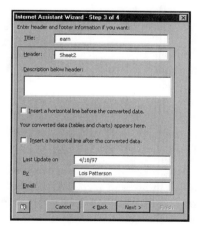

The text you enter in the Title box appears at the top of the browser. The text you enter in the Header box appears as the first text in the document and is in large, bold letters. You can enter text below the header and above the table if you want (this text can be explanatory in nature or can contain other information). You can choose whether to have horizontal bars above and below the table. The entries Last Update On, By, and Email appear at the bottom of your document. Click Next to go to the fourth dialog box of the Internet Assistant Wizard.

The Just an HTML Table Option

If, in the Step 2 dialog box, you chose to have your HTML file appear in an already-created HTML document, you see the dialog box shown in Figure 20.10.

Figure 20.10.
The third step of the Internet Assistant Wizard—for creating an HTML table.

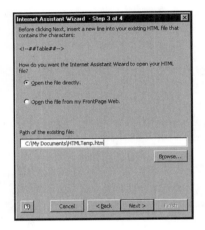

You now have to open your HTML file—in either a text editor or your preferred HTML editor—and enter the character string `<!--##Table##-->` wherever you want the table to appear. You don't have to close Excel to do this—just open the text editor or HTML editor separately.

You can then choose to have the file opened directly, or you can choose to have the file open from the FrontPage Web. You use the latter option only if you have a FrontPage Web server. For more information about FrontPage, refer to the Microsoft FrontPage site at `http://www.microsoft.com/FrontPage`.

Enter the pathname of the existing HTML file you want to use (the one you just modified) in the Path of the Existing File box.

Click Next when you have finished selecting options in the third step of the Internet Assistant dialog box to display the fourth dialog box.

20

The Fourth Step of the Internet Assistant Wizard

After you click Next in either of the Step 3 dialog boxes, the Step 4 dialog box of the Internet Assistant Wizard appears (see Figure 20.11).

From this dialog box, you can choose the code page you want to use. Usually, you want the default US/Western European code page (unless you are creating Web pages with a different character set, such as Cyrillic, Chinese, or one of several other options). A *code page* represents the characters in the character set you are using. The typical character set used by English-speaking users is Latin-1; the default US/Western European code page means that the Latin-1 character set is used with the Web page you are creating.

Figure 20.11.

The fourth step of the Internet Assistant Wizard.

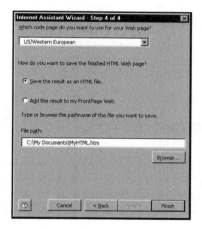

You can either save the file as an HTML file or add the result to your FrontPage Web, if you are using a FrontPage Web server.

Enter the file path for the new HTML document. You can use the same pathname as the HTML file you specified in the third dialog box, if you want to modify your original file.

Click Finish when you have made all your choices.

You can then upload the file to your Internet site as you would any other HTML file. If you want to keep your file local, you can do that as well. To see what your Excel worksheet looks like in your browser, you can enter the pathname in the text box at the right end of the Web toolbar.

You can modify the HTML file created by the Internet Assistant Wizard just as you can any other HTML file. However, any changes you make to the HTML file do not affect the Excel file. If you want to avoid the "split-source" problem that arises when you have different versions of the same document, make changes only to the Excel document and re-create the HTML file when necessary. If you are not concerned with the split-source problem, go ahead and make whatever modifications you see fit directly to the HTML file.

What Happens to Charts and Graphic Objects

If you convert an Excel worksheet containing a chart and include the chart as one of the items you want to convert in the first Internet Assistant Wizard dialog box, the chart is converted automatically to a GIF file, and the GIF file is placed in the same directory as the HTML file.

JUST A MINUTE

> Internet Assistant does not convert graphic and drawing objects; it converts only data and charts. If you want a specific graphics file in your HTML document, you must edit the text of the HTML file with a text or HTML editor and add the link to the graphic. If the graphics file is not in the correct format, you must convert it. In general, most browsers support graphics files in GIF or JPEG format.

Putting Excel Workbooks Directly on the Web

You can upload your Excel worksheets in their original format to your Web site without converting them to HTML or any other format. Those users who have Excel 97 can view your files precisely as they look to you. For users who do not have Microsoft Excel, the Excel 97 Viewer Program is available free from Microsoft. The Viewer can be downloaded from `http://www.ftp.com/product/keyv2.html`. Note that the Viewer program allows you only to view the Excel worksheet; you cannot modify the data contained within the worksheet with the Viewer.

Remember, however, that not all your Web site visitors will have the appropriate platform to use this viewer and many will not want to bother downloading it. Saving your Excel worksheets as HTML files ensures the widest cross-platform compatibility. But even if you convert your worksheets to HTML files, you should be aware that some users probably will not have browsers that support tables.

Summary

You can access World Wide Web documents or documents on your computer or network directly from the Web toolbar. Your default browser opens HTML files, whether they are local or on the Web, when you enter the URLs or pathnames in the text box at the right end of the Web toolbar. If you open documents in other formats using the Web toolbar, these documents open up in their associated applications.

20

The Internet Assistant Wizard facilitates the process of saving your Excel documents as HTML files. The wizard can convert charts and data but not graphics and drawing objects. You can then upload the files to your Web site using your standard procedure. You can also upload original Excel worksheets to your Web site, although you restrict the audience that can view them if you do so.

Workshop

Term Review

code page The character set used by a particular application or document.

hyperlink A "clickable" link: If you click the text of a hyperlink, a new document opens up. A hyperlink can be a link to another file on your system or on an external system, or it can be a link to a particular cell or range reference.

start page The page that opens by default when you open your Web browser.

URL Universal Resource Locator. A document address that follows the addressing system developed by the World Wide Web Consortium. Hyperlinks to World Wide Web files follow this convention.

Q&A

Q How can you access World Wide Web sites?

A Make sure that the Web toolbar is displayed. Enter the URL by typing the address in the text box at the right end of the toolbar and press Enter.

Q Why would you want to put Excel workbooks—either converted to HTML files or as-is—on a Web site?

A Internet users from anywhere in the world can access your data if you make it available on your Web site. If you convert your Excel documents to HTML format, the files are accessible to more users than if you put Excel files on your Web site unaltered.

Exercise

Try converting one or more of the workbooks you created in preceding hours to an HTML file using the Internet Assistant Wizard. You can choose either to create a separate HTML file or incorporate data from your workbook into an already existing HTML file if you have one.

20

Hour **21**

Sharing Workbooks and Consolidating Data

Why would you want to share a workbook with other users? If your workbook also functions as a database, there may be very good reasons why it must be accessible to more than one person at a time. One person may be retrieving data from it; another person may be adding data to it.

You may also have a workbook that requires input from several people. For example, you may prepare a forecast of anticipated product sales for the next quarter for one product, a colleague may fill in his forecast for a different product, and the entire file may then go to a manager for her revisions and approval.

These are just two of many reasons why you might want to share workbooks with different users. Keep in mind, however, that sharing workbooks can compromise data, particularly if you are not careful about who has authority to review and accept changes.

To work along with the examples in this hour, you should create a simple workbook with a few entries. Of course, you can also use a workbook you have previously created.

CAUTION

> Much of this chapter will not be applicable if you are not working on a network.

Setting Up a Workbook for Sharing

Here's how to set up a workbook for sharing with other users:

1. Open the workbook you want to make accessible to other users.

2. Choose Tools | Share Workbook from the main menu to display the Share Workbook dialog box, shown in Figure 21.1. Select the Editing tab if it is not visible.

   Notice that your name and the date are listed in the Who Has this Workbook Open Now field.

Figure 21.1.

The Share Workbook dialog box.

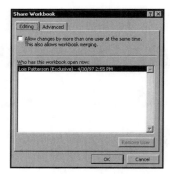

3. Check the Allow Changes by More than One User at the Same Time box.

4. Click OK.

5. You are prompted to save the file. Save the workbook to your network drive so that other users can access it.

JUST A MINUTE

> You can tell whether a workbook can be shared because [Shared] appears on the title bar along with the filename.

TIME SAVER

Any users who have access to the shared workbook will want to make sure that their names are set up properly in their personal copies of Excel. Otherwise, the **change history** (the record of the different changes made by different users) will be incorrect. Choose Tools | Options from the main menu and select on the General tab in the Options dialog box. Change your name as required and click OK.

Limitations of the Shared Workbook

You can see who is using a workbook at any given time by opening the workbook, displaying the Share Workbook dialog box, and looking at the Editing tab. The users who have the workbook open are listed in the Who Has this Workbook Open Now field.

Every user who has the workbook open can customize the view to suit his or her preferences. However, you are subject to a number of restrictions when using a shared workbook. You cannot create or edit charts, pictures, objects, hyperlinks, pivot tables, data tables, macros, scenarios, or data restrictions. You cannot change or edit passwords, nor can you add password protection (although any password scheme in place before the workbook was shared remains in place). You cannot delete worksheets, individual cells, or most groupings of cells, although you can insert or delete entire rows or columns.

Advanced Options

You can specify options for how long a change history should be kept, how frequently changes should be saved, and how conflicts between data input by various users should be handled.

To see the advanced options available, choose Tools | Share Workbook to display the Share Workbook dialog box and then select the Advanced tab (see Figure 21.2). The following sections describe the options available on this tab.

Figure 21.2.
The Advanced tab of the Share Workbook dialog box.

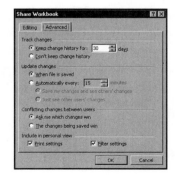

Tracking Changes

You have two options when it comes to tracking changes: You can keep a change history for a specified number of days, or you can decide not to keep a change history at all.

When you have multiple users working on one Excel workbook (or even if you are the sole user), you may want to keep a log of any changes made to the file. A change history can be particularly useful if you have complicated formulas that may become nonfunctional when you make certain changes. If you keep a history of the changes made to the file, you can figure out where you went wrong.

On the other hand, keeping a change history for days, weeks, and months greatly expands the size of your file. After a certain amount of time, you may see little need to keep track of changes made a long time ago.

To set a change history for a particular number of days, select the Keep Change History for X Days radio button and then select the value for X from the control. To keep no change history at all, select the Don't Keep Change History button.

Updating Changes

The options for updating changes let you determine when the file should be saved. You can specify that the file should be updated with any changes only when the file is saved. Alternatively, you can specify that the file should be automatically updated with any changes after a specified time interval has elapsed.

If you share your workbook with other users, you can also determine whether you want to see the changes others make when the file is being saved by selecting the Save Changes and Let Me See Others' Changes option. To see only the changes of other users, select the Just See Other Users' Changes option.

Resolving Conflicts between Users

When you share a file with other users, it is quite possible that there will be conflicts between information entered by two or more users. For example, if you enter data in cell F8, and another user enters different data in cell F8 of the same worksheet, you cannot both "win." Excel must make a choice between the value you entered and the value entered by the other user.

You can choose to be prompted about which changes "win" (that is, which changes are to be incorporated into the file), or you can choose to have the changes being saved win.

As noted in the section, "Making Revisions and Highlighting Changes," later in this hour, you can also choose which changes to accept or reject from the entire change history.

Modifying Personal Views

With a shared workbook, each user can have his or her own print and filter settings. To make these selections, check the boxes at the bottom of the Share Workbook dialog box.

21

The Print Settings option is in respect to preserving the settings for your default printer in Excel. The Filter Settings option is in respect to displaying or hiding particular rows and columns of data. One user may prefer to hide the top 100 rows of a worksheet, for example, because those rows have nothing to do with her interest in the worksheet. Another user may prefer to hide everything except 10 particular rows. Each user's filter choices can be preserved by him or her by checking this box.

The Protect Shared Workbook Options

You can set up a workbook for sharing and prevent other users from removing the change history. Recall that the *change history* lets you see what changes have been made by which users. If the change history is removed, it's difficult to be sure of the integrity of your data—particularly with a large worksheet. As the reviewer, you want to make sure that no stray errors have crept in by looking at the change history, particularly because the worksheet may be too large to scan visually.

Choose Tools | Protection | Protect and Share Workbook from the main menu to display the dialog box shown in Figure 21.3. Select the Sharing with Track Changes box. Enter a password if you want to protect the workbook with a password. Note that a password is only as secure as you make it. If you or other users give out the password to others, those people can access the workbook as well.

Figure 21.3.

The Protect Shared Workbook dialog box.

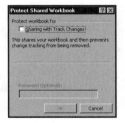

Removing a Workbook from Shared Use

Suppose that you've set up a workbook to be shared by more than one user. But now that everyone has had their chance to work on it, you want to have it revert back to single usage again. Here's how to make those changes:

1. Open the shared workbook.

2. Choose Tools | Share Workbook from the main menu and select the Editing tab.

   You should be the only person listed in the Who Has this Workbook Open Now field. If other people are listed in this field, ask them to save their work and close the file.

21

3. Click the Allow Changes by More than One User at a Time box so that no checkmark appears in it and click OK. The confirmation dialog box shown in Figure 21.4 appears.

4. Click Yes if you want to have the workbook revert to exclusive user status *and* you want to clear the change history. As mentioned earlier in the section "The Protect Shared Workbook Options," losing the change history prevents you, as the reviewer, from determining what changes have been made to a file.

Figure 21.4.

Removing a shared user.

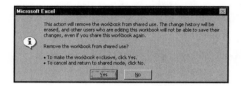

Making Revisions and Highlighting Changes

Excel 97 allows you to keep track of any revisions made to a workbook. In many situations, workbooks are handled by more than one person; keeping track of who does what to a file is very important if you want your data to be accurate.

Follow these steps to turn on the option to track changes so that you can see right away which cells have been altered:

1. Select Tools | Track Changes from the main menu and then choose Highlight Changes to display the Highlight Changes dialog box shown in Figure 21.5.

Figure 21.5.

The Highlight Changes dialog box.

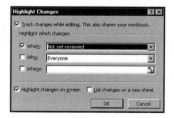

2. Select the Track Changes while Editing checkbox. This choice enables your workbook to be shared (just as choosing Tools | Share Workbook causes the workbook to be shared).

3. Choose your preferred tracking options: When, Who, and Where.

21

For the When and Who options, make selections from the drop-down list:

☐ For the When option, you have several suboptions: Since I Last Saved, All, Not Yet Reviewed, and Since Date.

☐ For the Who option, you have the following options: Everyone, Everyone But Me, *Name of User1*, *Name of User2, etc.* (note that Excel lists the names of every user with access to the shared workbook).

☐ For the Where option, click the Collapse Dialog icon and select the range of cells for which you want to highlight changes.

4. Check the Highlight Changes on Screen box if you want each user's changes to appear in a different color and you want a small triangle to appear in the upper-left corner of any cell that has had changes made to it. Select the cell containing such a triangle to see an accompanying comment that gives the revision history (see Figure 21.6).

Check the List Changes on a New Sheet box if you want the cell references for the changes you make to be listed on a new worksheet rather than be indicated on the active worksheet. The List Changes on a New Sheet option is available only if you have saved the workbook as a shared workbook.

Figure 21.6.

A comment showing the change history.

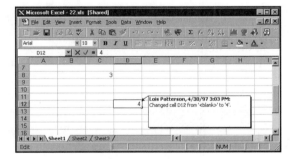

Accepting and Rejecting Revisions

You can decide at any point in the process whether you want to accept or reject the changes that have been made. In a hypothetical situation, one person may create the worksheet and enter some data, and then hand the workbook to the next person who makes some changes. Then a reviewer looks at the workbook and decides whether or not to keep the changes made by the second person.

You can deal with each worksheet in the workbook separately. You can also accept or reject changes for each cell individually. Here's how to accept or reject the changes that have been made to a worksheet:

1. Choose Tools | Track Changes | Accept or Reject Changes from the main menu to display the Select Changes to Accept or Reject dialog box (see Figure 21.7).

21

Figure 21.7.

The Select Changes to Accept or Reject dialog box.

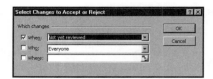

2. Specify the changes you want to review by making the appropriate choices for the When, Who, and Where options.

☐ For the When option, you can choose the date after which you want to review the changes, or you can choose to see all changes that have not been reviewed.

☐ For the Who option, you can choose to review your own changes, those of other users excluding yourself, or the changes of everyone (the default).

☐ For the Where option, you can select the specific cell or range for which you want to view the changes and decide whether to accept or reject the changes.

3. Click OK when you have made your choices. The Accept or Reject Changes dialog box shown in Figure 21.8 appears.

Figure 21.8.

The Accept or Reject Changes dialog box.

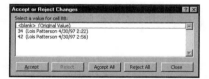

4. You can process the changes for one cell at a time. From the list of changes in the Accept or Reject Changes dialog box, select the value you want the cell to have and click Accept. Excel searches for the next revised cell and displays the Accept or Reject Changes dialog box for that change. You are given the opportunity to accept or reject every change that has been made. The revision process looks at the cells in order from left to right, and from top to bottom.

If you want to accept all the changes made, without reviewing them individually, click Accept All; the revised versions of all the cells are accepted. If you want to reject all the changes made, without reviewing them individually, click Reject All; none of the changes made is accepted. Note that if you choose this option, you reject all the changes without viewing each change individually.

5. Click Close to terminate the entire operation.

The Reviewing Toolbar

The Reviewing toolbar lets you made changes and alterations to a worksheet or workbook. You can use this toolbar to add, edit, or delete comments to each of the revised cells.

21

To see the Reviewing toolbar, choose View | Toolbars | Reviewing from the main menu. The Reviewing toolbar is shown in Figure 21.9.

Figure 21.9.

The Reviewing toolbar.

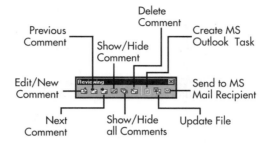

If you have turned on Tracking Changes and are highlighting changes on-screen, you will see the tiny markers indicating which cells have been revised. If you run your cursor over these cells, you see a comment telling you when and what the change is and who made it. You can edit these comments by clicking the Edit Comment tool on the Reviewing toolbar. The comment box appears so that you can make your changes.

You can move between the comments by clicking either the Previous Comment or Next Comment tool. You can show or hide particular comments (or show or hide all the comments at once) by clicking the appropriate tool on the Reviewing toolbar. You can also delete comments.

In addition, you can create a Microsoft Outlook task, update the file, or send the workbook to a Microsoft Mail recipient.

Merging Workbooks

Excel includes a feature for merging different workbooks together. You can use this feature when you have more than one reviewer working on a file. Each reviewer opens his or her own copy of the file and works on it independently. When all the different copies are complete, you can merge them into a single copy. You can then review the change history generated by this process and determine which changes by which reviewers you want to keep. This process works very well if the reviewers have been given different sections of a workbook to work on. With the merge option, there is no question of losing changes because of a conflict between two or more reviewers.

There is a two-step process involved here. You must first prepare separate copies of the file and then, when the reviewers have finished their work, merge the copies together.

21

To prepare the separate copies of the workbook, follow these steps:

1. Create the workbook.
2. Make the workbook a shared workbook by choosing Tools | Shared Workbook from the main menu to display the Share Workbook dialog box.
3. Check the Allow Changes by More than One User at the Same Time box on the Editing tab.
4. Click the Advanced tab and choose a number of days for the change history. Make sure that the time period you specify is long enough for all of the reviewers to do their work. It's safer to specify too many days than too few because you cannot merge files if the change history tracking time has expired.
5. Click OK to close the dialog box.
6. Save the file as usual.
7. Choose File | Save As from the main menu and save the file again, this time using a different filename. This step creates a copy of the file for another reviewer.
8. Repeat step 7 as many times as necessary to create enough copies of the original file for all the reviewers.

The reviewers can now get to work on their respective files for a period of days, weeks, or months. Just remember that the time period you specified in step 4 is the deadline by which you must merge the reviewed files.

When you want to compare and combine the changes from the various reviewers to make a final document, you merge the files together as follows:

1. Open one copy of the workbook.
2. Choose Tools | Merge Workbooks from the main menu. Save the file if you are prompted to do so. The Select Files to Merge into Current Workbook dialog box appears (see Figure 21.10).
3. Select the file—recalling the different names under which you saved the files in the first step of the process—you want to merge with the active workbook. You can enter the filename or browse through the directories.
4. Click OK when you have made your selections. The dialog box closes and the selected files are merged into the open workbook.

So, which workbook wins out when you merge two workbooks? The active workbook is the one that has its cells changed; the workbook you choose from the Open dialog box is the one whose cell contents are accepted.

21

Figure 21.10.

The Select Files to Merge into Current Workbook dialog box.

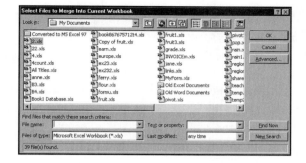

Suppose that you have the workbook region.xls open and you choose to merge the region1.xls file with it. The changes in region1.xls win out. The result is the region.xls worksheet open on your screen with the contents of region1.xls. You can then review the changes—as you would with any other document—as described earlier in this hour in "Accepting and Rejecting Revisions."

If you want to merge more copies of the document, repeat the preceding process for each document. Keep in mind that the final document merged is the one whose changes are displayed. However, the change history tells the story of what has happened, and you can accept or reject any of the many changes made to the original document.

You can also merge all the copies of the files at the same time. Refer to step 3 of the preceding steps; if you want to select more than one file to merge into the active workbook, press and hold the Ctrl key (to select nonadjacent files) or the Shift key (to select adjacent files) and select the various files. Otherwise, continue the steps as described.

Summary

Excel includes a number of features to facilitate sharing workbooks among different users. If you are working in a networked environment, you can make the workbook files accessible on the network. You can protect the workbooks if you want by locking cells or by setting up password protection. Hour 6, "Formatting and Protecting Worksheets," gives you more information on protecting your worksheets.

Workshop

Term Review

change history   The record Excel keeps (if you have turned on this option) of the changes made to a file by particular users within a particular period of time.

21

Q&A

Q **What does *sharing workbooks* mean?**

A When you "share a workbook," it means that two or more users can access a workbook file simultaneously.

Q **Why would you want to share workbooks?**

A If the data contained in the workbook is important, more than one person may need to have access to it. Several people may need to work together on a single file.

Q **What is the change history?**

A You can turn on the Change History feature so that all the changes made to a workbook are preserved. You can then accept or reject these various changes.

Q **How do you merge workbooks?**

A First you create two or more copies of a file, making sure that sharing is turned on and that the change history is being preserved. Then the various reviewers work on their own copies of the workbook. When all the reviewers are finished, you can combine the files together with the Merge Workbook feature.

21

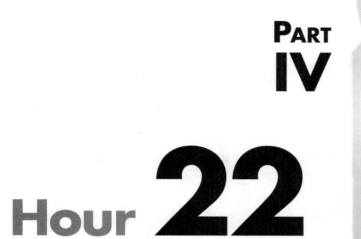

Hour 22

Creating and Running Macros

What is a *macro*? It is a small program that does a specific task automatically. Some people, when they hear the word *program*, freeze up in fear. Don't worry—macros are no more than a recorded series of steps. If you know how to do a task in the first place, a macro is just a way of doing it again. Macros are written in a programming language called Visual Basic for Applications. However, the way Excel has set up the process of macro creation, you need never see the actual code—at least for relatively simple macros.

You can devise macros to automate tasks such as the following:

- ☐ Automatically generate particular headers or footers.
- ☐ Make bold a particular range of cells.
- ☐ Choose a particular selection of cells and print it.
- ☐ Search and replace a number of different words or phrases.

☐ Copy and paste information from a cell containing a particular formula to another worksheet.

☐ Color a cell a particular color and AutoFit it so that it is wide enough for the contents.

A macro is like a recording. It executes all the keystrokes for a particular task—and you don't have to do anything while it operates. You can play the macro over and over again as necessary.

Macros can save you keystrokes, and they can also be used to make a difficult and intricate task foolproof. If you create the macro correctly in the first place, you can run it without having to worry about errors.

In this hour, you do not get into heavy-duty programming with Visual Basic for Applications (VBA)—that would fill a book of its own. But you should know that Excel does offer you the opportunity to create full-scale applications with VBA if you want to do so.

JUST A MINUTE

Macros are not the only way you can automate specific tasks. You can use *templates*, as described in Hour 7, "Using Excel Worksheet Templates," to save particular formats for use over and over again.

Creating a Macro

Suppose that you want to create a macro that will automatically place a header on a worksheet. With macros, you can create a header once and then insert it instantly into any of your documents. Suppose that you are responsible for more than one department at your company, and each department has its own specific header for its worksheets. You can create a macro for each department so that the appropriate header is inserted for the worksheets.

To start recording a macro, choose Tools | Macro | Record New Macro from the main menu to display the Record Macro dialog box shown in Figure 22.1.

Figure 22.1.
The Record Macro dialog box.

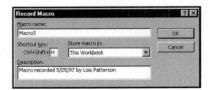

22

Naming the Macro

You can name the macro whatever you want. However, you cannot have a name of more than 255 characters, and you are limited to numbers, letters, and the underscore character; you cannot include spaces in the macro name. You cannot begin the name with a number or the underscore character. Type the name in the Macro Name text box in the Record Macro dialog box. In this example, the name Macro3 is used.

Choosing a Keyboard Shortcut

You can also choose a keyboard shortcut for your macro, although this is optional. Excel has a number of keyboard shortcuts for performing various tasks, as described in Hour 3, "Introduction to the Excel Environment." If you type a lowercase **a** in the Shortcut Key field of the Record Macro dialog box, you can later run the macro by pressing the Ctrl and the A keys together. If you type an uppercase **A**, you can later run the macro by pressing the Ctrl, the Shift, and the A keys together.

In this example, the purpose of the macro is to create a header, so we'll type **H** in the Shortcut Key field. This means that we can later activate this macro by pressing the Ctrl, Shift, and H keys together.

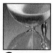

CAUTION

> If you use a keyboard shortcut for your macro, the keys you specify will override any preexisting Excel keyboard shortcut. Either choose a keyboard shortcut that isn't already used by Excel, or choose one that you rarely or never use.

For this example, choose the default This Workbook option from the Store Macro In drop-down list. Later in this hour, you learn how to make macros available in some or all of the workbooks in your files.

Adding a Description

Excel includes a default description in the Description field of the Record Macro dialog box that shows the date the macro was recorded and the owner of the Excel program used to create the macro. Change the text in the Description field to something descriptive to help you or your fellow users remember the purpose of the macro.

Once you have made all your choices in the Record Macro dialog box, click OK. The Stop Recording toolbar appears on the screen (see Figure 22.2).

Figure 22.2.

The tiny Stop Recording toolbar.

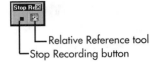

— Relative Reference tool
— Stop Recording button

Recording the Macro

You can now start to record the steps of the macro. Press the keystrokes necessary to do a particular task. For this example, you want the macro to add a header to an Excel file. Perform these steps to record them in the macro:

1. Choose View | Header and Footer from the main menu. The Page Setup dialog box appears.

2. Use the Page Setup dialog box to create the header as you normally would. When you are finished defining the header, click OK to close the dialog box.

3. Click the Stop Recording button to end the macro.

You can now resume working with your worksheet as you normally do—entering data, drawing graphics, doing charts, or whatever you want to do.

The macro you have created will work for all the worksheets in your current workbook. To find how to make your macro applicable to all Excel worksheets, refer to the section "Saving a Macro to Use in Other Workbooks," later in this hour. Because this macro does not operate on a specific cell, absolute or relative cell references don't matter here. However, for many macros, the type of cell reference you use is significant. Refer to the section "Absolute and Relative References with Macros," later in this hour.

TIME SAVER

If you are typing text in your macro, make an error, and then delete the unwanted text, Excel does not include these missteps in the macro. Similarly, if you open a dialog box and then cancel out of it, Excel does not record that mistake either.

Be sure to click the Stop Recording button when you are finished with the macro. If you forget to click this button, the macro continues to record your activities within the worksheet. The macro grows larger and larger, and will be useless because you will not want to use the extra steps it is recording in other macros.

Saving the Macro

If you choose This Workbook from the Store Macro In drop-down list in the Record Macro dialog box, the macro you create in a particular workbook is saved when you save the workbook. The macro is available only for that particular workbook.

22

If you choose `New Workbook` from the Save Macro In drop-down list, you are prompted for the name of a new workbook in which to store your files. If you choose this option, the macro is available only for that particular workbook.

Saving a Macro to Use in Other Workbooks

The sample macro you created in the preceding exercise is limited to use in the workbook in which you created it or saved it. If you want to use a macro in other workbooks, you can specify that in the Record Macro dialog box. From the Save Macro In drop-down list, you can choose to save the macro in a new workbook or in a personal macro workbook.

If you choose `Personal Macro Workbook`, the macro you create will be available in all your workbooks. What happens is that Excel creates a workbook called `PERSONAL.XLS` and stores it in your `C:\Program Files\Microsoft Office\Office\XLStart` directory (assuming that you installed Excel in the default directory). `PERSONAL.XLS` is opened every time you open Excel, although it is hidden from view.

Absolute and Relative References with Macros

The macro you created earlier inserts a header into a document. It does not refer to particular cells. However, many—perhaps most—of the macros you create refer to specific cells. For these macros, the question of whether to use absolute or relative references is significant.

Suppose that you want to create a macro that finds the difference between numbers in the two cells above the cell in which the macro is located. Here's how you would create that macro using the default absolute references:

1. Choose Tools | Macro | Record New Macro from the main menu. Enter a name for the macro, such as `subC`, and specify a shortcut key if you want.

2. Select cell C3 and enter the formula `=C2-C1`.

3. Click the Stop Recording icon to stop recording the macro.

Try applying this macro to another worksheet in your workbook. Type some numbers in cells C1 and C2 and run the macro. It won't matter where your cursor is when you run the macro; the result of the formula is automatically placed in cell C3 and will be based on the values in cells C1 and C2.

However, you may want the macro to find the difference between two numbers directly above the active cell, wherever that active cell happens to be. To have the macro do that, you must use relative cell references. To create a macro so that it works with relative references, follow these steps:

1. Begin the macro as usual by choosing Tools | Macro | Record New Macro from the main menu.

2. Type the name of the macro and specify a shortcut key if you want.

3. Click the Relative Reference tool, located on the right side of the Stop Recording toolbar.

4. Enter your formula as you did before: Select cell C3 and enter the formula =C2-C1.

When you run this version of the macro, it looks at the cells that are one and two cells above the selected cell—whatever that cell is—and calculates the formula based on those numbers. The macro places the formula result in the selected cell. For example, if you select cell F9 and run the macro, the formula calculates the result of F8–F7.

Using a Macro

If you created a macro and assigned it a shortcut key, you can execute the macro by pressing Ctrl+*key*. You can also run the macro by choosing Tools | Macro | Macros from the main menu and clicking the name of the macro you want to run.

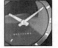

JUST A MINUTE

To stop a macro while it is running, press the Esc key.

TIME SAVER

Save your work before creating or executing a macro. It's possible that a poorly designed macro can cause you to exit from Excel or make the system crash (although these results are unlikely with very simple macros). Nevertheless, it's always best to back up your data by saving it.

To delete a macro, choose Tools | Macro | Macros from the main menu. In the Macro dialog box that appears, highlight the macro you want to delete and click the Delete button.

Editing a Macro

If you have done some programming, or if you are interested in doing so, you may prefer to work directly with the macro code. Excel macros are written in the language Visual Basic for Applications (VBA). When you create macros with the Record Macro dialog box, you are insulated from actually seeing the Visual Basic code. However, you can choose to see and edit the code for yourself if you want to make changes to the code. This section does not describe the VBA syntax in detail. If you want to find out more about using Visual Basic for Applications, check the Excel online help and find the Microsoft Excel Visual Basic Reference.

22

To look at the code of a macro and edit it, choose Tools | Macro | Macros from the main menu and click the Step Into button on the Macro dialog box. The Visual Basic code that makes up the macro appears.

Changing Macro Options

When you create a macro, you may find later that you want to make changes to it. Perhaps you think that a different shortcut key is more appropriate, or that the description is incorrect (as may be the case if you are changing someone else's work to suit your own preferences). With Excel, you can change the shortcut key assigned to a macro as well as the description for the macro.

Choose Tools | Macros | Macro from the main menu to display the Macro dialog box. Click the Options button to display a dialog box similar to the one in Figure 22.3. Make the required changes to the macro's description or shortcut key and click OK.

Figure 22.3.

The Macro Options dialog box.

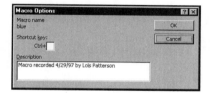

Attaching a Macro to a Graphic or Button

With many computer applications, you press or click buttons or pictures to achieve particular effects. For example, within an Excel worksheet, you can click the Print tool in the Standard toolbar, which resembles a printer, to print a file. Similarly, when you are creating forms in Excel, you can create macros that are associated with graphical images. When you click the image, the macro is activated. For example, you may have a macro that calculates mortgage payments. You can attach that macro to a picture of a house to form a logical connection between what the macro does and the graphic that activates the macro.

To assign a macro to a graphic, first draw or insert the graphic on the worksheet. Right-click the graphic and select Assign Macro from the popup menu. Select the macro you want to associate with the graphic.

You can move the graphic around just as you would any other graphic object. Many designers like to attach macros to graphic objects that look like pushbuttons for both aesthetic appeal and functionality.

Understanding Macro Viruses

As millions of computer users share information, there is a growing danger of malicious people creating viruses that can destroy data. A macro *virus* is a macro written to be destructive. Macro viruses, which can be programmed to infect various Office 97 applications, are a growing plague, but you can take steps to help prevent data loss on your system. Some macro viruses are cute—they do things such as put a little message at the bottom of each page. Other viruses are malicious and can destroy all the data on your hard drive. In any event, macro viruses can be designed to infect all your Excel files. If your files are infected with a macro virus, you must use antivirus software to kill it.

When you open a file that contains macros, whether it is one you created or one you received from someone else, you see the dialog box shown in Figure 22.4. If you are sure that the macros contained in the file are safe, click Enable Macros. However, if the file is from a "foreign" source—even if it's from a trusted friend or business associate—the file may contain a virus.

Figure 22.4.

Opening a workbook
that contains macros.

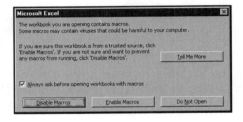

You can find more information about the latest Excel viruses at this Web site:

`http://www.microsoft.com/excel/productinfo/vbavirus/emvolc.htm`

You can download Excel add-ins from Microsoft that can detect and clean Excel viruses from the Web page. You can find these add-ins at the following URL:

`http://www.microsoft.com/excel/productinfo/vbavirus/add_in.htm`

Creating a Macro Toolbar

Now that you have worked with Excel for a while, you have become very familiar with toolbars. You can create your own macro toolbars to do specific tasks. Creating your own

22

toolbars was discussed in Hour 4, "Data Entry and Editing in Excel." This section discusses how to make toolbars for your macros.

First, create the toolbar by following these steps:

1. Choose Tools | Customize from the main menu to display the Customize dialog box shown in Figure 22.5.

Figure 22.5.

The Customize dialog box for toolbars.

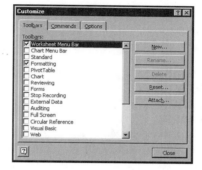

2. Click the New button and enter a name for your toolbar. For this example, type **Header** and click OK.

3. Now add commands to the toolbar: Select the Commands tab in the Customize dialog box and choose Macros from the Categories list.

4. Drag the happy-face Custom Button into the toolbar, as shown in Figure 22.6.

Figure 22.6.

Dragging the happy-face button into your newly created toolbar.

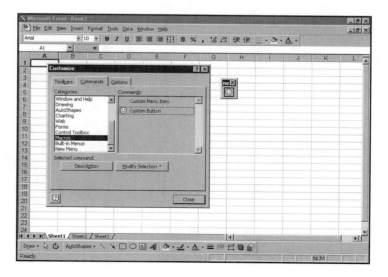

5. Right-click the happy-face button and choose Assign Macro from the popup menu (see Figure 22.7). The Assign Macro dialog box appears.

Figure 22.7.

The popup menu for the macro toolbar.

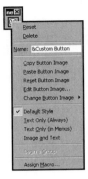

6. From the Assign Macro dialog box, click the name of the macro you want to assign to the happy-face button.

7. Click Close to close the Customize dialog box.

The happy-face icon, cute as it may be, is not always the best graphic for business applications. In most cases, you would do better to use a specially created graphic with an associated macro if you feel the urge to add visual appeal to your worksheets.

To change from the happy-face icon, right-click the icon and choose Change Button Image from the popup menu. The menu of options shown in Figure 22.8 appears. Click an image, and the toolbar button then displays that image.

Figure 22.8.

The choices for changing the macro button image.

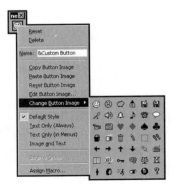

22

Creating Web Forms

If you have a World Wide Web site, you know the value of soliciting user input. You may even have a business or personal site set up to elicit specific information. Online forms are used to take purchase orders, technical support requests, and other information. You can use Excel to create these forms.

To use the Forms feature, you must have CGI support on your Web site, or you must be running the Microsoft Internet Information Server with the Internet Database Connector. CGI stands for Common Gateway Interface and refers to your site's capability of running programs on the Web server. If you are not familiar with the World Wide Web, ask your system administrator for assistance before you begin the following exercise, particularly with steps 3 through 6.

First, you must create your form so that it contains the controls you need for the user to enter the data you require. When you create a form, you decide which choices the user will be able to make; you make these choices available to the user with controls such as option boxes, list boxes, radio buttons, checkboxes, and so on. The labels on the blanks in the form correspond to the field names in the database.

The form used in the following example is a T-shirt order form, which offers different options for color and neckline styles. Keep in mind that Web forms are of limited usefulness because users who access your form on the Web must have Microsoft Excel on their systems in order to fill out the form.

Once you've created the form in your Excel worksheet, follow these steps to turn it into a Web form:

1. Choose Tools | Wizard | Web Form from the main menu.

   If you don't see the Web Form Wizard on the Wizard submenu, you must install it. Choose Tools | Add-ins from the main menu, select the Web Form Wizard checkbox, and click OK. Once the wizard is installed, choose Tools | Wizard | Web Form from the main menu to display the first dialog box of the wizard. (This dialog box is purely informational.)

2. Click Next to display the second dialog box of the Web Form Wizard (see Figure 22.9). This dialog box contains the various controls you can add to your form. The option buttons that are part of the Excel worksheet—such as style Option Button 2—are each listed by name. Of course, you can also use other types of controls such as checkboxes, list boxes, and so forth from the Forms toolbar.

Figure 22.9.

Step 2 of 6 in the Web Form Wizard, along with a typical form.

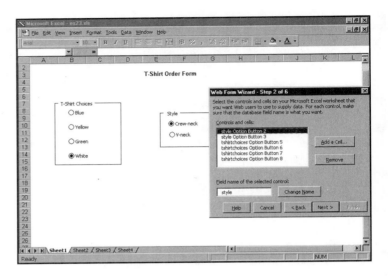

3. If you want to change the name of a control, do so in the Field Name of Selected Control box. You may want to change the name of a control if you want the control to have a different name on the Web than it does on the worksheet. Click Next to display the third dialog box of the Web Form Wizard.

4. In the third dialog box, select the type of Web server you have and click Next to display the fourth dialog box of the wizard.

5. Decide whether you want to save the Web form as a Microsoft Excel file (which is what you do in most situations) or to save it to your FrontPage Web (which you can do if you are using Microsoft FrontPage, of course). Enter the pathname in the File Path field and click Next to display the Step 5 dialog box of the Web Form Wizard (see Figure 22.10).

Figure 22.10.

Step 5 of the Web Form Wizard.

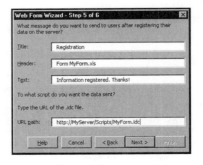

22

22

6. Specify the message you want your users to see after they submit the data in the online form. This message requires a *title*, which is displayed in the Windows 95 title bar. The *header* is displayed in large, bold text at the top of the page. The text of the page comes below the header. The purpose of this message is to let users know that the data has been entered and received. Type the title, header, and text you want and enter the URL that the .idc file is to have. Click Next to display the final dialog box of the wizard.

7. The final dialog box gives some general information about placing the files on your server. The wizard has created all the files you need for the online form; you must upload them to the server to make them available to other users. Click Finish to end the wizard. The files you need to upload all have the same name as the .xls file. For example, if the file is myform.xls, all the other files also begin with myform. For more information on how to set up the files on the Web server, search the Online Help topics for Web Form Wizard.

Summary

In this hour, you have learned the basics of creating and running macros. Macros are programs written in Visual Basic for Applications that work within Excel to do specific tasks. Ordinary users can create and use macros without having to do any programming. You can capture the keystrokes required to do a specific task, save the sequence of keystrokes, and then run the macro to reproduce the keystrokes whenever you need to do so.

Another programming task Excel can do is to create a Web form (and the associated files you need to implement it) for use on World Wide Web sites. The Web Form Wizard streamlines the process so that you don't have to do any programming.

Workshop

Term Review

macro   A usually small program you can create by recording a series of keystrokes. You can then run the macro as often as necessary to repeat those keystrokes. You can save a macro in the current workbook, a new workbook, or make it available for use in all your Excel workbooks.

keyboard shortcut   Two or three assigned keys that, when you press them together, perform a particular task, such as running a macro or saving a file.

virus   A usually malicious program that can be attached to macros or other executable files.

form   In Excel, a form is a part of a worksheet in which the user can enter particular data that is then stored in a database.

Q&A

Q What are macros used for?

A Macros are used to automate time-consuming and repetitive tasks. If you use a correctly designed macro to do a task that would otherwise take a number of steps, you can be sure of getting it right the first time.

Exercises

☐ Create a macro that colors a column of cells blue.

1. Select Tools | Macros | Record New Macro from the main menu.
2. Enter a name for the macro—**blue** is an appropriate choice—and click OK.

3. Click the Relative Reference tool on the Stop Recording toolbar.
4. Select a column in the worksheet (it doesn't matter which one).
5. Choose Format | Cells from the main menu to display the Format Cells dialog box and select the Patterns tab.
6. Select the color blue you prefer and click OK.
7. Click the Stop Recording button.

☐ Run the macro you just created.

1. Select a cell in the column you want to color.
2. Choose Tools | Macros | Macro from the main menu to display the Macro dialog box.
3. Select the **blue** macro and click Run. The selected column will turn blue.

☐ For extra credit, create an icon with the **blue** macro attached. A natural choice is a blue circle.

1. Create a blue circle.
2. Select the circle and right-click it to display the popup menu.
3. Choose Assign Macro.
4. Select the **blue** macro and click OK.
5. Run the macro attached to the blue circle: Select a cell in the column you want to color and then click the blue circle graphic. The selected column will turn blue.

22

Hour 23

Using Custom Controls, Forms, and Data Validation

In the preceding hours, you have learned different ways to control the appearance of worksheets with different colors, fonts, graphics, borders, and patterns.

Controls, forms, and data validation are other ways you can control the appearance and behavior of your worksheets. You can set out the type of data each cell will accept and use the controls to facilitate the entry of this data. Data forms are a way to facilitate data entry.

The Forms Toolbar

You can use the Forms toolbar, shown in Figure 23.1, to place various sorts of controls on your worksheets. A *control* allows you to perform particular tasks within Excel. A control can be a button, a checkbox, a list box, or something similar that allows the user to make choices within a form.

Figure 23.1.

The Forms toolbar.

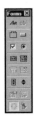

In your use of dialog boxes, you have seen many of these controls. For example, many dialog boxes use checkboxes so that you can check or uncheck an option. Similarly, you can use the checkbox control to provide those who use your worksheet with the same easy way to enter data.

Here are the various types of controls you can place on a worksheet:

Control	Description
Label	Use this control for a simple text box.
Group Box	You can group two or more controls together into a single area. This control is useful for option boxes, as discussed in "The Option Box Control," later in this hour.
Button	You can assign a macro to a button graphic that executes when the button is clicked.
Checkbox	You can select a single option or not by checking the box.
Option Box	Also called a *radio button*. You can choose one—and only one—of a list of choices.
List Box	Contains a list of items from which you can choose.
Combo Box	Contains a drop-down list of items from which you can choose.
Scrollbar	You can scroll through a list of options, or click the scroll arrows to move through the list of options.
Spinner	For numeric values only. By clicking the spinner arrows, you increase or decrease the value in the text box.

Using the Controls on the Forms Toolbar

To use a tool on the Forms toolbar, click it. Then position the mouser pointer in the worksheet where you want the control to go, click, and drag the mouse until the control is the size you want it. Each of the controls makes a rectangular shape; you can control how big the rectangle is and what proportions it has.

23

The Label Control

Label controls do not "do" anything. In most cases, you are better off entering a label into an Excel cell as usual and then formatting it as you want. You cannot use labels created with the label tool in formulas, nor can you format them. However, with the label tool, you can create labels that overlap parts of cells in a way you cannot do with text in an actual Excel cell.

Click the tool and then click the worksheet where you want to place the control. Drag the pointer until the label control is the size you want. Once you have drawn the label, click inside the box to edit the text.

The Checkbox Control

You use a checkbox control, as its name implies, to check a box if you want a certain option; you uncheck the box if you do not want that option.

Click the checkbox tool in the Forms toolbar and drag a checkbox control on your worksheet. To edit the text of the checkbox, select the control and then right-click it to display the popup menu. Choose Edit Text from the popup menu. Change the text of the checkbox to something that makes sense in context. For example, if you are creating a customer survey form, you might want the text of the checkbox to be `Check here to be added to our mailing list`.

You may want to change the settings of the checkbox so that it is either checked or not by default. Choose Format | Control from the main menu to display the Format Control dialog box and select the Control tab. You can set up the checkbox so that its default value is Checked, Unchecked, or Mixed. If you choose Mixed, the box is grayed out so that neither the checked nor unchecked state is preferred.

Choose the Cell Link option to link to the cell reference you want to control. The cell you specify will be given the value `TRUE` if the checkbox is checked; it will be given the value `FALSE` if the checkbox is unchecked. The cell reference does not have to be in the same worksheet or the same workbook. In practice, you can use the `TRUE` or `FALSE` value in other formulas to determine a particular result. Suppose that you are creating an order form. The checkbox control asks users whether they want their e-mail addresses added to a mailing list. A possible formula could look at the value of the cell link; if the cell's value is `TRUE` (indicating that the user has checked the box and wants to be added to the mailing list), the formula then looks at the e-mail address entered by the user (elsewhere in the worksheet) and copies this e-mail address to another worksheet.

Each of the other tabs on the Format Control dialog box affects certain properties. You can change the following with each of the other tabs:

☐ Use the Colors and Lines tab to change the appearance of the checkbox
☐ Use the Size tab to change the size of the checkbox

☐ Use the Protection tab to change whether or not the control is locked

☐ Use the Properties tab to determine the interaction of the control with other cells in the worksheet

The Option Box Control

Option boxes are used when you want to offer at least two options but you want the choices to be mutually exclusive. For example, on an order form, you may want to offer three color choices for an item. For each item, however, only one of those color choices can be selected. The option box control is perfect for this situation because it allows only one of the group of boxes to be selected at a time. Option boxes are also called *radio buttons*.

In Figure 23.2, three option box controls are drawn and the appropriate text has been inserted. (To edit the text associated with each option box, right-click the control and choose Edit Text from the popup menu.) Each control also has a cell link to cell F13. To specify the cell link, select each option box in turn, display the Format Control dialog box, and click the Control tab. Enter the cell reference in the Cell Link field.

Figure 23.2.

An example showing three option boxes.

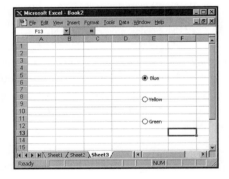

You can control the appearance of an option box by displaying the Format Control dialog box, selecting the Colors and Lines tab, and choosing the fill and line options you want from the dialog box.

You can group option box controls that are logically linked together by selecting the group box tool from the Forms toolbar (it's the tool with the letters XYZ on top of the square) and drawing a box around the controls you want to group together. If you do not use a group box control to group a set of option boxes together, all the option boxes in a worksheet are linked together, no matter where they are located.

Click inside the group box to edit the text. You may want to put a title at the top to indicate what the option boxes are about. If you want to edit the text of the option buttons themselves, right-click a button and choose Edit Text from the popup menu.

23

The value in the cell referred to by the Cell Link reference depends on the numerical position of the selected option box. If you select the first option, the value 1 appears in the linked cell. If you select the second option, the value 2 appears in the linked cell, and so on.

You can specify whether you want the option box controls to have a default value of Checked or Unchecked by displaying the Format Control dialog box and selecting the Control tab. Only one option box in a group can be checked, so if you try to choose Checked for more than one of the option boxes in the group, only the latest one is selected.

If you use group boxes, you can have as many groups of option boxes as you want. If you do not group your option buttons, all the ungrouped option boxes in the worksheet belong to the same group—meaning that only one option box in the entire worksheet can be selected.

TIME SAVER

You do not have to position the option boxes in a line in your worksheet, but in most cases, there is an obvious advantage in terms of appearance if you do so.

The Scrollbar Control

The scrollbar control is used to scroll through sequential integer values. (Note that a *scrollbar control* differs from the *scrollbars* that appear along the side or bottom of the screen in Excel to help you navigate a document.) Draw the control using the scrollbar tool from the Forms toolbar in the usual way. Most designers create scrollbar controls that are relatively small, but you can make them as large as you want. You determine whether the scrollbar is horizontal or vertical when you first draw the control.

To set the values through which the scrollbar can operate, display the Format Control dialog box and click the Control tab (see Figure 23.3). Use the minimum and maximum fields to set these values for the scrollbar.

Figure 23.3.

The Format Control dialog box for the scrollbar control.

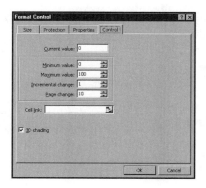

The Incremental Change setting allows you to specify the increment that each click on the arrow bar causes. The default increment is 1, but you can specify that each click on the scrollbar causes the value of the scrollbar control to increment or decrement by 2, 5, 10, 100, or any number you want.

The Page Change setting controls how much the value of the scrollbar changes when you click in between the arrows on the scrollbar.

Indicate the cell reference for the cell you want to control with the scrollbar in the Cell Link field. In most cases, you want to place the scrollbar control next to the linked cell so that the connection between the two is apparent to the user. In Figure 23.4, the cell link is B15 because that is an obvious location for the answer to the question. The Incremental Change value for the scrollbar control is 5, and the Page Change value is 10. Note that the user can still type the number directly if he or she wants to do so; the user is not bound by the increment value when typing a specific value. That is, the user can type 12 even though the scrollbar control permits entries of only 10 and 15.

Figure 23.4.

The scrollbar control in action.

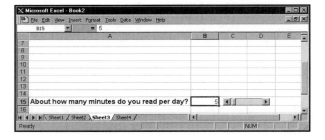

The Spinner Control

The spinner control is similar to the scrollbar control except that the spinner control is oriented vertically. In addition, the spinner control has no space between the arrows and has no Page Change setting to specify. Otherwise, you specify the Current Value, the Minimum Value, the Maximum Value, and the Incremental Change value in the same way you do for the scrollbar control: from the Control tab on the Format Control dialog box.

JUST A MINUTE

The 3D Shading option is available for both the spinner and scrollbar controls. The shading of the two options differs; the 3D controls are shaded to look like 3D objects and the 2D controls are shaded to look like they are flat on the screen. The 3D controls are more visible than the 2D controls. In general, however, it is a matter of aesthetic choice whether you want 2D or 3D controls.

23

The List Box Control

You can create a list box control that allows the user to choose a particular item from a menu of choices.

First, you must create the list of choices and place it in a range of cells in the worksheet. For example, if you want your list box control to offer the options Hot Fudge, Strawberry, Caramel, and Plain, you enter these text values in a range of cells.

Next, you draw the list box control by selecting the list box tool from the Forms toolbar and dragging the rectangle around the range containing the options you just typed.

Display the Format Control dialog box; in the Input Range field, enter the range reference for the list of choices. In the Cell Link field, type the cell reference where you want the value selected from the list to appear.

The value that appears in the linked cell is not the actual value chosen from the list but a value that denotes the numerical position of the choice. For example, if Hot Fudge is first in the list and is the option chosen, the number 1 appears in the Cell Link reference. In practice, you will probably use this value in a formula. In Figure 23.5, Plain is selected, and the number 4 would appear in the Cell Link reference.

Figure 23.5.

A list box control.

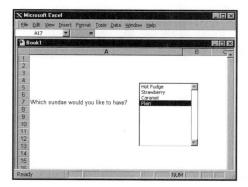

TIME SAVER

Cell Link references for any of the controls do not have to refer to a cell in the same worksheet as the control—or even in the same workbook. If you want, you can hide the cell referenced by the Cell Link, just as you can hide any other cell.

The Combo Box Control

The combo box control is much the same as the list box control, but it creates a drop-down list rather than showing all the available options at once. You enter the Input Range and Cell Link values for the combo box control in the same way as you do for the list box control: Display the Format Control dialog box, click the Control tab, and enter the desired values.

You can control how many of the entries are visible at one time by specifying the desired value in the Drop Down Lines field on the Control tab of the Format Control dialog box.

The Button Control

The button control is very versatile; you can use it to activate any macro you have created.

Draw the button on the worksheet by selecting the button tool from the Forms toolbar and dragging the button shape on the worksheet. You can format the button with the Format Controls dialog box so that it has the appearance you want.

To change the appearances and properties of the button, right-click *the border* of the button and select Format Control from the popup menu. If you right-click *inside* the control, you can specify the actual text that appears on the button.

To assign a macro to the button, right-click the border of the button and select Assign Macro from the popup menu. The Assign Macro dialog box appears. Enter the name of the macro, or record one, as described in Hour 22, "Creating and Running Macros." The Macros In field on the Assign Macro dialog box lets you control which workbooks are affected by the choice. Now when the user clicks the button, the macro operates automatically.

You can set up a button that calculates how much the user owes based on some other values entered in the worksheet, or that performs a subtotal calculation for an order form, or that does any of the myriad things you can do with macros.

COFFEE BREAK

Deciding which Control to Use

You can achieve similar effects with different types of controls. For example, you can have two option buttons do the work of one checkbox. However, in many situations, one choice will be preferable to another, for aesthetic or functional reasons.

If your list of choices changes fairly often, it's probably easier to use a list box control rather than an option box control to present the list of options because it's easier to add a value to the list or edit a value in the list than it is to add an option box control to a group.

23

Other Tabs on the Format Control Dialog Box

As you have undoubtedly noticed, the Format Control dialog box differs for each type of control. However, certain tabs are present for all the different controls: Size, Protection, Properties, and Control.

You use the Size tab to rescale a control—shrink it, expand it, and change its proportions. You can also change the size of a control by clicking the border of the control and dragging the handles until the control is the size you want.

You use the Protection tab to protect particular controls from being altered by the user. To protect the control, you must first protect the worksheet, as described in Hour 6, "Formatting and Protecting Worksheets." You can choose to protect the worksheet with a password if you want. After protecting the worksheet, you can either protect or unprotect a particular control by selecting the control, displaying the Format Control dialog box, and clicking the Protection tab. The Format Control dialog box differs for each type of control—choose the options you want for the particular control you are formatting.

You use the Properties tab to make choices regarding the positioning of the control. You can specify whether or not the control should move with the underlying cells, if those are moved, and whether or not the control should be resized if the underlying cells are resized.

Managing Controls and Other Objects

You may have a control that you want to place on top of a graphic, or you may want a graphic to cover up part of a control. You can determine the position of objects in relation to each other, whether they are controls or graphic objects.

Suppose that two or more objects occupy some of the same area, and you want to move one to the front or one to the back. Select one of the objects and right-click. Select Order from the popup menu and then choose from the various options on the submenu: Bring to Front, Send to Back, Bring Forward, and Send Backward. Bring Forward and Send Backward move the object forward or backward one level; Bring to Front and Send to Back move the object to the front or back of all the objects. With these four commands, you can manipulate each of the objects so that it occupies the position you want.

You may want to draw a rectangle that holds all the controls within it, leaving the rest of the worksheet free. You could create all the controls first, move them into the positions you want, and then draw a rectangle with the Rectangle tool from the Drawing toolbar. Then select the rectangle, right-click it to display the popup menu, and choose Order | Send to Back to send the rectangle object behind all the other control objects.

COFFEE BREAK

Worksheet and Form Design

With all the different controls you can use, worksheet design can be a little tricky. It's easy to throw together a bunch of different colors, controls, graphics, and fonts—but the result will be a rather wild-looking and somewhat inscrutable worksheet.

The design principle to keep foremost in your mind is this: **Keep it simple**. Your worksheet will work best if you include appropriate blank space and use color and graphics sparingly.

Gridlines are not necessary for most forms. When designing the form, however, you may want to have gridlines in place to help you determine cell references and cell links. You can always remove the gridlines later.

If you are designing your worksheets and forms for other users, seek their advice to see whether your work meets their needs.

Using Data Forms

When you create a data list (remember that a *list* is an internal database within Excel, as described in Hour 14, "More Data Manipulation"), you generally add data to it as time goes by. For example, if you have a list of customers and their purchases, some data in that list is likely to change (for example, when a customer's address changes) and the list is likely to need additions (for example, to add new customers and new products). Using a data form makes the process easy.

To create a data form that adds information to a data list in your worksheet, follow these steps:

1. Start by creating the list, making sure that the column labels are in place. You don't have to add all the data to the list—that's what the data form is for.

   A typical list is shown in Figure 23.6. You can use the data form to add, delete, and edit the data in that list.

2. Select any cell in the list.

3. Choose Data | Form from the main menu to display the dialog box shown in Figure 23.7.

   This is the data form you use to add, delete, or edit the information in the data list.

To navigate through the records, use the scrollbar to scroll up and down through the data list. You can also jump from record to record by clicking the Find Next or Find Prev button.

Figure 23.6.
A typical data list.

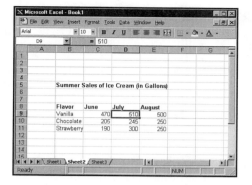

Figure 23.7.
A data form.

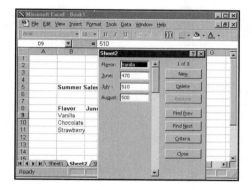

Adding a Record

To create a record, display the data form and click New. A new data form dialog box appears with all the labels in place, but with the data fields blank. Type information in each of the fields in the data form as you want the data to appear in the data list. Press Tab or Enter to move between fields in the data form. When you have entered all the information for the record, click the Close button to add the record to the data list, directly below the last record (row) in the data list. When you click Close, the data form dialog box closes and you return to the worksheet.

Figure 23.8 shows a data form dialog box with information for a new record. When you click Close, this information is added to the data list just as if you had entered the data directly to the worksheet.

Deleting a Record

To delete a record, open the data form dialog box and scroll through the records in the data list until you locate the record you want to delete. Click the Delete button.

Figure 23.8.

Adding a record to a data list.

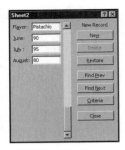

CAUTION

> If you use the data form to delete a record from your data list, you cannot get the record back. If you think you may have to restore a deleted record, you should delete the record directly in the worksheet; if you then have to restore the deleted record, click Undo or press Ctrl+Z.

Searching for and Finding Records

If your data list is particularly lengthy and you have to search for specific records within that list, you may find it easier to use the data form than to scan the list manually. To find a particular record in the data list, display the data form dialog box and click the Criteria button. A blank form appears. Enter the character string or numerical value you want to locate in a particular field and press Enter (or click Find Next). You return to the worksheet; the next available record that fits the specified criteria appears in the record form.

For example, if you are using the data list shown in Figure 23.6 and want to search for a particular quantity of ice cream sold in a specific month, first display the data form dialog box and then click the Criteria button. Now enter 300 in the July field (or whatever value you are looking for in a particular field) and press Enter or click Find Next. The Strawberry record is highlighted because that is the only record in the data list that has the value 300 in the July column.

If you want to search backwards from the current position of the cursor in the data list, display the data form dialog box, click the Criteria button, and then click the Find Prev button rather than clicking Find Next or pressing Enter.

You can also precede the value you want to search for with a relational operator. Table 23.1 shows the relational operators you can use.

23

Table 23.1. Relational operators.

Operator	Meaning
=	equals
<	less than
>	greater than
<=	less than or equals
>=	greater than or equals

23

Again using the data list in Figure 23.6, display the data form dialog box and click the Criteria button. Enter `<400` in the June field and click Find Next. The `Chocolate` record appears in the record form. If you click Find Next again, the `Strawberry` record appears in the record form.

Validating Data

Why do you have to validate data? Suppose that users enter data that is of the wrong type or that is out of range. The result is that the rest of your worksheet may be rendered useless. You may be the one responsible for creating worksheets, templates, and forms, but other people may be the ones who actually use them to enter data. If the wrong type of data is entered, formulas won't work, charts won't work, and the data won't mean anything. If your user enters `1000` where he or she should have entered `Tennessee`, you have a problem. Unfortunately, it's difficult to validate your data to ensure that the actual data is correct. Getting the right *type* of data is a good start, however. You can ensure that dates are entered in a cell that is supposed to have dates, and that text is entered in a cell that is supposed to list surnames, for example. However, you can't ensure that the date is correct for the date cell, nor can you ensure that the surname is correct for the surname cell. Excel validates the data as you enter it—as soon as you attempt to exit a cell in which you have entered the incorrect type of data, you get an error message.

Start by selecting the cells for which you want to control the type of data that is entered. Consider Figure 23.6 again (the list with the sales of various ice cream flavors). In this example, you may want to ensure that users enter integer values between `1` and `1000` for cells C9 through E11.

After selecting cells C9 through E11, choose Data | Validation from the main menu to display the Data Validation dialog box. For this example, choose `Whole Number` from the Allow drop-down list. You can set the possible values to be those between `1` and `1000`, as shown in Figure 23.9.

Figure 23.9.

The Data Validation
dialog box with criteria
set.

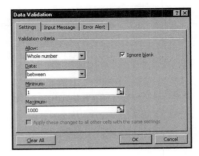

If you want, click the Input Message tab so that you can enter a message that users will see when they select a cell in the selected range. For this example, a good message would be `Enter a number between 1 and 1000`. You can also enter a title if you want. When you enter data in a cell that has an accompanying input message, a popup box appears with the specified title at the top of the box and the input message in the middle, giving you instruction as to what type of data to enter in the cell.

Select the Error Alert tab to create a customized warning dialog box that appears when the data the user enters is out of the specified range. For this example, a good title for the dialog box would be `Error - Out of range`; a good error message would be `Enter a number between 1 and 1000`. The error dialog box displays two buttons: Retry and Cancel. The user can click Retry to return to the cell to enter the data correctly. Figure 23.10 shows both the input message and the error alert dialog box.

Figure 23.10.

A sample input message
and error alert dialog
box.

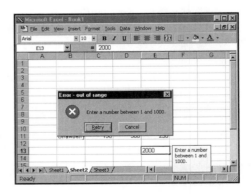

In the Data Validation dialog box, you can use the `Decimal`, `Date`, and `Time` options from the Allow drop-down list in the same way you used the `Whole Number` option in the preceding example. You can choose `Text Length` from the Allow drop-down list if you want to make sure that a particular entry is at least a certain number of characters and no more than a certain number of characters. For example, you may want to set an allowed text length value of 15 for a last name field.

23

Setting up data validation is much the same as formatting cells. The difference is that when you format cells, you can still enter a value that does not correspond with the format chosen for that cell (nothing stops you from entering text in a cell that has been formatted for dates, for example). But if you set up the cell with the Data I Validation command, that cell accepts only date values and rejects all other values. Of course, the user can still make factual errors or typos. And, as mentioned later in the hour, custom validation, in particular, is imperfect when it comes to screening out entries that aren't applicable.

List Validation

As just noted, the validation features offered by Excel are somewhat limited. You can control the *type* of data placed in a cell, but you cannot ensure that the user enters the *right* data.

With the List Validation option (note that the term *list* as used here is unrelated to the list box control or the meaning of *list* as an internal database), you have greater control over what the user places in the cell—although it's still possible to make errors. What you do is create a list of possible values and validate the cell contents against those values. Thus, there are only a finite number of possibilities for the data the cell can contain. Suppose that the only valid entries for a particular cell are California, Oregon, and Washington. You can set up a range that contains these three text values and specify that range as the validation range.

Here's how to validate a cell entry by reference to a list (these steps assume that you have already entered the valid values in a range in the worksheet):

1. Select the cell or cells for which you want to restrict the values.
2. Select Data I Validation from the main menu to display the Data Validation dialog box. Click the Settings tab if you have not done so already.
3. Choose List from the Allow drop-down menu.
4. Enter the range that contains the valid values in the Source field. If you entered the three valid state names in the range A2:A4, you would enter =A2:A4 in the Source field. You can also type the names directly in the Source field, separating them with commas, like this: California, Oregon, Washington.

If you select the In-Cell Dropdown checkbox, the cells will have an icon next to them. In that case, the user can click this icon to display a drop-down list from which he or she can select the correct entry.

If you select the Ignore Blank checkbox in the Data Validation dialog box, the user can leave the selected cells blank. Otherwise, the cells must have some data entered in them to avoid an error message.

Custom Validation

For custom validation, you use an Excel formula. Suppose that you want to enter a value in cell C2 only if cell B2 contains a positive number, and you want to be sure that the value in cell C2 is a positive number also.

Here's how you would set this validation rule for a particular cell or range:

1. Select the cell or range for which you want to set the validation rule. For this example, cell B3 is a convenient choice, but you can choose whatever cell you want.

2. Choose Data | Validate from the main menu to display the Data Validation dialog box. Click the Settings tab, if you have not already done so. Choose Custom from the Allow drop-down list.

3. Enter a formula in the Source field that results in either a TRUE or FALSE value. For this example, the formula to enter is =IF(B2>0,C2>0).

   This formula says, in effect, "If you enter a negative value in B2 and then try to enter a value in C2, you will be unsuccessful."

   However, you can still enter a text value in cell C2, which may not be what you want.

4. Check the Apply these Changes to All Other Cells with the Same Settings box, to change the input and error messages for all the cells you are validating with the same data validation formula.

Here is another example of a custom validation: Suppose that you want all the cells in column C to be subject to a particular restriction depending on the values of the cells in column B. For example, you can only enter a positive value in cell C2 if cell B2 has a value greater than zero; you can only enter a positive value in cell C3 if cell B3 has a value greater than zero, and so on. Relative references make it easy to apply custom validation to a range of cells. Here's how to make this example of custom validation work:

1. Select the range of cells in column C whose entries you want to restrict.

2. Choose Data | Validation from the main menu to display the Data Validation dialog box. Click the Settings tab, if you have not already done so.

3. In the Source field, enter the formula =IF(B2>0,C2>0) and click OK.

   If you select any cell in the specified range in column C and then select Data | Validation, you will see that the formula in the Source field has been adapted automatically to that particular cell.

Data validation does not conflict in any way with the use of data forms and controls, other than to ensure that the data entered is correct.

23

Summary

Creating and using custom controls in your worksheets can make your worksheets look like data entry forms. You can use various types of controls: checkboxes, option boxes, list boxes, scrollbars, and spinners. Each has a specific purpose and is ideally suited for particular types of data entry.

Data forms are a way to enter data in a list. You can use data forms to create new records, to edit already existing records, and to find records that meet particular criteria.

Data validation ensures that the data entered into a specific cell or cells is of a specific type or falls within a certain range. Data validation is no guarantee of accuracy, but it helps catch egregious errors.

Workshop

Term Review

checkbox   A type of control you use to select, or not select, a single option. A checkmark appears in the control if the option is selected.

control   A movable object that allows the user to make particular choices about the data entered. Controls can take a number of different forms.

data form   A dialog box that lets you enter data for a record in an organized fashion.

form   An Excel worksheet that allows the user to make particular selections or choices.

label control   A text box you can format that can be placed anywhere within an Excel worksheet.

list box   A control that allows you to choose from a list of choices.

scrollbar   A control that uses scrollbars and scrollbar arrows to select a particular numeric value.

spinner   A control that uses arrows you can click to move through a range of numeric values.

Q&A

Q What are custom controls?

A Custom controls give the user options about making particular choices when entering data. Custom controls can be in the form of checkboxes, option buttons, scrollbars, and so on.

Q What does validation do?

A You can validate cells or ranges so that only specific types of data can be entered in them. A cell validated only for dates cannot have unrelated text placed in it, for example.

Exercises

☐ Create a worksheet similar to the one shown in Figure 23.11.

1. Create a title at the top by using the Merge and Center button on the Formatting toolbar.

2. Create a list of values for the T-shirt Colors drop-down list; these values are Blue, Yellow, Green, and White. Place these list values in the range M1:M4.

3. Create two option box controls for the style of T-shirts and place a group box control around these two option boxes.

4. Use a scrollbar control for the number of T-shirts to purchase. Set the Cell Link reference to cell B16.

5. Set the columns to the correct width by selecting Format | Column | AutoFit from the main menu.

6. Color the cells in the T-shirt order form gray and remove the gridlines so that the worksheet looks rather like a dialog box.

7. Use data validation so that cell B16 (the one indicating the number of T-shirts) can have only an integer value.

Figure 23.11.

A T-shirt order form.

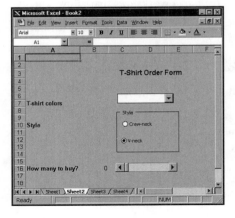

23

☐ Set up the list shown in Figure 23.12. Enter only the labels in row 5 and use data forms to enter the rest of the data.

Use data validation to ensure that only text can be entered in the Name field, that only dates can be entered in the Date of Birth field, and to ensure that only M or F can be entered in the Sex field. Set the text length in the Name field to a maximum of 25 characters. Set the Date of Birth column so that the minimum and maximum values are between January 1, 1901, and January 1, 1990.

23

Figure 23.12.

A simple data entry form.

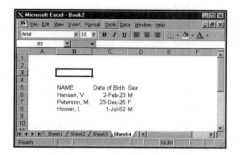

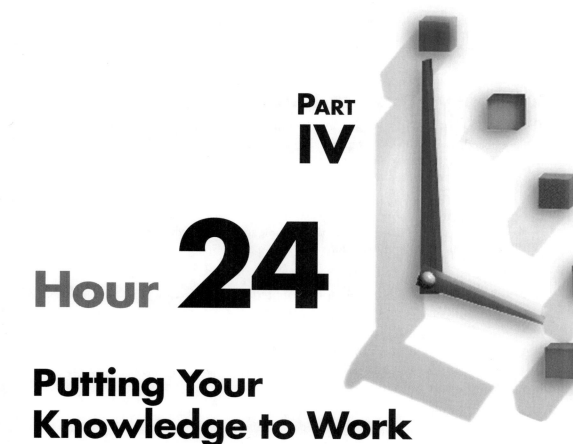

Hour 24

Putting Your Knowledge to Work

Although you've learned many of the various features of Excel in the last several hours, putting all those elements together to form a coherent application can take more than a little time and effort. Excel is so powerful that it's easy to forget its many capabilities. As mentioned in earlier chapters, the Baarns Publishing Web site at http://www.baarns.com/ and the Microsoft Excel Web site at http://www.microsoft.com/excel/ are both useful stops if you want some ideas of the numerous applications you can create with Excel and the ways you can manipulate data.

In this hour, you create two different applications. The first is a lottery-number selector, and the second is a financial report.

A Lottery-Number Selector

Many states have a lottery game: Players purchase tickets for which they have chosen six numbers between 1 and 49. Some players base these numbers on intuition, family birthdays, or other personal choices, but many players prefer to select the numbers at random. You can use Excel to create your very own random-number selector for such a game.

If you don't have a 6/49 game (the lottery game in which you pick six numbers between 1 and 49) where you live or if you don't play the lottery, you can adapt this application to your own purposes later. For now, follow this example and envision what you could do if you won a few million dollars for your efforts.

What do you have to do to create such an application? Here are the steps:

1. Create the worksheet with the relevant text labels in place.
2. Create a macro to select six randomly selected numbers.
3. Create a graphic object that looks like a button or other pushbutton device and attach the macro to that graphic.
4. Delete the extraneous worksheets from the workbook and rename the active worksheet to reflect its significance.
5. Save the file.

Figure 24.1 shows the final result.

Figure 24.1.

A lottery-selector application created in Excel.

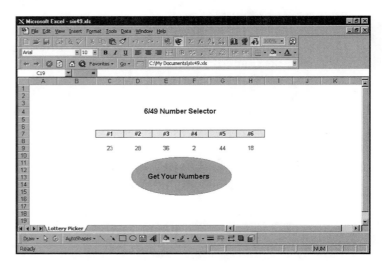

You can design the worksheet so that it fits your aesthetic preferences, but here's how to create an application like the one shown in Figure 24.1:

1. Start Excel and open a blank workbook.

2. Choose Tools | Options from the main menu to display the Options dialog box. Select the View tab and clear the Gridlines checkbox.

   Now you can enter the text.

3. Enter the labels #1 and #2 in a convenient location on the worksheet. In this example, the labels have been entered in cells C7 and D7.

4. Select the cells containing the labels #1 and #2. Select the AutoFill tool and drag it across the row until all six labels are in place, from #1 to #6.

5. Format the labels. The cells in Figure 24.1 have had their alignment, patterns, font, and border altered:

   ☐ Select all six label cells and choose Format | Cells from the main menu to display the Format Cells dialog box.

   ☐ Center the contents of the cells: Click the Alignment tab in the Format Cells dialog box and select Center for the Horizontal value.

   ☐ Apply a color to color all the cells (in the figure, they are light green): Click the Patterns tab of the Format Cells dialog box and select the color you want the cells to be.

   ☐ Change the font of the labels (in this example, the only change made was to make the text bold): Click the Font tab of the Format Cells dialog box and select Bold for the Font style. You can make any other changes you want.

   ☐ Add borders around and between the cells: Click the Border tab of the Format Cells dialog box and choose the type of border you want for the cells. In this example, Outline was selected.

   ☐ Click OK to close the Format Cells dialog box and apply all the changes to the selected cells.

Creating the Title

In this sample worksheet, you want the title to appear centered above all six labels. Here are the steps to follow:

1. Two rows above the row that contains the labels, select the six cells above the labels.

2. Click the Merge and Center tool on the Formatting toolbar.

3. Type the text for the title and press Enter. The text will be centered above the labels.

To change the font style for the title, select the cell containing the title. On the Formatting toolbar, click the Bold tool to change the title to bold. Now click the arrow next to the Font box to see the drop-down list of available fonts. Select one to change the font of the title. If you want to change the size of the text, click the arrow next to the Size box and select a point size from the drop-down list of available sizes.

Creating the Button

Once you have the title and labels in place, the worksheet is starting to take shape. Now you have to create the button the user clicks to generate the random lottery numbers:

1. Display the Drawing toolbar by choosing View | Toolbars | Drawing from the main menu.

2. Create the type of button you want. If you like, you can even insert a clipart graphic, or a graphic you have created in another program.

   In this example, the button is an oval. To draw an oval, click the Oval tool on the Drawing toolbar. Then click in the worksheet where you want to start drawing the oval and drag the cursor to get the size and shape you want.

3. Fill the oval. First, select the shape. Then select the Fill tool from the Drawing toolbar and choose the color you want.

4. Write text inside the oval. First right-click the shape to display the popup menu. Choose Add Text and then type the text you want to appear in the oval. You can format this text the same way you format text outside the oval: Use the tools on the Formatting toolbar.

Removing Extra Worksheets and Renaming the Current Worksheet

In this application, you do not need Sheet 2 and Sheet 3 of the workbook. To tidy up the presentation, delete these two sheets and rename the remaining sheet to be more descriptive:

1. Delete Sheet 2 by selecting its tab, right-clicking to display the popup menu, and selecting Delete from the popup menu. Repeat this process to delete Sheet 3.

2. Rename Sheet 1 to something more descriptive: Right-click the Sheet 1 tab and choose Rename from the popup menu. Type the new name.

3. When finished, press Enter to return to the worksheet.

Creating the Macro

Once the button is in place, you have to create the macro that picks the six random numbers. First of all, consider what you will need. Let's look at the functions you will use outside the context of this particular application.

24

The random-number generator function that gives you random numbers is called RAND. You use this function in a cell like this:

```
=RAND()
```

When you select the cell and press Enter, this function generates a randomly generated number between 0 and 1. In practice, you never get either 0 or 1, only the numbers in between.

How do you randomly generate a number between 1 and 49? If you multiply the random number by 49, you get a number that is between 0 and 49, although once again the number will not, in practice, be either of those numbers, but will fall in between those two limits. The resulting number will not be a whole number either.

In marches the INT function to the rescue. If you turn the result of multiplying the randomly generated number by 49 into an integer, you can then add 1 to it. All numbers between 1 and 49 are then possible. The formula you use looks like this:

```
=INT(49*RAND())+1
```

The INT function rounds down a number to the next-lowest integer. Both 2.9 and 2.1, for example, are rounded down to 2 with the INT function.

Suppose that this formula generates the random number 0.25. When this number is multiplied by 49, rounded down to the next integer, and added to 1, the result is 13. Similarly, if the randomly generated number is 0.75, the result is 37.

The result of this function is as random as is technically possible.

This macro has to make the random numbers appear in the cells beneath the labels. In the example in Figure 24.1, the labels are in row 7, but the random numbers are placed in row 9. You may have a different preference, but the principle is the same.

Here's how you create the macro:

1. Right-click the graphic object (the oval button), and choose Assign Macro from the popup menu. Enter the name of your new macro in the Macro Name field (a descriptive name possibility is getnumbers). Click Record.
2. Select cell C9. Type the formula =INT(49*RAND()) in the cell and press Enter.
3. Use the AutoFill tool to drag this formula into cells D9 through H9.
4. Click the Stop Record button on the Recording toolbar.

Everything is now in place. When you created the macro, you automatically caused six random numbers to be generated. To generate another six random numbers, click the oval button.

COFFEE BREAK

Trouble in Paradise

Note that this lottery-number selector is imperfect. At times, two or more of the same numbers appear in the set of six numbers—when, of course, the six numbers you choose for a lottery are all different.

How can you resolve this problem? That's left as an exercise for you to solve! Here are a couple of hints. Look at the IF function. Compare values of cells using the not equals (<>) operator. You can create a sophisticated macro that looks at the values of the cells already generated to determine whether the newly generated value has already been used. If the number already exists, the macro creates a new random number.

Saving the File

This step should have been mentioned earlier. You should save the worksheet file early and often to help prevent loss of data.

 Choose File | Save from the main menu. Type a descriptive name for the workbook file, such as lottery, and click OK. You can also save a file by using the keyboard shortcut Ctrl+S or by clicking the Save tool in the Standard toolbar.

Similar Applications and Exercises for the Reader

What are some applications you can create that are similar to this lottery example? Well, instead of generating lottery numbers, you can set up a dice game.

Create a graphic that looks like a die. Assign a macro to the graphic that generates random numbers between 1 and 6. If you really want to go all out with this, you can create six separate pictures of the die, showing all six faces (the first face has a single dot on it; the second face has two dots on it; and so on). You can then arrange for the appropriate picture to be inserted in the worksheet depending on the value generated.

The random-number generator is always good for a bit of fun. Try some tricks with it and see what you come up with.

Creating a Final Report

This exercise walks you through the creation of a Product Sales Summary, the creation of a chart and a map to represent the data, and the creation of a Web document from the workbook. When you start this exercise, all you have are the state names and the sales figures for the various products by state. Excel does the work of calculating totals and creating a map,

24

chart, and HTML file almost automatically. Your input is necessary at crucial stages, however; you are also the one who decides what data should go into the map, chart, and HTML file, and how it should be presented.

The Product Sales Summary is shown in Figure 24.2. The following sections explain how to create this document.

Figure 24.2.

The Product Sales Summary example.

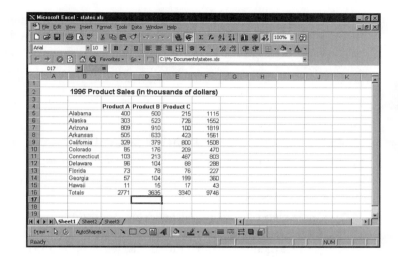

Entering the Labels and Data

To begin with, you must enter the labels and data for this summary sheet. Then you can format the information.

1. Type the labels **Product A**, **Product B**, and **Product C** in cells C4, D4, and E4. Although you don't have to enter data in the same cells as shown in Figure 24.2, the rest of the discussion will be easier to follow if you do.

2. Enter the state names in column B.

If you have a list of states you want to use, you do not have to enter the names in alphabetical order. You can use the Sort Ascending feature to alphabetize them. Once you have listed the states in column B, select one of the cells and click the Sort Ascending tool in the Standard toolbar.

3. Enter the sales data. Don't enter the data for the Totals row—those figures will be generated later. Put the Totals label in place—just don't type anything in that row.

You do not have to follow the steps in the order just presented, but the order I have given is reasonable. There are usually several ways to get to the same goal.

Adding the Title

Once you have the data and labels in place, you can add the title:

1. Select the cell range A2:G2. Click the Merge and Center tool on the Standard toolbar.
2. Enter the text of the title.
3. Format the title as you want. This example uses a 12-point bold Arial font. To format the cell in this way, choose Format | Cells from the main menu to display the Format Cells dialog box.
4. Click the Font tab.
5. Select the formatting options you want.
6. Click OK.

Getting the Totals and Saving the File

The data you have entered for each of the states can be totaled in at least three ways. You can calculate the total sales for each state, the total sales for each product, and the total sales for all the products in all the states.

To calculate the total product sales for Product A, select the cell C16. Click the AutoSum tool on the Standard toolbar. The values in cells C5:C15 are added together. To calculate the total product sales for Product B, select the cell D16 and click the AutoSum tool. Similarly, to calculate the total product sales for Product C, select the cell C16 and click the AutoSum tool.

To get the total sales for all the products, select cell F16 and click the AutoSum tool.

If you want the total sales for all products for each state, select the cells F5:F15 and click the AutoSum tool.

Choose File | Save from the main menu to save the file; enter an appropriate filename and click OK.

Creating a Chart

Creating a chart for this worksheet will liven up your data and make the meaning of the numbers more apparent.

Because a chart showing all the values for Products A, B, and C by state would be unwieldy, a reasonable alternative is to make the chart show only each state and the total value of products sold for each state. A bar or column chart is likely the most appropriate choice, but you can decide differently if you like.

24

Here's one way to make a chart using the data in Figure 24.2:

1. Select the two columns you want to include in your chart. For this example, choose column B (which lists the states) and column F (which lists the total sales). Select the states in column B as you normally select a range of cells; then press and hold the Ctrl key and select the totals in column F. Do not select the Totals label in column B or the totals value in column F.

2. Choose Insert | Chart from the main menu. The first dialog box of the Chart Wizard appears.

3. Select the type of chart you want to create. Either the bar chart or the column chart is a reasonable choice for this example. You can preview different types of charts by selecting them and then clicking the Press and Hold to View Sample button. If you want to create a bar chart, you may want to select the Clustered Bar option for the chart subtype; if you want to create a column chart, the Clustered Column with a 3D effect is also a reasonable choice, as is a plain 3D column.

4. Click Next to see Step 2 of 4 of the Chart Wizard dialog box. (The remaining steps are based on creating a clustered column chart.)

5. If you want the state names to appear along the bottom axis of the chart, accept the default Series In Columns option. If you want the bottom axis to represent the totals—with a different color column for each state and a legend explaining which state corresponds to which color—select the Series In Rows option. Select both options to see the difference in the chart. You do not have to make any changes in this dialog box if you do not want to.

6. Click Next to see Step 3 of 4 of the Chart Wizard dialog box.

7. Type a title for the chart. For this example, enter **1996 Product Sales (in thousands of dollars)**.

8. Enter a label for the Category (X) axis. **States** is a reasonable label for this example.

9. Enter a label for the Value (Y) axis. **Units (thousands of dollars)** is a descriptive choice.

10. Click Next to display the fourth and final dialog box of the Chart Wizard.

11. Choose either to insert the chart as an object on the current worksheet or to place it in its own separate worksheet. For this example, specify that you want the chart on its own worksheet.

12. Click Finish to close the Chart Wizard dialog box and create the chart.

The chart for this example is shown in Figure 24.3; you can resize it as necessary.

24

Figure 24.3.

A column chart of the states and total sales for each state.

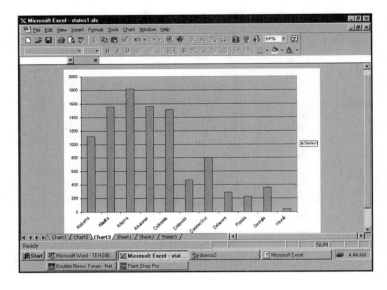

You can use the Goal Seek feature with this chart to figure out various scenarios. Try dragging one of the values in the chart—for example, the sales figures for Alaska—to a different value. Suppose that you want the total sales for Alaska to be 1600. Drag the Alaska bar to the 1600 mark. The Goal Seek dialog box, shown in Figure 24.4, appears. Cell F6 contains the total value for Alaska; you can change the value in cell C6, D6, or E6 to achieve this value.

Figure 24.4.

The Goal Seek dialog box.

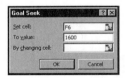

You can also create a chart that compares the total sales for Products A, B, and C. You may want to create this kind of chart if you want to compare the popularity of each product, for example. For more information about formatting charts, refer to Hour 9, "Creating Excel Charts."

Creating a Map

Now let's create a simple map for the data in Figure 24.2:

1. Select all the state names in the range B5:B15, just as you did when creating the chart in the preceding section.

2. Press and hold the Ctrl key and select all the sales totals in the range F5:F15, just as you did when creating the chart in the preceding section.

24

3. Select Insert | Map from the main menu. The mouse pointer changes to a crosshair, which you can use to draw a map inside the active worksheet.

4. Drag the shape of the map to the size you want (you can resize it later).

5. After you set the initial size of the map, you see the Multiple Maps Available dialog box. Choose either United States (AK & HI Inset) or United States in North America. For this example, the map with the inserts will probably work better. Make your choice and click OK.

A map like the one shown in Figure 24.5 appears in your worksheet. The states are shaded differently, depending on the total sales amount for each.

Figure 24.5.

A map created from the Product Sales Summary worksheet.

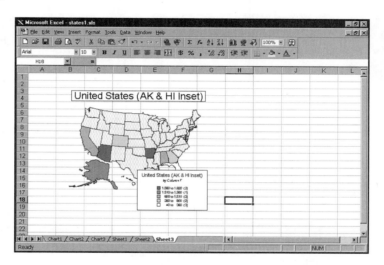

You can alter the legend, color scheme, and other characteristics. You can also insert "stick pins" in different states (for example, you may want to mark the states in which you plan to sell your products next year). You can choose to resize the map if you want. For more information about formatting maps, refer to Hour 10, "Using Excel's Map Features."

Creating a Web Document

Once you have your Excel worksheet the way you want it, you may want to think about creating a Web page from it.

To create a Web document from the file you have been developing in the second part of this hour, follow these steps:

1. Choose File | Save as HTML from the main menu to display Step 1 of the Internet Assistant dialog box.

2. Choose the ranges and charts you want to convert to HTML format (the format required by Web documents). Select the ranges you want to convert. You can always come back to convert the other components.

3. Click Next to display Step 2 of the Internet Assistant dialog box.

4. Specify whether you want the Web page to be created as a separate file or you want to insert the table into a Web page file that already exists. For this example, specify that you want to create a separate file.

5. Click Next to display Step 3 of the Internet Assistant dialog box.

6. Choose the title, header, description, and other information for the Web page.

7. Click Next to display Step 4 of the Internet Assistant dialog box.

8. Specify which character code you want to use. In most cases (and certainly for this example), choose US/Western European. Specify whether you want to save the document as an HTML file or add it to an existing FrontPage Web file. Enter the pathname you want for this file.

9. Click Finish to close the dialog box and create the Web page.

In Hour 20, "Excel and the World Wide Web," you learned about the process of creating Web pages from your Excel worksheets in more detail.

Summary

In this hour, you learned how to create two separate applications. Any time you have a task that involves calculating numbers or presenting data, Excel can likely play a role. You can use Excel for tasks that you may not have even thought of yet. You can set up a simplified tax-simulation model to see the effects of earning more or less income. You can calculate the calories you consume in a day, a week, or a month, presuming that you have the data about food quantities and their associated calories. You can look at what would happen to your earnings potential if you worked five hours more or less per week. How would your earnings change if you made 50 cents more per hour? Thinking of creative applications is more than half the fun of using Excel.

24

Workshop

Q&A

Q What are the two most important things to remember when using Excel?

A These are the main points to remember when you use Excel:

☐ Save your files regularly. You can also set up the AutoSave add-in to save your files automatically every 10 minutes (or whatever time interval you prefer).

☐ Use Excel's online help and the Office Assistant. You can get instant answers to just about any problem you may encounter from these two sources. Of course, it won't hurt to take a look at this book's index, either!

24

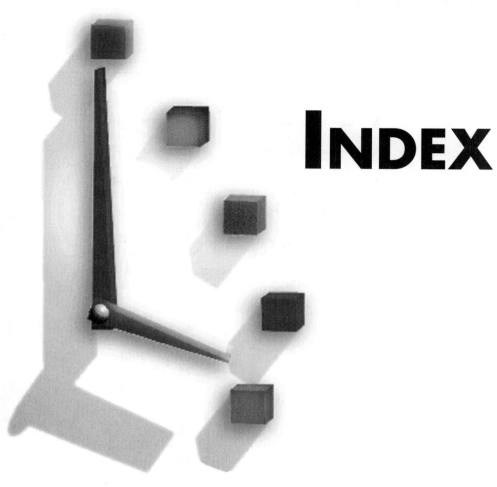

INDEX

exclamation mark (!)
HYPERLINK function,
328
exclusive rights (shared
workbooks), reverting,
341-342
exiting Excel 97, 46
expanding outlines (Auto
Outline), 237
Explorer, opening work-
books, 33
exponents, formatting, *see*
scientific notation
expressions (logical),
evaluating, 195
extending cells keyboard
shortcut, 32
External Data Range
Properties dialog box, 317
external databases (Query
Wizard), 314

F

FACT function, 212
false values (logical functions), 213
FALSE( ) function, 213
favorites (WWW sites),
adding to, 322, 326
Features command (Map
menu), 172
fields, 226
   Access
     converting, 306
     Form Wizard, 308-309
     Report Wizard, 310
   field names, 226
     see also labels

pivot tables
   amount setting, 247
   creating, 243
   naming, 245
   see also columns
File Conversion command
(Tools menu), 278
File Conversion Wizard,
278-279
File Conversion Wizard
Report dialog box, 279
File menu commands
   Close, 40, 158
   New, 32
   Open, 33
   Open Binder, 295
   Page Setup, 183
   Print, 186
   Print Binder, 297
   Print Preview, 180
   Properties, 83
   Save, 38
   Save As, 39
   Save as HTML, 329
   Save Workspace, 40
File menu commands
(Binder)
   Binder Page Setup, 297
   Binder Print Preview, 297
   Save, 297
   Save As, 297
files, 274
   Binder
     adding, 296-297
     deleting, 297
     editing, 297
     moving, 297
     printing, 297
     saving, 297
   graphics, 138
   linking worksheets, 325

printing to, 187
replacing, installation,
19-20
saving (Text Import
Wizard), 277
sharing, converting
formats, 278
shortcuts, creating, 289
Fill Down keyboard
shortcut, 30
Fill Right keyboard shortcut, 30
Fill tool (Drawing toolbar),
128, 386
Filter Data dialog box, 316
Filter menu commands
   Advanced Filter, 230
   AutoFilter, 226
filtering
   advanced filters, 230-231
     copying lists, 231
     criteria, 231
     in-place filtering, 231
   AutoFilter tool, 226-227
     Bottom values, 228
     customizing, 228-230
     deselecting, 228
     multiple filtering, 230
     specific values, 227
     Top-10 filter, 228
   shared workbooks,
     341-348
filters, installing, 15
financial functions, 210
Find command (Edit
menu), 63
Find dialog box, 63
Find keyboard shortcut, 30
finding
   find/replace, 63
   functions, 209

H

Header and Footer command (View menu), 86
Header and Footer dialog box, 86
Header dialog box, 86
headers
  customizing, 86-87
  displaying, 86-87
  printing setup, 185
height (rows), 67
Help
  About Microsoft Excel, 45
  Contents and Index, 43-44
  functions, entering, 222
  installing, 15
  Lotus 1-2-3, 45
  Microsoft Map, 166
  Office Assistant, 41-43
    accessing, 41
    appearance, changing, 42
    asking questions, 42
    Clippity, 42
    customizing, 42-43
    functions, 209
    positioning, 42
  print previewing, 181
  Web site, 44
  What's This, 44
Help menu commands
  About Microsoft Excel, 45
  Contents and Index, 29, 43
  Lotus 1-2-3, 45
  Microsoft Map Help Topics, 166

Hewlett-Packard Graphics Language file extensions, 138
HEX2BIN function, 216
Hide command (Window menu), 79
hiding
  columns/rows, 78
  comments, 102
  graphics, 135-136
  gridlines, 57
  legends, 156, 171
  Microsoft Map Control, 173
  tables, 156
  toolbars, 26
  workbooks, 79
  worksheets, 79, 94
Highlight Changes dialog box, 342-343
hints (Solver tool), 262
horizontal alignment (cells), 64
horizontally displaying (workbooks), 82
HTML converting, 329-330
  charts, 334
  code pages, 333-334
  separating files, 331-332
  tables, 332
Hyperlink command (Insert menu), 324
HYPERLINK function, 327-328
  cell insertion, 327
  friendly_name, 327
  link_location, 327
  pathname referencing, 328
hyperlinks, *see* links

I

IDs, 11
IF function, 214-215
Image Control tool (Picture toolbar), 139
images, *see* graphics
IMCONJUGATE function, 216
Import Spreadsheet Wizard (Acess), 305
importing
  objects, 290
  text, 275-278
in-place editing (OLE), 293-294
in-place filtering (advanced filters), 231
indenting cells, 75-76
Information functions, 215
Insert Cells dialog box, 75
Insert dialog box, 293
Insert Hyperlink dialog box, 325
Insert Hyperlink keyboard shortcut, 30
Insert Hyperlink tool, 324
Insert menu commands
  Cells, 75
  Chart, 145, 391
  Columns, 75
  Hyperlink, 324
  Map, 165, 393
  Object, 137, 291
  Picture, 136
  Rows, 75
  Worksheet, 79
Insert menu commands (Word; Object), 292

X-Y

Z

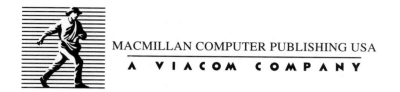

MACMILLAN COMPUTER PUBLISHING USA

A VIACOM COMPANY

Technical Support:

If you need assistance with the information in this book or with a CD/Disk accompanying the book, please access the Knowledge Base on our Web site at **http://www.superlibrary.com/general/support**. Our most Frequently Asked Questions are answered there. If you do not find the answer to your questions on our Web site, you may contact Macmillan Technical Support **(317) 581-3833** or e-mail us at **support@mcp.com**.

Teach Yourself Microsoft Word 97 in 24 Hours

Linda Jones & Ruel Hernandez

Written in a straightforward, easy-to-read manner, *Teach Yourself Microsoft Word 97 in 24 Hours* enables the reader to become productive quickly with Word 97. From very basic concepts such as opening new and existing documents to more complex features such as using styles and macros, beginning users quickly learn how to use the new features of the most popular word processing application.

Includes coverage of concepts relating to the Office 97 suite—how applications relate to each other as well as how to interface with online resources

Price: $19.99 USA/$28.95 CAN　　　User Level: Casual—Intermediate
ISBN: 0-672-31115-1　　　　　　　400 pp.　　　　　　Word Processing

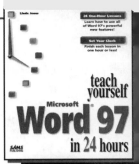

Teach Yourself Microsoft PowerPoint 97 in 24 Hours

Alexandria Haddad & Christopher Haddad

Teach Yourself Microsoft PowerPoint 97 in 24 Hours is an introductory tutorial enabling the reader to quickly create dynamic, captivating presentations. Beginning users quickly learn how to use the new features of PowerPoint 97 with the easy, task-oriented format—the material is presented in manageable one-hour lessons.

Practical, easy-to-follow exercises walk the reader through the concepts.

Sections on free informational resources (templates, graphics, and so on) are included.

Price: $19.99 USA/$28.95 CAN　　　User Level: New—Casual
ISBN: 0-672-31117-8　　　　　　　400 pp.　　Design/Graphics—Business Graphics

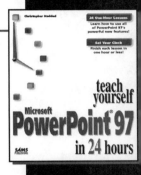

Teach Yourself Access 97 in 24 Hours

Timothy Buchanan, Craig Eddy, & Rob Newman

As organizations and end users continue to upgrade to NT Workstation and Windows 95, a surge in 32-bit productivity applications—including Microsoft Office 97—is expected. Using an easy-to-follow approach, this book teaches the fundamentals of a key component in the Microsoft Office 97 package: Access 97. Users learn how to use and manipulate existing databases, create databases with wizards, and build databases from scratch in 24 one-hour lessons.

Price: $19.99 USA/$28.95 CDN　　　User Level: New—Casual
ISBN: 0-672-31027-9　　　　　　　400 pp.　　　　Databases

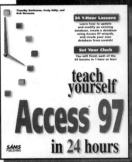

Teach Yourself Microsoft Outlook 97 in 24 Hours

Brian Proffitt & Kim Spilker

Microsoft Office is the leading application productivity suite available; in its next version, it will have Outlook as a personal information manager. Using step-by-step instructions and real-world examples, readers explore the new features of Outlook and learn how to successfully integrate Outlook with other Office 97 applications—painlessly.

Each hour focuses on working with Outlook as a single user as well as in a group setting.

Price: $19.99 USA/$28.95 CAN　　　User Level: Casual—Intermediate
ISBN: 0-672-31044-9　　　　　　　432 pp.　　　　Integrated Software/Suites

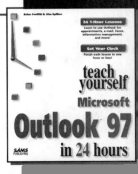

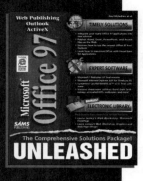

Microsoft Office 97 Unleashed, Second Edition

Paul McFedries, et al.

Microsoft has brought the Web to its Office suite of products. Hyperlinking, Office Assistant, and Active Document Support let users publish documents on the Web or an intranet site. Microsoft Office also completely integrates with Microsoft FrontPage, making it possible to point-and-click a Web page into existence. This book details each of the Office products—Excel, Access, PowerPoint, Word, and Outlook—and shows the estimated 22 million registered users how to create presentations and Web documents.

Describes the various Office Solution Kits and how to use them.

CD-ROM includes powerful utilities and two best-selling books in HTML format.

Price: $39.99 USA/$56.95 CDN   *User Level: Accomplished—Expert*
ISBN: 0-672-31010-4   *1,370 pp.*   *Office Suites*

Teach Yourself Web Publishing with Microsoft Office 97 in a Week

Michael Larson

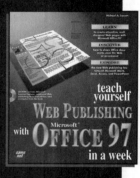

Using a clear, step-by-step approach and practical examples, this book teaches users how to effectively use components of Microsoft Office to publish attractive, well-designed documents for the World Wide Web or an intranet.

Explains the basics of Internet/intranet technology, the Microsoft Internet Explorer browser, and HTML. CD-ROM is loaded with Microsoft Internet Explorer 3.0 and an extensive selection of additional graphics, templates, scripts, ActiveX controls, and multimedia clips to enhance Web pages.

Price: $39.99 USA/$56.95 CDN   *User Level: New—Casual—Accomplished*
ISBN: 1-57521-232-3   *480 pp.*   *Internet/Web Publishing*

Teach Yourself Microsoft FrontPage 97 in a Week

Donald Doherty

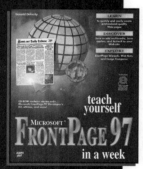

FrontPage is the number-one Web site creation program on the market, and this book explains how to use it. Everything from adding Office 97 documents to a Web site to using Java, HTML, wizards, VBScript, and JavaScript in a Web page is covered. With this book, readers learn all the nuances of Web design and use the step-by-step examples to create an entire Web site using FrontPage 97.

CD-ROM includes Microsoft Internet Explorer 3.0, ActiveX and HTML development tools, plus additional ready-to-use templates, graphics, scripts, Java applets, and more.

Price: $29.99 USA/$42.95 CDN   *User Level: New—Casual*
ISBN: 1-57521-225-0   *500 pp.*   *Internet/Web Publishing*

Add to Your Sams Library Today with the Best Books for Programming, Operating Systems, and New Technologies

The easiest way to order is to pick up the phone and call

1-800-428-5331

between 9:00 a.m. and 5:00 p.m. EST.
For fastest service please have your credit card available.

ISBN	Quantity	Description of Item	Unit Cost	Total Cost
0-672-31115-1		Teach Yourself Microsoft Word 97 in 24 Hours	$19.99	
0-672-31117-8		Teach Yourself Microsoft PowerPoint 97 in 24 Hours	$19.99	
0-672-31027-9		Teach Yourself Access 97 in 24 Hours	$19.99	
0-672-31044-9		Teach Yourself Microsoft Outlook 97 in 24 Hours	$19.99	
0-672-31010-4		Microsoft Office 97 Unleashed, Second Edition (Book/CD-ROM)	$39.99	
0-672-31039-2		Paul McFedries' Windows 95 Unleashed, Professional Reference Edition (Book/CD-ROM)	$59.99	
1-57521-232-3		Teach Yourself Web Publishing with Microsoft Office 97 in a Week (Book/CD-ROM)	$39.99	
1-57521-225-0		Teach Yourself Microsoft FrontPage 97 in a Week (Book/CD-ROM)	$29.99	
		Shipping and handling: See information below.		
		TOTAL		

Shipping and Handling: $4.00 for the first book and $1.75 for each additional book. If you need to have it immediately, we can ship your order to you in 24 hours for an additional charge of approximately $18.00, and you will receive your order overnight or in two days. Overseas shipping and handling cost an additional $2.00 per book. Prices subject to change. Call for availability and pricing information on latest editions.

201 W. 103rd Street, Indianapolis, Indiana 46290

1-800-428-5331 — Orders   1-800-835-3202 — Fax   1-800-858-7674 — Customer Service

Book ISBN 0-672-31116-X